Analysis of Neurogenic Dis[...]
Discourse Production

Analysis of discourse production among speakers with acquired communication disorders is an important and necessary clinical procedure. This book provides a comprehensive review and discussion of aphasia and its related disorders, their corresponding clinical discourse symptoms that speech-and-language pathologists should address, and the different methods of discourse elicitation that are clinically and research oriented.

This edition has been thoroughly updated throughout to include the latest research, including advances in word retrieval and discourse production, cognitive and multicultural aspects of disordered discourse production, application of technology to understand and evaluate spoken discourse, and evidence-based intervention of discourse impairments. Contemporary issues related to disordered/clinical discourse elicitation are added. Recent advancement in discourse analysis is covered and discussions of various treatment options of discourse symptoms are provided. Finally, the manifestation of discourse symptoms as a function of speakers' multilingual/multicultural status and specific considerations related to clinical assessment and remediation are explored.

As the only introductory text to include comprehensive coverage of basic knowledge of neurogenic disordered discourse, it is a must-read for students, clinicians, and researchers in various fields. Readers will also benefit from plenty of examples that provide a connection between the theoretical contents presented in the text and application to real-life contexts of discourse production.

Anthony Pak-Hin Kong is a professor and research scientist specialized in aphasiology at The University of Hong Kong. He is a world-renowned scholar in speech-and-language pathology and is currently Section Editor (Linguistics Section) of PLOS ONE and Editorial Board Member of Perspectives of the American Speech-Language-Hearing Association (ASHA) Special Interest Groups.

Analysis of Neurogenic Disordered Discourse Production

Theories, Assessment and Treatment

Second Edition

Anthony Pak-Hin Kong

Routledge
Taylor & Francis Group

NEW YORK AND LONDON

Cover image: © Getty images

Second edition published 2022
by Routledge
605 Third Avenue, New York, NY 10158

and by Routledge
4 Park Square, Milton Park, Abingdon, Oxon, OX14 4RN

Routledge is an imprint of the Taylor & Francis Group, an informa business

© 2022 Anthony Pak-Hin Kong

First edition published by Routledge 2016

Library of Congress Cataloging-in-Publication Data
A catalog record has been requested for this book

ISBN: 9781032184845 (hbk)
ISBN: 9781032184821 (pbk)
ISBN: 9781003254775 (ebk)

DOI: 10.4324/9781003254775

Typeset in Bembo
by Newgen Publishing UK

To my parents, Imalda and Simon

To my niece, Meredith, and nephew, Anakin

To my grandma, PorPor

and

To my feline companions, Tiger and Boney

This edition of the text was prepared, updated, and finalized during the time I was under COVID-19 lockdown and quarantine in two different places – the United States and Hong Kong. The global spread of COVID-19 has posed challenges to every one of us, and particularly those with acquired or developmental communication disorders as well as their caregivers. We have all demonstrated our strong determination and resilience in overcoming these difficulties. I would like to dedicate this work to people who have been affected by this pandemic, physically, psychologically, socially, economically, or beyond.

Contents

About the Author

Dr. Anthony Pak-Hin Kong earned a B.Sc. in Speech and Hearing Sciences and a Ph.D. in Aphasiology from The University of Hong Kong. As an internationally-known and dedicated research scholar in speech-and-language pathology, Dr. Kong has a long and solid line of international research, teaching, and consultation work. His research focuses on discourse production by individuals with aphasia, development of assessment tools of aphasia and related cognitive disorders, and gesture production and neurogenic communication disorders in multi-lingual speakers. Other research interests include distinctive linguistic properties and prosodic features of speakers with aphasia, community support to individuals with aphasia and their families, the relationship between bilingualism in aphasia and language recovery and processing, and clinical application of technology to manage aphasia, dementia, and other related cognitive-communicative disorders.

Dr. Kong has provided research, clinical, or professional consultations to many international agencies, such as Aphasia United, Hong Kong Hospital Authority, Self Help Group for the Brain Damaged, The Hong Kong Association of Speech Therapists, The Hong Kong Society for Rehabilitation, and Project BRIDGE (Building Research Initiatives by Developing Group Effort). He has been actively engaged with a broad cross-section of the healthcare community in the greater Orlando area that offers community speech therapy-related services to those with aphasia and related cognitive communicative disorders, such as Orlando Veterans Affairs Medical Center, Veterans Affairs Hospital, Veterans Health Community Living Center, Central Florida Brain Injury Support Group, and Share the Care. In 2013, Dr. Kong received the Certificate of Recognition for Outstanding Contribution in International Achievement from the American Speech-Language-Hearing Association (ASHA). Dr. Kong is currently Section Editor (Linguistics Section) of PLOS ONE and Editorial Board Member of Perspectives of the ASHA Special Interest Groups.

Preface

Analyzing oral discourse produced by speakers with acquired language disorders is an important and necessary clinical procedure. However, systematic and adequate discourse analyses are often limited to research investigations rather than being incorporated in daily clinical situations. In addition, the topic of discourse analysis for the clinical population is usually not extensively covered in the training of speech–and–language pathologists, for two main reasons: (1) the relatively restricted amount of research done in this area, as compared to other aspects of communication disorders, and (2) the lack of appropriate teaching materials.

In the last decade, there was a healthy growth in research pertaining to disordered discourse analyses; this has in turn promoted clinical application of these reported evidenced-based assessments. Preparing professionals to deal with the complex nature of discourse deficits among speakers with acquired communication disorders is a daunting task. *Analysis of neurogenic disordered discourse production: Theories, assessment and treatment* is a tool to help prepare graduate students, speech–and–language pathologists, related clinical professionals, and researchers in various fields to serve people with deficits in discourse production. Readers who want to learn the background and techniques of conducting discourse analysis, to refresh acquired knowledge on discourse production, to update their knowledge about options for assessing and managing discourse production, as well as to learn about contemporary issues around computerized discourse annotation and analyses will find this book a valuable resource.

Chapter 1 of the book provides a comprehensive overview and discussion of aphasia and related disorders, including traumatic brain injury, right hemisphere damage, and dementia. The corresponding clinical symptoms and characteristics associated with these disorders at the discourse level, for which speech–and–language pathologists and related healthcare professionals should address, are also summarized. Chapter 2 presents different methods of eliciting discourse samples. Practice guidelines that can facilitate clinicians' collection and subsequent processing of these samples are also discussed.

Chapters 3 and 4 feature detailed information on various analytic systems or frameworks that are clinically feasible and research oriented, respectively, for quantifying disordered discourse. The strengths and weaknesses of these systems or frameworks are also explained, so as to assist readers to evaluate their clinical and research values. Chapter 5 addresses the use of multi-linear transcriptions and includes illustrations to explain how this approach can facilitate the analysis of oral discourse. Chapter 6 describes the novel approach of adopting a multi-modal and multi-level analysis of oral discourse. Specific information regarding the advantages of considering non-verbal behaviors as well as prosodic features that accompany oral language is provided. Chapter 7 reviews a number of clinical studies on intervention strategies addressing discourse symptoms found in speakers with aphasia as well as individuals with acquired cognitive communication disorders. A systematic discussion of various traditional and contemporary treatment options in relation to discourse symptoms is provided. Chapter 8 focuses on the description about manifestation of discourse symptoms in the bilingual or multilingual populations. How a language is impaired as a function of the status of bilingualism or multilingualism and specific considerations related to clinical assessment and intervention are explored. Finally, Chapter 9 is devoted to highlighting some directions for conducting future investigations on clinical discourse analyses.

It is believed that with a comprehensive coverage of topics around discourse analysis, this text will provide readers with a thorough understanding on the nature, assessment, and remediation of discourse deficits associated with aphasia and related disorders. Readers will benefit from carefully selected examples that aim to provide a connection between the theoretical contents presented in the text and their application to real-life contexts of discourse production. It is hoped that this book may add to our current knowledge of neurogenic discourse impairments and will inspire research that continues to enrich our conceptualization, understanding, and management of disordered discourse production.

Abbreviations

AAMAS	Asian American Multidimensional Acculturation Scale
AMAS	Abbreviated Multidimensional Acculturation Scale
APT	Attention Process Training
BAT	Bilingual Aphasia Test
CA	Conversation analysis
CAPPA	Conversation Analysis Profile for People with Aphasia
CAT	Communication Awareness Training
CHAT	Codes for the Human Analysis of Talk
CHI	Closed head injury
CIAT	Constraint-induced aphasia therapy
DELAD	Database Enterprise for Language And speech Disorders
ECP	Everyday communication partner
GVT	Gestural + verbal treatment
IPR	Interpersonal process recall
LCM	Linguistic Communication Measure
MAE	Multilingual Aphasia Examination
MCA	Main Concept Analysis
MCT	Multi-modal Communication Training
MLU	Mean length of utterance
NARNIA	Novel Approach to Real-life communication: Narrative Intervention in Aphasia
NER	Named Entity Recognition
NLP	Natural Language Processing
NNLA	Northwestern Narrative Language Analysis
OHI	Open head injury
OLA	Open Language Archives Community
QAR	Question asking reading
SCA	Supported Conversation for Adults with Aphasia
SFA	Semantic feature analysis
SOLO	Strategies of observed learning outcomes

SPPARC	Supporting Partners of People with Aphasia in Relationships and Conversation
SSG	Social skills group
SST	Social skills treatment
tDCS	Transcranial direct current stimulation
TMS	Transcranial magnetic stimulation

Chapter 1

Acquired Language Deficits Associated with Aphasia and Related Disorders

Chapter Objectives

The reader will be able to:

1. understand the evolution of scientific research of **aphasia** and related language disorders
2. define aphasia and identify major clinical characteristics of the disorder
3. discuss various methods for classification of aphasic syndromes
4. describe the symptoms of **discourse** in aphasia
5. describe the symptoms of discourse in **traumatic brain injury (TBI)**
6. describe the symptoms of discourse in **right hemisphere damage (RHD)**
7. describe the symptoms of discourse in **dementia**
8. compare and contrast the common clinical assessment procedures of aphasia and other related language disorders.

Historical Review of Aphasia

Our concepts about aphasia have developed in the course of the last two centuries. Gall (1825) proposed that separate organs existed in the cerebral cortex of human brains. Each of these organs was claimed to sub-serve a specific intellectual, moral, or spiritual faculty. This view of arguing language to be localized in the brain was greatly challenged during the first half of the nineteenth century, when scientific connections between aphasic symptoms and localizations of brain damage areas were made (Code, 2011). The later classic research reports by Broca (1865) and Wernicke (1874), who discussed two distinctive types of aphasia, have shaped the way we understand and think about aphasia, with reference to two major features related to language impairment – auditory comprehension and verbal expressive abilities.

Broca's (1865) description about a clinical case of "Mr. Tan," who had a stroke about 20 years prior to the report, was known for his relatively good

DOI: 10.4324/9781003254775-1

verbal comprehension but extremely limited and non-fluent oral expression. He was only able to say "tan tan" for oral production after his stroke. Post-mortal examination of Mr. Tan revealed lesions in the postero-external part of the left anterior lobe. Broca then declared that the left hemisphere controls human's speaking and the Broca's area, a localized center in this hemisphere, is a functionally specific site for articulation of speech.

Another patient who showed a language pattern very different from Mr. Tan was reported by Wernicke (1874). Unlike Mr. Tan, this patient's verbal expression was not scarce, halting, nor effortful, but his verbal comprehension was severely impaired. Other reported clinical characteristics included fluent articulation and normal intonation pattern with the exception that the patient's language content did not make sense to listeners. Autopsy results indicated an infarct in the posterior area of the left temporal gyrus (or the Wernicke's area), which was then claimed to be the area for auditory comprehension.

Research and clinical studies on aphasia started to emerge more rapidly after the end of the First World War because a large number of young soldiers were wounded and left with different degrees of language disorders that were long-lasting. Team members of the rehabilitation programs in military hospitals at that time included neurologists, psychologists, and speech pathologists (Basso, 2003), but major emphasis on the assessment and treatment of aphasia had primarily been focused on auditory comprehension and oral production of language at the single word to sentence level. Extremely little has been examined and, therefore, researched on the post-sentential performance among these returning troops.

What Is Aphasia?

Many definitions of aphasia have been proposed in the literature during the past few decades. For example, Luria (1964) was among the first few researchers who defined aphasia as a disorder characterized by the disturbance of the sound system (speech and phonemes), semantic organization, and syntactic coding of language. Specifically, destruction of any zone in the cerebral cortex could interfere with speech processes, which could subsequently lead to disintegration of functional systems of verbal output.

Contemporary behavioral investigations on aphasia have advanced our conceptions of aphasia, with more recent definitions emphasizing the loss or impairment of the power to use or comprehend words. In addition, disturbance of language functions commonly involve both reception and expression, which may manifest itself in various ways including difficulties in listening, reading, speaking, and writing. This later definition is considered to be more comprehensive in a sense that it covers different modalities of language processing, including the verbal and written aspects of language. Note that the term "dysphasia" has historically been used interchangeably with "aphasia." To avoid potential confusion in the broader medical community, an international group of aphasiologists affiliated to Aphasia United (www.aphasiaunited.org/) has advocated to eliminate the use of the term "dysphasia" (Worrall et al., 2016) to enhance consistency of describing the disorder across scholarly publications, websites of consumer organizations, clinical guidelines to manage aphasia, and different clinical professionals.

A summary of existing definitions of aphasia in the literature, based on the following perspectives – neurological, neuro-linguistic, cognitive, and functional – was summarized by Papathanasiou et al. (2022):

- From a neurological perspective (e.g., Goodglass & Kaplan, 1983), aphasia is acquired from a focal brain lesion in the absence of other cognitive, motor, or sensory impairment. This acquired language deficit can affect one or more language components (including phonology, morphology, syntax, semantics, and pragmatics) and can manifest in one or more modalities (listening, speaking, reading, writing, and signing).
- From a neuro-linguistic perspective (e.g., Lesser, 1987), a focal lesion can impair the functioning of a specific language domain within the language system. An intact language system typically includes an auditory, a visual, and a written input as well as a spoken and a written output.
- From a cognitive perspective that commonly considers language as one of the domains of **cognition** (e.g., Davis, 2012; Ellis & Young, 1988), aphasia is defined as the selective breakdown of the processing for comprehending and formulating language, which can be intertwined with the underlying cognitive system covering other cognitive skills (such as memory, attention, executive function, and visuospatial ability).
- Finally, from a functional perspective of language use (e.g., Kagan, 1995; Kagan & Simmons-Mackie, 2013), aphasia is a communication breakdown that masks inherent competence of verbal interactions and affects a speaker's skills of conversational information exchange, social functioning, and quality of life.

The World Health Organization (WHO) has also provided the framework of International Classification of Functioning, Disability, and Health (ICF; WHO, 2001) to assess, conceptualize, and define aphasia. This ICF classification defines disability with reference to three major levels that are multi-dimensional, including "impairment of body function," "activities limitation," and "participation restriction." Therefore, according to what the WHO emphasizes, defining aphasia using the ICF framework should be related to the ultimate goal of intervention in aphasia, which is to maximize quality of life (Simmons-Mackie & Kagan, 2007). Specifically, in terms of "impairments," aphasia refers to the disordered language system. Examples of impairment of "body function" associated with aphasia may include difficulty with word finding (i.e., **anomia**) or difficulty attending to auditory-verbal information (i.e., attentional deficits). In terms of "activities limitation," aphasia can be defined as a communication breakdown that reduces one's personal activities. Difficulty understanding own medication schedule and problems with completing a job application document are examples of activity limitations commonly found in aphasia. Finally, in terms of "participation restriction," aphasia is a condition that can lead to reduced involvement in life situations. Examples of participation restrictions associated with aphasia include one losing the ability to manage own health care or one not holding a job. Due to the fact that the functioning and disability of an individual with aphasia occurs in a context (or life situation), the ICF also includes a list of environmental and contextual factors that impede or facilitate body function and participation.

Regardless of which approach mentioned above one uses to understand and conceptualize aphasia, it is important to realize that one element that has been commonly agreed in defining aphasia is its center on how the condition impedes language functions. In other words, no matter how a clinician defines aphasia, the critical component in an examination is to measure how a patient's ability in using language is affected, which will be crucial for subsequent language remediation.

Causes, Prevalence, and Common Clinical Characteristics of Aphasia

Aphasia is commonly found in someone with a brain injury. Causes of sudden-onset aphasia include stroke, which occurs when blood (and therefore oxygen) supply is unable to reach the part of the brain responsible for language function, or severe blows to the head, such as open or closed head injury (CHI). There are also cases when aphasia can develop gradually, such as in the case of brain tumors, brain infections, or other progressive neurological diseases, including dementia and **Parkinson's disease**. Gradual onset of aphasia can lead to increasing level of difficulties for someone to communicate over time.

According to the National Aphasia Association (2021), aphasia currently affects about two million people in the United States; this is in contrast to the estimated one million people by the National Institute on Deafness and Other Communication Disorders (NIDCD, 1997). The NIDCD (2017) has also reported an increase of approximately 180,000 new cases of aphasia every year in the nation; compared to the estimated 80,000 annual new cases in 2008 by National Stroke Association back in 2008 (National Stroke Association, 2008), an increasing number of Americans are facing the unique challenges of aphasia. Internationally, about five million people experience a stroke-induced aphasia every year (Robb, 2015). While stroke is the most common cause of aphasia, the incidence of post-stroke aphasia reported in the literature has ranged between 17% and 43% (Kadojić et al., 2012; Kotila et al., 1984; Reinvang, 1984; Wade et al., 1986; Worrall & Foster, 2020). Up to 31% of stroke survivors exhibit symptoms of depression that can impede functional recovery (Hackett & Pickles, 2014). Advancing age has increased the risk for aphasia, with an estimated prevalence rate of 15% among individuals aged 65 years and 43% among those who are 85 years of age (Engelter et al., 2006). Although there is a lack of gender differences in aphasia incidence, three aphasia syndromes – Wernicke's, global, and anomic aphasias – were found to be more common in women. Broca's aphasia, on the other hand, occurs more frequently in men (Hier et al., 1994).

Instead of viewing aphasia as a single disorder, it is more appropriate to consider it as a family of disorders involving varying degrees of impairments across auditory and reading language comprehension as well as spoken and written expression. Depending on the type and severity of the disorder, common symptoms associated with aphasia may include:

- impaired ability in comprehending spoken words or sentences
- word production errors (e.g., semantic or phonological paraphasias **perseverations, neologisms**, or **jargons**)
- word-finding difficulties (anomia)
- impaired ability to verbally repeat single words, phrases, or sentences
- speech dysfluency
- impairments of reading
- problems in using written language.

In fact, anomia has been described as the "core" symptom of aphasia by a number of aphasiologists (e.g., Benson, 1988; Fridriksson et al., 2007; Helm-Estabrooks et al., 2014) because word retrieval problems can occur across conditions from probing for specific single words, to constructing sentences, as well as to producing a **narrative** discourse. In particular, the total number of words produced and appropriate measures of specific parts of speech (such as **open-class words** of nouns, verbs, or adjectives versus functors) may help infer word retrieval difficulties in connected speech (Kavé & Goral, 2017). The level of difficulty in retrieving a specific lexical item also ranges from mild to severe depending on the psycholinguistic properties of the target such as age of word acquisition, frequency of occurrence in the language, length and phonemic complexity of words, emotional valence, semantic class of words, and part-of-speech (Laganaro et al., 2006; Wepman et al., 1956). Even a very mild degree of aphasia can lead to compromised accuracy and/or efficiency in retrieving words during an expressive language task. Although a speaker with aphasia often retains relatively intact non-linguistic cognitive skills, the brain damage in connection to the aphasic condition may sometime lead to comorbid cognitive deficits, such as dysfunction in memory, attention, or executive functions. Presence of selective sensory deficits, including visual field deficits or **agnosia** (visual or auditory), is rare but not uncommon. This is particularly the case among individuals who are in still in the acute or early stage of aphasia (i.e., the first few days to few weeks post-onset of aphasia).

Syndromes of Aphasia and Their Discourse Symptoms

Categorizing aphasia subtypes may sound easier said than done clinically. The traditional syndrome-based taxonomical approach has received challenges on its discrepancy between the clinical presentations of aphasic symptoms and the "absolute" relationship mapping of an aphasia type to lesion site(s) of the brain. With reference to the linguistic profiles of impaired and preserved language skills, a clinical classification of aphasia syndromes (or generally referred to as the "Boston classification system" because it was developed by a group of Boston-based aphasiologists back in the 1960s) can be conducted by careful and detailed assessment of the following skills in a speaker: fluency of verbal expression, auditory comprehension, repetition, and word retrieval (Goodglass, 1993; Helm-Estabrooks & Albert, 1991). Specifically, an examiner identifies the current linguistic skills and functioning of an examinee with aphasia and determines the examinee's aphasic syndrome based on the salient differences as compared to other speakers with aphasia. Figure 1.1 illustrates the decision tree for the clinical classification process. The first decision to make is about the presence of naming problems. As mentioned above, anomia is a hallmark of, and is almost always present in, aphasia. One without word finding difficulties will not be considered as aphasic. The second step is to determine whether a speaker is fluent or non-fluent according to samples of conversational speech and narrative discourse, typically elicited by a picture description task (see Chapter 2 for more details on discourse elicitation options and procedures and see Chapter 3 for information about methods of clinical discourse evaluation). Successively, the examiner evaluates whether the auditory comprehension skills are good or poor. This classification process ends with a final estimation of how well the oral repetition skills are. Each syndrome of aphasia has both specific and unique clinical characteristics that vary within the "fluent – non-fluent" dichotomy. In other words, overlapping of aphasic features across syndromes is commonly seen in reality. The summary in Table 1.1 illustrates the characteristics of the seven major aphasia syndromes.

Discourse largely refers to units of language larger than a sentence (see Chapter 2 for more details on how discourse is defined). Researchers proposing the above-mentioned syndrome-based taxonomical approach have very limited discussion on the relationships between symptoms at the discourse level and brain lesion locations. Although it has long been recognized that individuals suffering from aphasia are compromised in producing

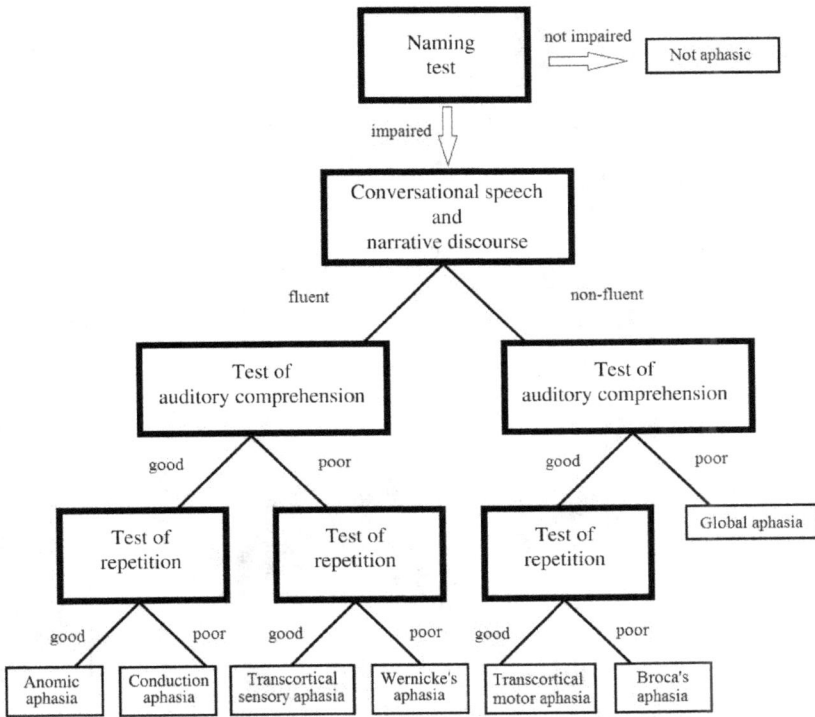

Figure 1.1 Decision tree for the classification of aphasia syndromes
Source: © Anthony Pak-Hin Kong, Ph.D.

well-formed sentences, decisions one makes when adapting the "Boston classification system" to assess spontaneous discourse production focuses mainly
on the degree of fluency only. Other important discourse characteristics,
such as syntactic complexity or sentence well-formedness, elaboration, and
error pattern, are often less attended during the diagnostic process. On top
of the impairment in retrieving appropriate lexical items or target words for
constructing sentences or a discourse (e.g., Kay et al., 1992; Lesser & Perkins,
1999), many speakers with aphasia demonstrate difficulties with the production of sentences (e.g., Cooper, 1990; Garrett, 1980, 1982), procedurals and
narratives (e.g., Bird & Franklin, 1996; Rochon et al., 2000; Saffran et al.,
1989; Ulatowska et al., 1981), as well as discourse with complex syntactic
structures (e.g., Damico et al., 1999). Specifically:

- For speakers with *anomic aphasia*, a milder form of fluent aphasia, the
  most prominent difficulty is in word finding. There is a tendency of

Table 1.1 Clinical characteristics of major syndromes of aphasia

General category	Syndrome	Naming	Conversational speech and narrative discourse	Auditory comprehension	Verbal repetition
Fluent	Anomic	Mild to severe word-finding difficulty	Syntactically close-to-normal verbal output; frequent circumlocutions	Mildly impaired	Mildly impaired
	Conduction		Frequent phonological paraphasias		Moderately to severely impaired
	Transcortical sensory		Frequent semantic paraphasias; occasional circumlocutions and neologisms	Moderately to severely impaired	Mildly impaired
	Wernicke's		Overuse of **jargon** and/or neologisms with varying degree of self-awareness; may talk excessively, frequent semantic and/or phonological paraphasias		Moderately to severely impaired
Non-fluent	Broca's	Mild to severe word-finding difficulty	Effortful, telegraphic, and agrammatic verbal output; imprecise articulation; occasional phonological paraphasias	Mildly to moderately impaired	Moderately to severely impaired
	Transcortical motor		Syntactically simplified utterances; occasional phonological paraphasias		Mildly impaired
	Global	Moderate to severe word-finding difficulty	Very limited or no spontaneous verbal output	Severely impaired	Severely impaired

overusing generic fillers in utterances, such as non-specific pronouns or nouns, and a higher proportion of **circumlocution**, where one describes and talks around a specific target lexical item, in the speech.

- Syndrome of *Wernicke's aphasia*, another type of fluent aphasia, is characterized by massive use of jargons, or nonsensical words and phrases, when one attempts to speak. Utterances of a speaker with Wernicke's aphasia typically retain grammatical sentence structure (i.e., good syntax) but lack meaning (i.e., poor semantics). "Press of speech" is also common, in which the individual may be talking excessively with being aware of how they are talking, even when they should pause to allow others to speak.

- The hallmark of *conduction aphasia* is its prominent deficit with repetition. Although limited with some difficulties in word finding, the speaker can usually express ideas verbally fairly well. However, he or she will demonstrate greater difficulty in repeating phrases, especially during instances when these phrases increase in length and/or complexity. They may also stumble over words that they are attempting to pronounce, manifested as phonological paraphasias or phonemic jargons, in their conversational speech or narrative discourse.

- As for the last fluent syndrome of *transcortical sensory aphasia*, the discourse patterns are fairly similar to Wernicke's aphasia, except for a stronger ability in verbal repetitions of words and phrases.

The greatest distinction between non-fluent and fluent aphasic syndromes is the abnormal speech **prosody** among non-fluent speakers. Some common features to define speech prosody include melody, intonation, and rhythm of the verbal input (see Chapter 6). That being said, each of the three non-fluent aphasic syndromes has its unique clinical discourse symptoms. Specifically:

- The dominant feature of *Broca's aphasia* is **agrammatism** (i.e., poor syntax). Spontaneous speech production is usually effortful, telegraphic, and halting and, therefore, short in length. The content words, such as nouns and verbs, may be preserved in the speech but due to the problems with grammar, sentences are difficult to produce. Grammatical devices or markers are often omitted or wrongly used, resulting in ungrammatical utterances in the oral output. In addition, the ability in repeating words and/or sentences is usually poor. In more severe cases, spontaneous speech may be limited to single words only and the speaker is generally aware of the problem.

- The discourse characteristics of *transcortical motor aphasia* are similar to that of Broca's aphasia, with the exception of stronger repetition skills. Spontaneously answering a question can be challenging for speakers with transcortical motor aphasia but repeating long utterances is usually less problematic.

- *Global aphasia* is the most severe form of non-fluent aphasia with impairment of both expressive and receptive skills. Usually associated with a large left hemisphere lesion, people with global aphasia often produce very limited or even no spontaneous verbal output but may be able to use alternative means, such as the use of gestures, facial expressions, or simple intonation, to express themselves.

To illustrate the discourse symptoms mentioned above, Boxes 1.1 to 1.3 include **transcripts** of three speakers with aphasia telling the Cinderella story (see Chapter 5 for more details about the process of preparing a transcript).

Box 1.1 A Language Sample of Telling the Cinderella Story by a Female Speaker with Anomic Aphasia

Case background

Mary, is a 49-year-old, right-handed, Caucasian female with anomic aphasia (Western Aphasia Battery aphasia quotient = 91.9 out of 100) who suffered an **ischemic stroke** involving the left middle cerebral artery area. She was about nine years post-onset at the time the language sample was collected. Her speech sample includes instances of anomia (e.g., long and short pauses between or within sentences as well as overuse of fillers "um" or "mm" throughout the description), semantic (e.g., "them" for "him") and phonological (e.g., "Cilnerella" or "Sunderella" for target "Cinderella") paraphasias. As compared to the other two samples (Boxes 1.2 and 1.3), there is also a higher variety of generic terms, as indicated by a high proportion of pronouns in the sample:

> Cilnerella (Cinderella), um... [long pause], wants to get the stepmother and [fingers showing "two"] stɛpstɔɪzəɹ (stepsisters). Okay. He's introducing them... him. Okay. (sighs) Okay. Um Cilnderella (Cinderella) want to go to the ball. stɛpstɜrstɜrs (stepsisters) wants to go... [head shaking "no"]. Um stɛpstɜrstɜrs (stepsisters) good at. No. Um coulded (could) [head shaking "no"], um [short pause] didn't want to go. [speaker shrugs] I dunno. Um, so she had a fairy go(d)mother? She help (helped), m..., her to go. She said she was... midnight around all those. Her says alright. She said mi(d)night [long pause] the spell wi(ll) be broken. Um. Sunderella (Cinderella) went to the ball. Um she left her glass slipper and the prince [short pause] was to find it. Um, um, all around town, um, um, she had, um, um... Once she got there she, um, tripped

the man bringin(g) it to her. She, Cinnerella (Cinderella), um, um [short pause] um... went um... Cinderella went um... Oh god, um um... Cinnereller (Cinderella) got it and the prince, um, happy she found him. [head shaking "no"] I dunno. [speaker laughs] Yeah sure.

Note: Remarks of use of extra-linguistic behaviors or transcriber's notes are given in [square parentheses]. Correct targets the speaker originally intended to use are given in (parentheses).

Box 1.2 A Language Sample of Telling the Cinderella Story by a Male Speaker with Wernicke's Aphasia

Case background

George is a 66-year-old, right-handed, Caucasian male with Wernicke's aphasia (Western Aphasia Battery aphasia quotient = 53.0 out of 100) who suffered a left **hemorrhagic stroke** involving left frontal-parietal craniotomy for decompression of the left intra-parenchymal hematoma. He was 17 years post-onset at the time the language sample was collected. His transcript contains more words and includes utterances that are longer and structurally more complex than the anomic transcript (Box 1.1). Instances of untranscribable mumbles or unintelligible speech content are present. Some utterances also contain problematic word order involving redundant word insertion (e.g., "We'll put you in a another ride") or disordering of sentential constituents (e.g., "she gets helped by a friend says" or "we can work you gettin(g) out there"), which reduce the overall meaning of the discourse:

Um there's a little, little people living in this town where children are. And they're going outside doin(g) their thing. And there's always a woman talking about what's goin(g) on with people. She would like to do certain things but everybody else had time for them and they're sayin(g). No you can't do that xxx (untranscribable mumbles/ unintelligible speech). Well xxx (untranscribable mumbles/ unintelligible speech) lookin(g) around things and such... gee... maybe there's a party comin(g) up so I could try to do that. Well somebody else is lookin(g).

[Hands doing a circular motion] Yeah I'm gonna change my clothes and everything else but you gotta work out here. You can't do anything. So everybody else have fun and this person just sittin(g) out there but then she th.. hears about somebody in the air [gesture showing a wand] in the air sayin(g). God I wish I could go that way and [one arm raises] she gets helped by a friend says. Look we can work you gettin(g) out there. Get some clothes, get some pretty xxx (untranscribable mumbles/ unintelligible speech) make your clothes look good. We'll put you in a another ride as a bɑɹsɪnəl (neologism). Ride the kids over here then you go to the party. And so this kid went out there and went to these parties and xxx (untranscribable mumbles/ unintelligible speech)… And the only real problem was you had to xxx (untranscribable mumbles/ unintelligible speech) by midnight. So up (un)til then you can do anything you want. And they were singin(g) and dancin(g) havin(g) a wonderful time. But all of a sudden she looks at the clock [looks at his watch] and it's supposed to be midnight and… Oh my god I change my clothes. She starts [gesture mimicking a running action] running running and squeaks. And she got there in the woods. And there everybody else was talking about things but she's after that… She gets home no chariot or nothin(g) she gets home. And she doesn't know what to do about that. Well the next day somebody comes out and says. They're lookin(g) for her shoes (be)cause she had (th)em, um, the kids. Then she had to drop (th)em. She gets the shoes and tries all kinds of different people. That didn't work that xxx (untranscribable mumbles). And knocked the door and they finally xxx (untranscribable mumbles) they said "I think this fits!" She tries the shoe on a chair [gesture mimicking fitting a slipper] with the family. And that's how the story was because with all her fun at the end she got a shoe match forever. And that's how the story was.

Note: Remarks of use of extra-linguistic behaviors or transcriber's notes are given in [square parentheses]. Correct targets the speaker originally intended to use are given in (parentheses).

What should be highlighted is that, in reality, the symptoms of a person with aphasia may not always fit neatly into one single aphasia syndrome mentioned above. This is particularly the case when these discourse symptoms co-exist with other motor-speech conditions such as **dysarthria** or **apraxia**

Box 1.3 A Language Sample of Telling the Cinderella Story by a Female Speaker with Broca's Aphasia

Case background

Anna is a left-handed Caucasian female who had a left basal hemor-rhagic stroke at the age of 28. Two and a half years after the onset of her stroke, she was diagnosed with a Broca's aphasia (Western Aphasia Battery aphasia quotient = 72.8 out of 100) and provided the language sample of the Cinderella story. As compared to the previous two fluent speakers (in Boxes 1.1 and 1.2), her speech comprised of primarily nouns and verbs, with a clear underemployment of other parts-of-speech such as grammatical markers or **function words**. The syntax is also characterized by reduced structural complexity and impoverished structure, resulting in discontinuity of topic with fragmented discourse structure. Lack of cohesive devices, such as the use of pronouns, also makes it hard for naïve listeners to get the gist of her description:

> Cinderella the mother, um, evil is… A man is g..gun is. [chuckles]
> Um [short pause] uh uh shoes. No, her shoes. xxx (irrelevant speech not transcribed). I don't know [speaker laughs]. Nn…
> He's [finger tracing a line] fies (flies) um… [head nodding "yes"] yeah [speaker chuckles]. Um, a ball. xxx (irrelevant speech not transcribed) xxx (irrelevant speech not transcribed) is [head shaking "no"] not working is… Es [finger tracing some letters] mm… I don't know [speaker laughs].

Note: Remarks of use of extra-linguistic behaviors or transcriber's notes are given in [square parentheses]. Correct targets the speaker originally intended to use are given in (parentheses).

of speech. Syndrome transformation, which is the shift of aphasia types over time, is also very common among speakers whose communication skills are improving as a result of positive responses to treatment or during the period of spontaneous recovery (the first three to six months post–onset of aphasia). Consequently, the classification that originally fits a patient's linguistic pro-file most accurately may change. Proper evaluation and objective documen-tation of any discourse symptoms is, therefore, clinically important for both the purposes of assessment and subsequent intervention.

Traumatic Brain Injury (TBI) and Its Discourse Symptoms

Traumatic brain injury (TBI) can lead to significant impairments of **cognitive-communication skills** and, therefore, disabilities in the lives of those affected. Cognitive-communication disorders generally refer to any communication disorders neurological in nature that are associated with cognitive deficits, including the domains of attention, memory, and executive functions (Ylvisaker & Szekeres, 1989). Impaired discourse is an important and clinically distinctive feature of post-TBI cognitive-communication disorder (Coelho et al., 1995). Other symptoms of TBI include the following:

- Cognitive symptoms: impaired attention, impaired memory, reduced planning and reasoning, lowered concentration, difficulties in new learning, impaired executive control and functions, decreased abstract thinking, lower speed of mental processing, impaired judgment, and decreased self-awareness (Coelho et al., 1995; Cook et al.; Creamer et al., 2005; Draper & Ponsford, 2008; Murdoch & Theodoros, 2001; Hux, 2011; Veterans Health Initiative, 2010).
- Behavioral and somatic symptoms: depression, social isolation, anxiety, agitation, irritability, impulsivity, and aggression (Bombardier et al., 2010; Cook et al., 2011; Galski et al., 1998; Lew et al., 2006; Snow et al., 1999; Veterans Health Initiative, 2010).
- Physical symptoms: apraxia, dysphagia, limb weakness, balance disorder, headache, seizure disorder, nausea, vomiting, dizziness, blurred vision, sleep disturbance, sensory loss, spasticity, and disorders of coordination (Bush & Funk, 2011; Gouvier, 1989; Katz et al., 1990; Lew et al., 2006; Murdoch & Theodoros, 2001; Hux, 2011; Veterans Health Initiative, 2010).

To fully appreciate the underlying cause(s) and diverse patterns of clinical presentation of cognitive-communication impairments associated with TBI, it is essential to understand the various types of TBI as well as the nature and effects of the traumatic event on neurologic damage. There are three general diagnostic categories of TBI (Hagen, 1981): (1) predominant language-specific disorders, such as aphasia, without cognitive impairment; (2) disorganized language secondary to cognitive impairment; and (3) predominantly residual cognitive impairment without language dysfunction. Another traditional approach to classify TBI is determining whether the injury involves penetration (i.e., open head injury) of the skull or not (closed head injury) (Ylvisaker et al., 2008). In the past two decades, blast-related TBI has received growing attention clinically because troops returning from the Iraq and Afghanistan wars have demonstrated different patterns of physical symptoms, frequently compounded by linguistic symptoms (due to impaired or loss of hearing or vision), impaired peripheral sensory and motor systems, as well as behavioral symptoms, such as Post-Traumatic Stress Disorder (PTSD) (Elder & Cristian, 2009; Taber et al., 2006). Mechanism of injury each of these TBI types and its effects to the brain tissues are variable (Table 1.2).

Discourse impairments associated with TBI have been suggested to relate to the disruption of executive functions (Ylvisaker & Szekeres, 1989). Aspects of executive functions critical for successful formulation of oral discourse and effective conveying of ideas through verbal communication include self-awareness, goal-setting, planning, self-directing and initiating, self-inhibiting, self-monitoring, self-evaluation, and flexible problem-solving (Lê et al., 2011; Ylvisaker & Szekeres, 1989). Compared to typical speakers without brain injury, TBI survivors show significantly more difficulty in conversational exchanges. Their discourse production is symptomatic in terms of being tangential, self-centered or self-focused, and disorganized (Coelho et al., 1991; Ehrlich, 1988). Because of the above-mentioned executive dysfunctions, when a TBI survivor is engaged in a conversation, his or her newly selected topic may sometimes show little or no relation to the preceding topic(s). In less severe cases, **topic shading** (Hux, 2011) may be present in which language output contains frequent inappropriate shifting of conversational topic(s) that relate in some manner to previous ones. Impaired speech pragmatics (McDonald, 1993; Ulatowska & Olness, 2007), such as poor topic selection, conversational turn-taking, and topic **maintenance**, have been considered as another important contributing factor to the tangential speech by TBI survivors.

Logorrhea, which is the excessive production of incoherent and repetitive speech that can be incessant and never-ending, may be found in some TBI survivors' spontaneous narratives (Hux et al., 2008). This is in contrast to some earlier studies that reported paucity of verbal output in TBI's albeit relatively spared linguistic form and content, based on the results of language batteries geared toward individuals with aphasia (Coelho et al., 1991). One explanation of this discrepancy is related to the role working memory, a form of short-term memory that stores information temporarily for linguistic processing, plays in discourse production. Specifically, it has been suggested that impairment in working memory can adversely affect TBI survivors' use of figurative language (Moran et al., 2006), syntactic processing (Turkstra & Holland, 1998), and narrative discourse (Chapman et al., 2006; Hux et al., 2008; Youse & Coelho, 1995).

As expected, deficits in word retrieval is also a prominent symptom among survivors of TBI (Barrow et al., 2006; King et al., 2006). One should also note that longer delay in response time at the single-word level is fairly common in TBI. Furthermore, there is a higher degree of semantic errors among TBI survivors when they perform confrontation naming tasks. However, this word-finding impairment at the discourse level becomes less apparent

Table 1.2 Classification and characteristics of brain traumas

Type	Subtypes	Causes	Impact characteristics	Effects
Open head injury (OHI) or penetrating injury	Low velocity	Blows to head or motor vehicle accidents (MVA)	Concentrated blunt force trauma to the skull causing a fracture (instead of a perforation)	A foreign object passes through the skull causing the *primary effect* of tissue destruction along the path of the object itself. *Secondary effects* include (1) tissue damage due to the pressure wave generated within the skull and (2) complications or infections of brain tissue due to presence of external materials embedded in the brain (such as remaining foreign object, skin, hair, or bone fragments)
	High velocity	Gunshots or explosions	Projectiles perforate or pierce the skull	
Closed head injury (CHI) or non-penetrating injury	Non-acceleration injury	Blows to head	Foreign substances do not penetrate brain tissue Unrestrained head is struck by a moving object	*Primary effects* occurring at the moment of impact include (1) contusion of cortex and (2) twisting or stretching forces created by angular acceleration, leading to diffuse axonal injury (DAI). *Secondary effects* in response to the primary effects include (1) edema (accumulation of fluid) and increased intra-cranial pressure and swelling and (2) laceration of blood vessels that may cause hemorrhages.
	Acceleration injury	Falls, blows to head, or MVA	Foreign substances do not penetrate brain tissue Unrestrained head is struck by a moving object or moving head strikes a stationary object	

Blast-related brain trauma or blast injury	Primary injury	Explosions	Head is struck by blast, overpressure waves, or shock waves from the explosion	Internal brain tissues are damaged. Blast waves may induce direct subdural hemorrhages of brain tissues and/or formation of air emboli in vessels supplying blood to the brain causing cerebral infarction. External injuries may be absent
	Secondary injury		Head is struck by fragmentation or other objects propelled by the explosion	Effects are similar to OHI, CHI, or a combination of both.
	Tertiary injury		Air displacement by the explosion creates a blast wind that blows a victim's head against solid objects	Effects are a combination of OHI and CHI
	Quaternary injury	Secondary injury sources such as flash burns or exposure to chemicals	—	Effects may vary and include all other injuries not included in the first three classes

because these individuals can often compensate the difficulty through strategies such as longer reflection time to organize the narrative or circumlocutory description to avoid problems in accessing specific words during a conversation (King et al., 2006).

In terms of the micro-linguistic abilities to formulate sentences, it is largely agreed that deficits among survivors of more diffused TBI (i.e., injury that involved more scattered lesion sites in the brain) are not as readily apparent as those demonstrated by speakers with aphasia or individuals with more focal brain damage. Generally speaking, sentence syntax is relatively preserved in TBI discourse (Body & Perkins, 2004), but micro-linguistic processing that taps into the total number of words produced, retrieval of specific lexical items, lexical efficiency of producing **propositions** (e.g., number of words needed to convey an idea), communication efficiency (e.g., messages conveyed per unit time), or quantity of propositions produced are more problematic (Ellis & Peach, 2009). Not only the semantic complexity but also the density of propositions per sentence tend to be lower in TBI discourse, both factors that directly decrease the speech clarity and negatively affect the overall organization of discourse structure.

Research in the TBI discourse literature has also reported that TBI survivors demonstrate varying extents of problems in maintaining proper **cohesion** and **coherence** of discourse. Specifically, oral discourse of TBI tends to be weaker in semantic links, such that employment of cohesive markers (e.g., personal or demonstrative pronouns), conjunctive markers, or synonyms is much improvised (or even impaired in more severe cases of TBI) (see Liles & Coelho, 1988). The degree in which individual utterances relate to immediately preceding utterances (i.e., local coherence) and to the overall topic of a narrative (i.e., global coherence) has a tendency to be lower in the verbal output of TBI survivors, as compared to speakers with no neurological impairments (Glosser & Deser, 1991; McDonald, 1993). Box 1.4 includes a transcript of telling the Cinderella story by a TBI survivor.

Right Hemisphere Damage (RHD) and Its Discourse Symptoms

Right hemisphere damage (RHD) largely refers to a group of deficits or changes in cognitive-communication abilities that are caused by damage to the right side of the brain, such as poor memory, impaired attention, and problems in reasoning (Myers, 1999; Tompkins, 1995). Researchers and healthcare professionals have used terms such as "right hemisphere disorder" or "right hemisphere dysfunction" interchangeably to refer to the same condition. Common etiologies of RHD include right hemispheric stroke, TBI, infection, surgery, toxicity, and tumor. Typically, RHD does not involve pure linguistic deficits because the left hemisphere is dominant in language processing. That being said, one should not be mistaken that the right hemisphere

Box 1.4 A Language Sample of Telling the Cinderella Story by a Male Speaker with a Single Closed Head Traumatic Brain Injury

Case background

Kent is a right-handed, Caucasian male who sustained a single closed head traumatic brain injury at the age of 26. One year and five months after the accident, he provided the language sample of the Cinderella story. Kent has completed high school. According to the results of the Western Aphasia Battery (aphasia quotient = 96.4 out of 100), he was not aphasic. His discharge notes stated that Kent did not have any history of dementia, brain tumor, stroke, drug abuse, alcoholism, or mental illness. He also did not demonstrate any severe problems with articulation, oro-motor control, voice production, or swallowing. His output was characterized by repetitive phrases with occasional word-finding difficulties. Some topic shading could also be found, further affecting his lexical and communication efficiency of production. Employment of cohesive markers was also relatively weak:

> Alright the door knocks and the… there's a… a… a… (an) older lady and two younger kids and they look… they all look mad and they look angry. And then they walk in to the other bride and groomsman to the wedding. And then they're getting. See this is where I get lost. [head shaking "no"] And then it seems they get into an argument about something. Then they all… they all… three come in and they look… they don't look happy. And then they… they go in and talk to the other kids and adults… or bride and groom… not the bride and groom, the other wedding people. And then the bride… the bride gets… the bride gets shown her wedding dress and she seemed to not like it… by the way it looks and her face. And then something happens. Oh the bride… the… is that what the girl is called? The bride, let's just say, the girl getting married is… seems to get in a scruffle (scuffle) with a couple ladies and she messes up the wedding dress. They rip a stap (strap) off. The bride then wishes for a… wishing… wishes something on… wishes something and she gets a fairy. And I guess she asks to get a wedding dress and then she gets her wedding dress she really likes… wished upon her. And then she goes to the castle to get married to the groom or the king. And they say their vows and everything. And that's it [speaker smiles].

Note: Remarks of use of extra-linguistic behaviors or transcriber's notes are given in [square parentheses]. Correct targets the speaker originally intended to use are given in (parentheses).

does not play any role in human communication. In fact, processing of para-linguistic elements of communication, including speech prosody as well as use or recognition of non-verbal behaviors such as gestures, facial expression, and body language, has been found to be mediated by the right hemisphere. Moreover, intact right hemispheric functions allow one to use visuospatial and mathematical skills accurately and ensure effective regulation of cognitive functions sub-serving language, such as **sustained attention** and **selective attention**, for effective and efficient communication. Whereas different etiologies of RHD may lead to different cognitive-communication deficits, when both the left and right hemispheres are damaged, such as in the case of multiple stokes, vascular dementia, or TBI, it is common to have deficits associated with left hemispheric damage (such as aphasia) present simultaneously with RHD.

Attentional problems are the most prevalent cognitive deficits associated with RHD. Visual neglect, or more specifically left-sided neglect, is a common symptom of RHD. In particular, RHD survivors may show reduced attention to input from their left side, reduced awareness and recognition of the left side of the body, and reduced use of left limbs. Since left-sided neglect is an attentional impairment, when an RHD survivor is undergoing a discourse assessment or is presented with pictorial or written materials, he or she may not notice objects or stimuli in the neglected area (Myers, 1999). This is different from the condition of **hemianopia**, which is a sensory impairment that affects one's ability to see something. Some secondary impairments of left-sided neglect include neglect dyslexia when someone misses or misreads the left side of a page or the left side of words (Ellis et al., 1987).

Hypoarousal can be observed in RHD survivors, meaning that they are less attentive, less oriented, and less alert (Davidson et al., 1992), resulting in a lower level of sensitivity and slower responses to visual and auditory stimuli. Increasing the intensity of stimulation or allowing a longer processing time can be beneficial to RHD. Some RHD survivors are also impaired in sustaining attention and remaining vigilant, by demonstrating a longer reaction time in linguistic or narrative tasks that require shifting of attention (Koski & Petrides, 2001). Finally, deficits of selective attention may hinder RHD survivors to screen out distracting stimuli and to attend to the most important aspects of diverse stimulation. It has also been suggested that an increase in the demand of selective attention within a task can complicate the syndrome of neglect (Riddoch & Humphreys, 1987).

Some survivors with RHD may present with deficits in non-verbal episodic memory, verbal episodic memory, verbal working memory, and spatial working memory (Tompkins et al., 2011). Executive dysfunction in the aspects of planning, reasoning, organization, and problem solving, may also be found in RHD (Klonoff et al., 1990). **Anosognosia**, or the impaired awareness (not denial) of deficits, for the left limbs with reduced function due to hemiplegia may occur after RHD. Anosognosia may improve over time but in most cases of RHD remains a long-lasting problem even beyond the acute stage of RHD.

Interpreting prosody for comprehension of emotional state of a speaker or emotional content of the speaker's verbal output has also been reported to be impaired among RHD survivors. Literal interpretation of a verbal message is common in RHD because of the difficulties in processing the prosodic component of speech. On the expressive side, the use of appropriate prosody to reflect various features of a speaker (e.g., emotional status or presence of irony or emphasis) or an utterance (e.g., statement vs. question vs. command) poses a great challenge to RHD survivors (Manasco, 2014; Weintraub et al., 1981; Tucker et al., 1977). Likewise, given the predominantly monotonous speech intonation in oral discourse, RHD speakers are often negatively perceived to be non-emotional or expressionless by their communication partners.

RHD does not necessarily cause disruption of language itself but may affect the overall ability for one to effectively communicate. As a result of the combined deficits mentioned above, most studies in the literature have emphasized the impact of RHD on conversation. Specifically, proper use of social context and speech dynamics crucial to maintain interactive and spontaneous communication is compromised in RHD. More complex discourse tasks may lead to poorer performance in RHD. To summarize, discourse symptoms of RHD may include the following:

- Problematic pragmatics: RHD speakers are characterized by reduced and problematic use of conversational rules and conventions. They may be impaired in identifying the communicative setting and purpose of conversation as well as impaired in understanding the role(s) of communication partners. The capacity to fully participate in conversation is often reduced because of reduced sensitivity to shared knowledge and appreciation of emotional content (Chantraine et al., 1998; Kaplan, 1990). RHD speakers who are verbose may further indicate the difficulty in figuring out what listeners need to know when they are engaged in conversation (Myers, 1999). Gist of spoken narratives may be limited. Understanding of implicit, intended, indirect, or implied meanings is also reduced.

- Disconnected content: RHD survivors tend to have greater difficulties in sustaining a dyadic communication because of the impairments in selective and sustained attention. However, unlike speakers with aphasia or TBI, speakers with RHD do not necessarily have anomia (Myers & Brookshire, 1996; Rivers & Love, 1980); the sources of the discourse breakdown seen in RHD should, therefore, not be difficulties in word finding. Instead, RHD speakers have reduced discourse coherence since the use of cohesive ties to maintain relations across sentences within a spoken text is weaker or impaired (Myers & Blake, 2008). In a single or sequential picture description task, TBI survivors' deficits in generating inferences about individual elements of pictured scenes have been reported to limit the overall organization of verbal discourse (Myers & Brookshire, 1996). These difficulties are also present in other discourse tasks (see Chapter 2 for more details about discourse elicitation methods).

- Abrupt and perceived as less sensitive to situational and affective cues: Attentional deficits in RHD may have cognitive consequences of showing limited appreciation of the visual and verbal cues available during conversation. Managing implicit or alternative meanings can be a challenge. Some RHD speakers may appear to be impatient, uninterested, or hypo-responsive during discourse tasks, with little or no facial expressions and physical animation (Myers, 1999; Trupe & Hillis, 1985). Difficulties in using appropriate prosody to express emotions may also lead to listeners' misinterpreting RHD speakers' tone of speech (Weintraub et al., 1981).

- Verbose and less informative: Due to reduced sensitivity to speech content significant to the relevant conversational context(s) and lower ability in comprehending verbal and non-verbal expressions, spontaneous speech may be characterized by unelaborated, tangential, egocentric, idiosyncratic, and excessive verbal output (Gardner et al., 1983; Roman et al., 1987). Overall information content is reduced and the ability to generate a central theme of oral production tends to be impaired. High proportion of irrelevant comments and limited **macrostructure** in spontaneous discourse is also not uncommon (Myers, 1999).

- Impoverished and unelaborated output: In some case of RHD, the overall spontaneous verbal output may be limited (Trupe & Hillis, 1985). Examples include fewer words and **content units** in a picture description task or fewer episodes in telling a story. Speakers may present themselves as uninterested, impatient, or perfunctory during face-to-face conversations.

- Less insightful and animated during communication: The ability to generate alternative meanings in discourse may be reduced. As a result of the impaired ability to make inferences of figurative language, idioms, sarcasm, humor, and indirect requests, usage of these language devices is extremely limited in RHD discourse (Brownell et al., 1983; Stemmer et al., 1994). Deficits in emotional communication, such as the reduced employment of facial expressions, gestures, and postures, presence of depression or confusion symptoms, and/or impaired speech prosody, further impede the dynamic of spontaneous discourse.

Dementia and Its Discourse Symptoms

Dementia is a general term for a decline in mental ability in the rate beyond normal ageing that is severe enough to interfere with daily functioning.

Dementia is not a specific disease; instead, it covers a wide range of symptoms associated with a decline in memory and other cognitive-communication skills. **Dementia of Alzheimer's type (DAT)** accounts for up to 80% of cases of dementia. Statistics in 2019 suggested that about 5.8 million people in the United States of all ages are currently suffering from Alzheimer's disease, 81% of whom are aged 75 years or older (Alzheimer's Association, 2019). These figures of dementia are projected to increase significantly because of the anticipated larger size of the older adult population in the nation (55 million people of 65 years of age in 2019 to an estimate of 88 million by 2050) (He et al., 2016). The general diagnostic criteria of dementia include (1) a negative change from a previous level of cognitive function, such as memory skills; (2) a disruption of daily life; (3) no disruption of consciousness; and (4) negative occurrence of situational stress or other mental disorders or conditions. The term "dementia" in the Diagnostic and Statistical Manual of Mental Disorders (DSM-IV) by the American Psychiatric Association (1994) has been replaced by "major neurocognitive disorder" and "minor neurocognitive disorder" in the DSM-V (Table 1.3; for details see American Psychiatric Association, 2011 and DSM-V (American

Table 1.3 Diagnostic criteria for neurocognitive disorder

DSM-V label of disorder	Description
Minor neurocognitive disorder	• Evidence of *modest* cognitive decline from a previous level of performance in one or more cognitive domains. • A decline in neurocognitive performance, typically involving test performance in the range of *one to two* standard deviations below appropriate norms on formal/standardized diagnostic batteries. • Cognitive deficit(s) are *insufficient* to interfere with independence, but greater effort, compensatory strategies, or accommodation may be required to maintain independence. • Cognitive deficit(s) do not occur exclusively in the context of a **delirium** and are not primarily attributable to another mental disorder.
Major neurocognitive disorder	• Evidence of *substantial* cognitive decline from a previous level of performance in one or more cognitive domains. • A decline in neurocognitive performance, typically involving test performance with *at least two* standard deviations below appropriate norms on formal/standardized diagnostic batteries. • Cognitive deficit(s) are *sufficient* to interfere with independence. • Cognitive deficit(s) do not occur exclusively in the context of a delirium and are not primarily attributable to another mental disorder.

Source: American Psychological Association (APA, 2013)

Psychiatric Association, 2013). In diagnosing the degree of neurocognitive disorder, one must determine the etiological subtype of the major or minor neurocognitive disorder, such as DAT, vascular neurocognitive disorder (vascular dementia), Lewy body dementia, frontotemporal neurocognitive disorder (frontotemporal dementia), neurocognitive disorder due to traumatic brain injury, Parkinson's disease, substance-induced neurocognitive disorder, or neurocognitive disorder due to **Huntington's disease**. Details of these dementia subtypes can be found in Bayles et al. (2020).

While memory impairment is the hallmark of dementia, it is commonly agreed that language deficits can be found in all stages of dementia (Bayles, 1982, 1984; Bayles & Tomoeda, 1994; Bourgeois, 2005; Murdoch, 1990). Language symptoms in the early stage are comparatively less obvious because cognitive decline is relatively subtle. Anomia and reduced functional expressive vocabulary are commonly reported (see review in Bayles, 1984). Speakers tend to produce more pronouns due to limited access to nouns and, therefore, resort to the production of more general terms instead; their underlying semantic deficit also causes decreased word length and a higher proportion of frequent words (that are typically more preserved and accessible) in spoken discourse (Kavé & Goral, 2016). Incidence of naming errors, manifested in the form of semantic paraphasias and perseverations, increases as dementia gets worse. Concerning DAT, speakers in the early stage are more impaired in the semantic and pragmatic aspects (Bschor et al., 2001), as evident by the difficulty in word finding in isolation (Forbes-McKay et al., 2005; Semenza et al., 2000) or in a divergent naming task (Alberca et al., 1999). Simplification of grammatical structures (Forbes-McKay & Venneri, 2005) and overuse of simple sentences in oral discourse (Croisile et al., 1996) has also been reported. Moreover, as the condition of DAT progresses over time, a decreased amount of information and increased semantic errors (Kavé & Levy, 2003), deterioration in production efficiency, as well as increased numbers of circumlocutions, revisions, and repetitions of ideas were found (Tomoeda & Bayles, 1993). This is in contrast to the relatively preserved morpho-syntactic and phonological aspects of language until later stages (Kavé & Levy, 2003; Schwartz et al., 1979).

Research also indicates that individuals with dementia display deficits in discourse that are different from the subtle deterioration observed in normal aging (March et al., 2003). Compared to healthy elderly speakers, the propositions of dementia oral discourse have been reported to be more impoverished and less cohesive (Chenery & Murdoch, 1994; Ripich & Terrell, 1988). The maintenance of conversation topics and the ability to relate new to older topics in a conversation has also been found to be poorer (Garcia & Joanette, 1997). These deficits are more evident in later stages as the condition progresses over time. Speakers in the late stage of dementia tend to commit a higher degree of production errors at the utterance level, including deficits in local coherence and cohesion, than those in the early and middle stages (Dijkstra et al., 2002). Discourse-level characteristics, such as global coherence (the pragmatic use of discourse markers to structure and organize a conversation) and elaborations on a topic, among individuals in the middle and late stages are also more impaired than those in the early stage. These problems are in contrast to the preserved macro-level discourse functions demonstrated by elderly controls in retelling stories, producing summaries and gists, and explaining story morals (Ulatowska et al., 1998). Box 1.5 displays a transcript of telling the Cinderella story by a male speaker with mild cognitive impairment.

Box 1.5 A Language Sample of Telling the Cinderella Story by a Male Speaker with Mild Cognitive Impairment (MCI)

Case background

Mild cognitive impairment (MCI) often refers to a transitional stage between the expected cognitive decline of getting older and the more serious cognitive decline of dementia. Mr. Cooper, an 83-year-old male who had 20 years of education in the US, was recently diagnosed with a subtype of MCI from a neuropsychological assessment. In the past year, he has experienced a small but noticeable decline in memory, language, and thinking skills. During the assessment, Mr. Cooper was asked to tell the Cinderella story. Compared to cognitively intact elderly counterparts, his output was fluent and grammatical but much weaker in content (e.g., fewer information units with more empty phrases and indefinite terms) and less cohesive. The sentences were also reduced in length and complexity, but the overall morphological and phonological aspects of the production were largely preserved:

It's based on a fairytale. A young girl... um... is thinking about a dress. Uh... she sees a picture of the dress or she sees a dress, somebody's... somebody's holding the dress up. And she's very excited about the dress. And now she's wearing the dress and she looks beautiful in it. The man comes and picks her up. The man is evidently a man of high position and he's a young man and he takes her to the dance. And they're dancing. [long pause] I forgot exactly what comes next. [long pause] Something happens to the dress, I'm not sure what. But the man takes the dress and has it repaired, fixed, whatever. And gives it to the girl who puts it on. And she kisses him and he kisses her and they fall in love and get married and ride off together and I believe that's the story.

Note: Remarks of use of extra-linguistic behaviors or transcriber's notes are given in [square parentheses].

Earlier reports have attempted to relate the linguistic deficits that exist in dementia to those found in aphasia. In particular, speakers at the early or early-mid stages of dementia demonstrate symptoms considerably similar to anomic aphasia, in terms of word-finding difficulties, reduced conciseness of speech, as well as reduced length of utterance and number of subordinate clauses (Hier at al., 1985). During the mid or mid-late stages of dementia, verbal output is generally hyper-fluent and incoherent with noticeable phonemic substitutions. Apart from the progressive increase in speech emptiness and paraphasias, expressive language continues to decline with a lower degree of speech conciseness and a reduced number of prepositional phrases. Together with the accompanied naming and comprehension deficits, these speakers parallel those with Wernicke's aphasia (Obler & Albert, 1981). If the repetition abilities were also included in the comparison, these speakers were considered to be more similar to those with transcortical sensory aphasia (Hier et al., 1985). Finally, in the late or end stages of dementia, these speakers' verbal output is usually characterized by being non-fluent, echolalic, or perseverative. Severe impairment in auditory comprehension and mutism is not uncommon. This favors the idea of describing them as "global aphasia-like". One should, however, note that these comparisons are based solely on minimal linguistic abilities in discourse production without the consideration of the embedded cognitive load involved. Some researchers have challenged this "comparison approach" of investigating dementia because the association could have complicated and/or distorted the relationship between aphasia and dementia syndromes (e.g., Bayles, 1984). Nevertheless, this approach of investigating language production in dementia is supported given its potential contribution to early detection of the disease and to differentiate dementia sub-types (see Hart, 1988; Murdoch, 1988).

Common Clinical Assessment Procedures of Aphasia and Related Disorders

To ensure effective and successful remediation of acquired language disorders, accurate diagnosis of linguistic and cognitive abilities, as well as identification of a speaker's communication strength and weaknesses, is essential. Components that should be included in the evaluation process are as follow:

- Gather background information on the individual with acquired language disorders, including but not limited to chief complaints, admitting diagnosis, past medical history, family history, social history, education and employment history, and psychosocial history. Appendices 1.1, 1.2, and 1.3 show three case history forms or intake questionnaires for use with aphasia, brain injury, and dementia, respectively.
- Build rapport between the clinician and the individual with acquired language disorders and/or their family members or caregivers.

- Describe and quantify all components of language functioning as well as factors that may affect language (such as cognitive complications, emotional status, or family support). Table 1.4 displays the linguistic and cognitive areas commonly assessed in speakers with acquired communication disorders, including expressive and receptive language, speech production, reading aloud and comprehension, writing, spelling, drawing, cognition, non-verbal communication, and metacognition. Note that written language deficits are generally similar in nature to

Table 1.4 Linguistic and cognitive areas commonly assessed in speakers with acquired communication disorders

Skills to assess	Assessment tasks and examples
Expressive language	• Lexical retrieval (e.g., confrontation naming) • Word fluency (e.g., "Name as many animals as you can in one minute") • Convergent naming (e.g., "What are dogs, cats, and horses?") • **Automatic speech** (e.g., counting from one to ten) • Sentence completion (e.g., "The grass is ___") • Responsive speech (e.g., "Where can you get stamps?") • Repetition (e.g., "Repeat these words. Say ___") • Sentence production (e.g., sentence making with given words) • Conversation (e.g., "Tell me what brings you here") • Discourse production (e.g., picture description or story telling)
Receptive language	• Object recognition/identification (e.g., picture-object matching) • Object function identification (e.g., "Point to the one that we use to cut paper") • Single word comprehension (e.g., auditory word-picture matching) • Yes/No questions (e.g., "Is your name Smith?") • Simple/Complex commands (e.g., "Point to the pen with the book") • Sentence comprehension (e.g., auditory sentence-picture matching) • Discourse comprehension (e.g., understanding a novel story)
Speech production	• Fluency (e.g., telling a story) • Intelligibility (e.g., estimating percentage of unintelligible words) • Prosody (e.g., recite "Baa, baa, black sheep (have)") • Speech rate (e.g., calculating number of word per minute) • Articulation (e.g., measuring articulation agility at the phoneme and syllable level)

(continued)

Table 1.4 Cont.

Skills to assess	Assessment tasks and examples
Oral reading	• Reading aloud single words • Reading aloud irregular words (e.g., "ache" or "debt") • Reading aloud non-words (e.g., "screll" or "chass") • Reading aloud sentences • Reading aloud paragraphs
Reading comprehension	• Reading comprehension of single words (e.g., written word-object matching) • Reading comprehension of sentences (e.g., written sentence-picture matching) • Reading comprehension of paragraphs (e.g., answering questions after reading a novel story)
Writing	• Copying words • Copying sentences • Writing regular words to dictation • Writing irregular words to dictation (e.g., "yacht" or "guide") • Writing non-words to dictation (e.g., "fess" or "munt") • Confrontation writing (e.g., written picture naming) • Spontaneous writing (e.g., narrative writing)
Spelling	• Oral spelling • Written spelling
Drawing	• Copying (e.g., copying a figure) • Functional use of drawing (e.g., Clock drawing. "Set the hands to 'ten after eleven'")
Cognition	• Orientation (e.g., "What is next month?") • Attention (e.g., serial 7) • Memory (e.g., immediate or delayed recall) • Problem solving (e.g., "What would you do if you had a noisy roommate?") • Reasoning (e.g., "How can you tell if your food is very hot?") • Visuospatial skills (e.g., symbol cancellation) • Organizational skills (e.g., "These cards tell a story, but they aren't in the right order. Put them in order so that they tell the story")
Non-verbal communication	• Use of gestures (e.g., "Wave goodbye") • Use of facial expressions (e.g., counting total number of inappropriate facial expression) • Use of body language (e.g., counting total number of appropriate use of proxemics)
Metacognition	• Awareness • Alertness • Concentration • Motivation • Emotional status

the spoken language deficits, but the severity of written and spoken language problems demonstrated by a particular individual with aphasia may not be exactly the same.

- Seek input regarding language rehabilitation and information on a support system outside the clinic.
- Establish an accurate diagnosis and determine the prognosis of the language disorder.
- Set preliminary rehabilitation goals with reference to the current language disorder and expectations of the individuals with acquired language disorders and/or their family members.

Administration of formal or standardized tests is a common and necessary clinical procedure that allows clinicians to obtain the maximum amount of information in the shortest period of time. In particular, results of a standardized **norm-referenced assessment** of aphasia and related cognitive-communication disorders inform us important aspects of an individual's language functioning and related cognitive skills sub-serving language. Clinicians will be able to determine the presence of deficits and their severity and characteristics. Clinicians can also obtain the baseline performance of their clients, which is critical for measuring progress (including improvement, regression, and stability) over time, setting target areas for treatment planning, and estimating prognosis for language recovery. A standardized test must be conducted following the standard procedures in the same way every time it is offered. The standardization of the existing formal tests ensures their **validity** and **reliability** for quantification of language and related cognitive strengths and weaknesses (Davis, 2007; Ivanova & Hallowell, 2013). A list of some commonly used standardized tests for evaluating different acquired cognitive-communication disorders can be found in Table 1.5. Depending on how the norms (i.e., normative data) are presented for test score interpretation, clinicians may be able to compare how far the impairment of an examinee is, relative to his or her age-, education-, and/or gender-matched controls. Comparison across examinees, within the same or across different clinical settings, is also possible, which may further help determine the priority of treatment candidacy.

When time is limited to conduct a formal battery, or if an examinee is not fit for receiving a standardized test, use of informal examination is in order. However, this will usually require a higher level of clinical skills on the part of the examiners because a higher degree of creativity, flexibility, and sensitivity is always needed (Helm-Estabrooks & Albert, 1991). A list of some commonly used screening tools is displayed in Table 1.6.

It should be noted that although selected tests listed in Tables 1.5 and 1.6 have considered the performance of narrative discourse, clinicians may not be able to conduct a full-scale appreciation of the discourse functioning

Table 1.5 Standardized assessment batteries for acquired communication disorders (in alphabetical order)

Target disorder	Battery	Approximate administration time	Author(s)	Publisher (Year)
Aphasia	Aphasia Diagnostic Profiles (ADP)	40 to 50 minutes	Helm-Estabrooks	Pro-Ed (1992)
	Boston Assessment of Severe Aphasia (BASA)	20 to 30 minutes	Helm-Estabrooks, Ramsberger, Morgan, and Nicholas	Pro-Ed (1989)
	Boston Diagnostic Aphasia Examination - Third Edition (BDAE-3)	35 to 45 minutes	Goodglass, Kaplan, and Barresi	Pro-Ed (2000)
	Boston Naming Test (BNT)	15 to 30 minutes	Kaplan, Goodglass, and Weintraub	Lippincott Williams & Wilkins (2007)
	Communication Abilities of Daily Living – Second Edition (CADL-2)	30 to 60 minutes	Holland, Frattali, and Fromm	Pro-Ed (1999)
	Comprehensive Aphasia Test (CAT)	45 to 100 minutes	Swinburn, Porter, and Howard	Psychology Press (2004)
	Discourse Comprehension Test	20 minutes	Brookshire and Nicholas	PICA Programs (1997)
	Examining for Aphasia: Assessment of Aphasia and Related Impairments – Fourth Edition (EFA-4)	30 to 60 minutes	LaPointe and Eisenson	Pro-Ed (2008)
	Functional Assessment of Communication Skills for Adults (ASHA FACS)	20 minutes	Frattali, Holland, Thompson, Wohl, and Ferketic	American Speech-Language-Hearing Association (2005)
	Porch Index of Communicative Ability-Revised (PICA-R)	60 minutes	Porch	PICA Programs (2001)
	Psycholinguistic Assessments of Language Processing in Aphasia	30 to 90 minutes	Kay, Lesser, and Coltheart	Psychology Press (1992)
	Western Aphasia Battery-Revised (WAB-R)	30 to 60 minutes	Kertesz	Pearson (2006)

Table 1.5 Cont.

Target disorder	Battery	Approximate administration time	Author(s)	Publisher (Year)
Traumatic brain injury	Birmingham Cognitive Screen (BCoS)	30 to 60 minutes	Humphreys, Bickerton, Samson, and Riddoch	Psychology Press (2012)
	Brief Test of Head Injury (BTHI)	20 to 30 minutes	Helm-Estabrooks and Hotz	Pro-Ed (1991)
	Cambridge Prospective Memory Test (CAMPROMPT)	25 minutes	Wilson, Shiel, Foley, Emslie, Groot, Hawkins, Watson, and Evans	Pearson (2005)
	Cognitive Linguistic Quick Test (CLQT)	15 to 30 minutes	Helm-Estabrooks	Pearson (2001)
	Kaufman Short Neuropsychological Assessment Procedure (K-SNAP)	30 minutes	Kaufman and Kaufman	AGS Publishing/ Pearson Assessments (1994)
	Rivermead Behavioural Memory Test –Third Edition (RBMT-3)	25 to 30 minutes	Wilson, Greenfield, Clare, Baddeley, Cockburn, Watson, Tate, Sopena, and Nannery	Pearson (2008)
	Scales of Cognitive Ability for Traumatic Brain Injury (SCATBI)	30 to 120 minutes	Adamovich and Henderson	Pro-Ed (1992)
Right hemisphere damage	Burns Brief Inventory of Communication and Cognition (Burns Inventory)	30 minutes	Burns	Pearson (1997)
	Cognitive Linguistic Quick Test (CLQT)	15 to 30 minutes	Helm-Estabrooks	Pearson (2001)
	Frenchay Dysarthria Assessment – Second Edition (FDA-2)	20 minutes	Enderby and Palmer	Pro-Ed (2008)
	Mini Inventory of Right Brain Injury – Second Edition (MIRBI-2)	30 minutes	Pimental and Knight	Pro-Ed (2000)

(continued)

Table 1.5 Cont.

Target disorder	Battery	Approximate administration time	Author(s)	Publisher (Year)
	Rehabilitation Institute of Chicago (RIC) Evaluation of Communication Problems in Right Hemisphere Dysfunction – Third Edition (RICE-3)	30 to 45 minutes	Halper, Cherney, and Burns	Rehabilitation Institute of Chicago (RIC) Academy Bookstore (2010)
	Test of Everyday Attention (TEA)	45 to 60 minutes	Robertson, Ward, Ridgeway, and Nimmo-Smith	Thames Valley Test Company (1994)
	Right Hemisphere Language Battery – Second Edition (RHLB-2)	30 to 60 minutes	Bryan	Whurr Publishers Ltd. (1995)
Dementia	Arizona Battery for Communication Disorders of Dementia (ABCD)	45 to 90 minutes	Bayles and Tomoeda	Pro-Ed (1993)
	Dementia Rating Scale – Second Edition (DRS-2)	15 to 30 minutes	Mattis	Psychological Assessment Resources (2001)
	Functional Linguistic Communication Inventory (FLCI)	30 minutes	Bayles and Tomoeda	Pro-Ed (1995)
	Ross Information Processing Assessment – Second Edition (RIPA-2)	45 to 60 minutes	Ross-Swain	Pro-Ed (1996)

and impairment. This is because of the fact that almost all of these discourse assessments are limited by their quick-and-easy, qualitative, and/or crude analyses. Chapter 3 of this book includes a more in-depth discussion of various approaches of discourse analyses. Depending on the symptomology of the individuals with acquired cognitive-communication disorders, clinicians will need to pay close attention to the relationship between these symptoms and their immediate environment. Use of items relevant to the examinees (such as their interest or occupation, and functional situations of using language) can be beneficial.

Table 1.6 Screening instruments for acquired communication disorders (in alphabetical order)

Target disorder	Battery	Approximate administration time	Author(s)	Publisher/Source (Year)
Aphasia	Bedside Evaluation Screening Test – Second Edition (BEST-2)	20 minutes	West, Sands, and Ross-Swain	Pro-Ed (1998)
	Mississippi Aphasia Screening Test (MAST)	10 to 15 minutes	Center for Outcome Measurement in Brain Injury	www.tbims.org/combi/mast (2005)
	Quick Aphasia Battery (QAB)	30 to 45 minutes	Wilson, Eriksson, Schneck, and Lucanie	https://langneurosci.org/qab/ (2018)
	Quick Assessment for Aphasia	10 to 15 minutes	Tanner and Culbertson	Academic Communication Associates (1999)
	Western Aphasia Battery-Revised (WAB-R) bedside form	15 minutes	Kertesz	Pearson (2006)
Traumatic brain injury	Awareness Questionnaire	10 minutes	Sherer, Boake, Levin, Silver, Ringholz, and High	http://tbims.org/combi/aq/index.html (1998)
	Functional Independence Measure (FIM)	5 minutes	Uniform Data System for Medical Rehabilitation	www.tbims.org/combi/FIM/ (1996)
	Montreal Cognitive Assessment (MoCA)	10 minutes	Nasreddine	www.mocatest.org/ (2003)
	Oxford Cognitive Screen (OCS)	10 to 20 minutes	Demeyere, Riddoch, Slavkova, and Humphreys	www.psy.ox.ac.uk/research/oxford-cognitve-neuropsychology-centre/oxford-cognitive-screening/tests (2013)
	The Rancho Levels of Cognitive Functioning (Revised)	5 minutes	Hagen	www.rancho.org/research/cognitive_levels.pdf (1998)
Right hemisphere damage	Quick Assessment for Dysarthria	10 to 15 minutes	Tanner and Culbertson	Academic Communication Associates (1999)

(continued)

Table 1.6 Cont.

Target disorder	Battery	Approximate administration time	Author(s)	Publisher/Source (Year)
Dementia	Alzheimer's Quick Test (AQT) Assessment of Temporal-Parietal Function	3 to 5 minutes	Wiig, Nielsen, Minthon, and Warkentin	Harcourt Assessment (2002)
	Global Deterioration Scale (GDS)	5 minutes	Reisberg, Ferris, De Leon, and Crook	Reisberg (1982)
	Mini–mental state examination (MMSE)	10 minutes	Folstein, Folstein, and McHugh	Pergamon Press/ Elsevier (1975)

Rationales for Discourse Analysis

The disruption of discourse production can inform us about the form and extent of expressive language impairment in brain-damaged individuals. It also helps researchers infer normal functioning of the language system in neuro-linguistic investigations. Yet, there is a great heterogeneity of how linguistic symptoms are manifested in different language tasks, especially when it comes to the level of narrative discourse. This has motivated researchers to develop various assessment tools, both clinically- and research-oriented ones, for studying language disturbance. However, only a small number of them were developed specifically for the clinical evaluation of narratives or connected speech in English. In most cases, clinicians may find it hard to provide objective comments about one's spontaneous language output because most assessment batteries lack comprehensive measures of narratives. The amount of time needed to conduct a detailed quantification of discourse disruption is also often clinically not feasible. Different degrees of subjectivity involved in the diagnostic process, with reference to the experiences on analyzing discourse-level impairments a clinician has, further makes comparisons across individuals or across raters a particularly difficult job. More importantly, in cases of TBI or RHD, where linguistic form and content are often spared, language batteries geared toward individuals with aphasia also fail to reflect the subtle discourse impairments in these disorders. The above limitations speak for the need to have more systematic and clinically oriented methods of discourse analysis.

One of the fundamental functions of communication is to convey messages across communication partners. A detailed and accurate evaluation of everyday talk of people with aphasia and related cognitive-communication disorders will provide clinicians with critical insights into the ICF disability classification of language impairment. The source of problems leading to "activities limitation" and "participation restriction" can be explained with careful analyses of discourse breakdown. Moreover, goals to address or remediate these deficits can be set specifically to one's need and desire. In the following chapters, a more comprehensive review of traditional and more contemporary discourse analytic systems will be provided, followed by discussion on issues clinicians should consider when applying these techniques in real-life clinical situations.

Conclusions

A review of the classification systems of aphasia, traumatic brain injury, right hemisphere disorder, and dementia is provided in this chapter. Along with the description of these disorders, information about their corresponding etiologies, types, and salient clinical characteristics was presented. The discourse symptoms of different acquired neurogenic communication deficits vary, depending on factors such as the type and severity of cognitive-communication disorders, as well as the demand of language production. The body of research about discourse analysis has been growing in the past two decades, which will lead to a more promising evidence-based practice of clinical assessment and management of discourse deficits in acquired communication disorders.

References

Alberca, R., Salas, D., Pérez-Gil, J. A., Lozano, P., & Gil-Neciga, E. (1999). Verbal fluency and Alzheimer's disease. *Neurologia, 14*, 344–348.

Alzheimer's Association. (2019). Alzheimer's disease facts and figures. *Alzheimer's & Dementia, 15*(3), 321–387.

American Psychological Association (APA). (1994). *Diagnostic and statistical manual of mental disorders (DSM-IV)*. Arlington, VA: American Psychiatric Association American.

American Psychological Association (APA). (2011). Guidelines for the evaluation of dementia and age-related cognitive change. *American Psychologist, 67*, 1–9.

American Psychological Association (APA). (2013). *Diagnostic and statistical manual of mental disorders (DSM-V)*. Arlington, VA: American Psychiatric Association.

Barrow, I. M., Hough, M., Rastatter, M. P., Walker, M., Holbert, D., & Rotondo, M. F. (2006). The effects of mild traumatic brain injury on confrontation naming in adults. *Brain Injury, 20*, 845–855.

Basso, A. (2003). *Aphasia and its therapy*. New York, NY: Oxford University Press.

Bayles, K. A. (1982). Language function in senile dementia. *Brain and Language, 16*, 265–280.

Bayles, K. A. (1984). Language and dementia. In A. L. Holland (Ed.), *Language disorders in adults: Recent advances* (pp. 209–244). San Diego: College-Hill Press.

Bayles, K. A., McCullough, K., & Tomoeda, C. K. (2020). *Cognitive-communication disorders of MCI and dementia: Definition, assessment, and clinical management.* San Diego, CA: Plural Publishing.

Bayles, K. A., & Tomoeda, C. K. (1994). *Functional Linguistic Communication Inventory.* Austin, TX: Pro-Ed.

Benson, D. F. (1988). Anomia in aphasia. *Aphasiology, 2,* 229–235.

Bird, H., & Franklin, S. (1996). Cinderella revisited: A comparison of fluent and non-fluent aphasic speech. *Journal of Neurolinguistics, 9,* 187–206.

Body, R., & Perkins, M. R. (2004). Validation of linguistic analyses in narrative discourse after traumatic brain injury. *Brain Injury, 18,* 707–724.

Bombardier, C. H., Fann, J. R., Temkin, N. R., Esselman, P. C., Barber, J., & Dikmen, S. S. (2010). Rates of major depressive disorder and clinical outcomes following traumatic brain injury. *The Journal of American Medical Association, 303,* 1938–1945.

Bourgeois, M. S. (2005). Dementia. In L.L. LaPointe (Ed.), *Aphasia and related neurogenic language disorders* (pp.199–212). New York: Thieme.

Broca, P .P. (1865). Sur le siége de la faculté du language articulé. *Bulletin d'Anthropologie, 6,* 377–393.

Brownell, H. H., Michel, D., Powelson, J., & Gardner, H. (1983). Surprise but not coherence: Sensitivity to verbal humor in right-hemisphere patients. *Brain and Language, 18,* 20–27.

Bschor, T., Kuhl, K., & Reischies, F. M. (2001). Spontaneous speech of patients with dementia of Alzhemier type and mild cognitive impairment. *International Psychogeriatrics, 13,* 289–298.

Bush, E. J. & Funk, T. M. (2011). Dysphagia associated with traumatic brain injury. In K. Hux (Ed.), *Assisting survivors of traumatic brain injury: The role of the speech-language pathologists* (pp. 255–292). Austin, TX: Pro Ed.

Chantraine, Y., Joanette, Y., & Ska, B. (1998). Conversational abilities in patients with right hemisphere damage. *Journal of Neurolinguistics, 11,* 21–32.

Chapman, S. B., Gamino, J. F., Cook, L. G., Hanten, G., Li, X., & Levin, H. S. (2006). Impaired discourse gist and working memory in children after brain injury. *Brain and Language, 97,* 178–188.

Chenery, H. J., & Murdoch, B. E. (1994). The production of narrative discourse in response to animations in persons with dementia of the Alzheimer's type: Preliminary findings, *Aphasiology, 8,* 159–171.

Code, C. (2011). Significant landmarks in the history of aphasia and its therapy. In I. Papathanasiou, P. Coppens, & C. Potagas (Eds.), *Aphasia and related neurogenic communication disorders* (pp. 3–22). Burlington, MA: Jones & Bartlett Learning.

Coelho, C. A., Liles, B. Z., & Duffy, R .J. (1991). The use of discourse analyses for the evaluation of higher level traumatically brain-injured adults. *Brain Injury, 5,* 381–392.

Coelho, C. A., Liles, B. Z., & Duffy, R .J. (1995). Impairments of discourse abilities and executive functions in traumatically brain injured adults. *Brain Injury, 9,* 471–477.

Cook, K. F., Bombardier, C. H., Bamer, A. M., Choi, S. W., Kroenke, K., & Fann, J. R. (2011). Do somatic and cognitive symptoms of traumatic brain injury confound depression screening? *Archives of Physical Medicine and Rehabilitation, 92,* 818–823.

Cooper, P. V. (1990). Discourse production and normal aging: Performance on oral picture description tasks. *Journal of Gerontology, 45,* 210–214.

Creamer, M., O'Donnell, M. L., & Pattison, P. (2005). Amnesia, traumatic brain injury, and posttraumatic stress disorder: A methodological inquiry. *Behaviour Research and Therapy*, *43*, 1383–1389.

Croisile, B., Brabant, M. J., Carmoi, T., Lepage, Y., Aimard, G., & Trillet, M. (1996). Comparisons between oral and written spelling in Alzheimer's disease. *Brain and Language*, *54*, 361–387.

Damico, J. S., Oelschlaeger, M., & Simmons-Mackie, N. (1999). Qualitative methods in aphasia research: Conversation analysis. *Aphasiology*, *13*, 667–679.

Davidson, R. A., Fedio, P., Smith, B. D., Aureille, E., & Martin, A. (1992). Lateralized mediation of arousal and habituation: Differential bilateral electrodermal activity in unilateral temporal lobectomy patients. *Neuropsychologia*, *30*, 1053–1063.

Davis, G. A. (2007). *Aphasiology, disorders and clinical practice*. Boston, MA: Allyn and Bacon.

Davis, G. A. (2012). The cognition of language and communication. In R. K. Peach & L. P. Shapiro (Eds.), *Cognitive and acquired language disorders: An information processing approach* (pp. 1–12). St. Louis, MO: Elsevier.

Dijkstra, K., Bourgeois, M., Petrie, G., Burgio, L. & Allen-Burge, R. (2002). My recaller is on vacation: Discourse analysis of nursing-home residents with dementia. *Discourse Processes*, *33*, 53–76.

Draper, K., & Ponsford, J. (2008). Cognitive functioning ten years following traumatic brain injury and rehabilitation. *Neuropsychology*, *22*, 618–625.

Ehrlich, J. S. (1988). Selective characteristics of narrative discourse in head-injured and normal adults. *Journal of Communication Disorders*, *21*, 1–9.

Elder, G. A., & Cristian, A. (2009). Blast-related mild traumatic brain injury: Mechanisms of injury and impact on clinical care. *Mount Sinai Journal of Medicine: A Journal of Translational and Personalized Medicine*, *7*, 111–118.

Ellis, A. W., Flude, B. M., & Young, A. W. (1987). "Neglect dyslexia" and the early visual processing of letters in words and nonwords. *Cognitive Neuropsychology*, *4*, 439–464.

Ellis, A. W. & Young A. W. (1988). *Human cognitive neuropsychology*. Hove, UK: Lawrence Erlbaum.

Ellis, C. & Peach, R. (2009). Sentence planning following traumatic brain injury. *Neurorehabilitation*, *24*, 255–266.

Engelter, S. T., Gostynski, M., Papa, S., Frei, M., Born, C., Ajdacic-Gross, V., & Gutzwiller, F. (2006). Epidemiology of aphasia attributable to first ischemic stroke: Incidence, severity, fluency, etiology, and thrombolysis. *Stroke*, *37*, 1379–1384.

Forbes-McKay, K. E., Ellis, A. W., Shanks, M. F., & Venneri, A. (2005). The age of acquisition of words produced in a semantic fluency task can reliably differentiate normal from pathological age related cognitive decline. *Neuropsychologia*, *43*, 1625–1632.

Forbes-McKay, K. E. & Venneri, A. (2005). Detecting subtle spontaneous language decline in early Alzheimer's disease with a picture description task. *Neurological Science*, *26*, 243–254.

Fridriksson, J., Moser, D., Bonilha, L., Morrow-Odom, K. L., Shaw, H., Fridriksson, A., Baylis, G. C., & Rorden, C. (2007). Neural correlates of phonological and semantic-based anomia treatment in aphasia. *Neuropsychologia*, *45*, 1812–1822.

Gall, F. (1825). *Sur les fonctions du cerveau et sur celles de chacune de ses parties*. Paris: Baillière.

Galski, T., Tompkins, C., & Johnston, M. V. (1998). Competence in discourse as a measure of social integration and quality of life in persons with traumatic brain injury. *Brain Injury, 12,* 769–782.

Garcia, L. J., & Joanette, Y. (1997). Analysis of conversational topic shifts: A multiple case study. *Brain and Language, 58,* 92–114.

Gardner, H., Brownell, H. H., Wapner, W., & Michelow, D. (1983). Missing the point: The role of right hemisphere in the processing of complex linguistic materials. In E. Perecman (Ed.), *Cognitive processing in right hemisphere* (pp. 169–191). New York NY: Academic Press.

Garrett, M. F. (1980). Levels of processing in sentences production. In B. Butterworth (Ed.), *Language production* (Vol. 1, pp. 177–220). London: Academic Press.

Garrett, M. F. (1982). Production of speech: Observations from normal and pathological language use. In A. W. Ellis (Ed.), *Normality and pathology in cognitive functions* (pp. 19–76). London: Academic Press.

Glosser, G., & Deser, T. (1991). Patterns of discourse production among neurological patients with fluent language disorders. *Brain and Language, 40,* 67–88.

Goodglass, H. (1993). *Understanding aphasia.* San Diego, CA: Academic Press.

Goodglass, H., & Kaplan, E. (1983). *The assessment of aphasia and related disorders.* Philadelphia, PA: Lea & Febiger.

Gouvier, W. D., Maxfield, M. W., Schweitzer, J. R., Horton, C. R., Shipp, M., Neilson, K., & Hale, P. N. (1989). Psychometric prediction of driving performance among the disabled. *Archives of Physical Medicine and Rehabilitation, 70,* 745–750.

Hackett, M. L., & Pickles, K. (2014). Part I: frequency of depression after stroke: An updated systematic review and meta-analysis of observational studies. *International Journal of Stroke, 9*(8), 1017–1025.

Hagen, C. (1981). Language disorders secondary to closed head injury: Diagnosis and treatment. *Topics in Language Disorders, 1,* 73–87.

Hart, S. (1988). Aphasia and dementia: Steps towards a new era in neuropsychology. *Aphasiology, 2,* 195–197.

He, W., Goodkind, D., & Kowal, P. (2016). U.S. Census Bureau, International Population Reports, P95/16–1, An Aging World: 2015. www.census.gov/content/dam/Census/library/publications/2016/demo/p95-16-1.pdf .

Helm-Estabrooks, N., & Albert, M. L. (1991). *Manual of aphasia therapy.* Austin, TX: Pro Ed.

Helm-Estabrooks, N., Albert, M .L., & Nicolas, M. (2014). *Manual of aphasia and aphasia therapy.* Austin, TX: Pro Ed.

Hier, D. B., Hagenlocker, R., & Shindler, A. G. (1985). Language disintegration in dementia: Effects of etiology and severity. *Brain and Language, 25,* 117–133.

Hier, D. B., Yoon, W. B., Mohr, J. P. & Price, T. R. (1994). Gender and aphasia in the stroke data bank. *Brain and Language, 47,* 155–167.

Hux, K. (2011). Cognitive-communication deficits. In K. Hux (Ed.), *Assisting survivors of traumatic brain injury: The role of the speech-language pathologists* (pp. 121–184). Austin, TX: Pro Ed.

Hux, K., Wallace, S., Evans, K., & Snell, L. (2008). Performing "Cookie Theft" content analyses to delineate cognitive-communication impairments. *Journal of Medical Speech-Language Pathology, 16,* 83–102.

Ivanova, M. V., & Hallowell, B. (2013). A tutorial on aphasia test development in any language: Key substantive and psychometric considerations. *Aphasiology, 1,* 891–920.

Kadojić, D., Bijelić, B. R., Radanović, R., Porobić, M., Rimac, J., & Dikanović, M. (2012). Aphasia in patients with ischemic stroke. *Acta Clinica Croatica, 51*(2), 221–225.

Kagan, A. (1995). Revealing the competence of aphasic adults through conversation: A challenge to health professionals. *Topics in Stroke Rehabilitation, 2*, 15–28.

Kagan, A., & Simmons-Mackie, N. (2013). From my perspective: Changing the aphasia narrative. *The ASHA Leader, 18*(11), 6–8.

Kaplan, J. A. (1990). The effects of right hemisphere damage on the pragmatic interpretation of conversational remarks. *Brain and Language, 38*, 315–333.

Katz, R. T., Golden, R. S., Butter, J., Tepper, D., Rothke, S., Holmes, J., & Sahgal, V. (1990). Driving safety after brain damage: Follow-up of twenty-two patients with matched controls. *Archives of Physical Medicine and Rehabilitation, 71*, 133–137.

Kavé, G., & Goral, M. (2016). Word retrieval in picture descriptions produced by individuals with Alzheimer's disease. *Journal of Clinical and Experimental Neuropsychology, 38*(9), 958–966.

Kavé, G., & Goral, M. (2017). Do age-related word retrieval difficulties appear (or disappear) in connected speech? *Aging, Neuropsychology and Cognition, 24*(5), 508–527.

Kavé, G., & Levy, Y. (2003). Morphology in picture descriptions provided by persons with Alzheimer's disease. *Journal of Speech Language and Hearing Research, 46*, 341–352.

Kay, J., Lesser, R., & Coltheart, M. (1992). *Psycholinguistic Assessment of Language Processing in Aphasia (PALPA)*. Hove, UK: Lawrence Erlbaum Associates Ltd.

King, K. A., Hough, M. S., Walker, M., Rastatter, M. P., & Holbert, D. (2006). Mild traumatic brain injury: Effects on naming in word retrieval and discourse. *Brain Injury, 20*, 725–732.

Klonoff, P. S., Sheperd, L. C., O'Brien, K. P., Chiapello, D. A., & Hodak, J. A. (1990). Rehabilitation and outcome of right-hemisphere stroke patients: Challenges to traditional diagnostic and treatment methods. *Neuropsychology, 4*, 147–163.

Koski, L. & Petrides, M. (2001). Time-related changes in task performance after lesions restricted to the frontal cortex. *Neuropsychologia, 39*, 268–281.

Kotila, M., Waltimo, O., Niemi, M. L., Laaksonen, R., & Lempinen, M. (1984). The profile of recovery from stroke and factors influencing outcome. *Stroke, 15*, 1039–1044.

Laganaro, M., Di Pietro, M., & Schnider, A. (2006). What does recovery from anomia tell us about the underlying impairment: The case of similar anomic patterns and different recovery. *Neuropsychologia, 44*, 534–545.

Lê, K., Mozeiko, J., & Coelho, C. (2011). Discourse analyses: Characterising cognitive-communication disorders following TBI. *The ASHA Leader, 16*(2), 18–21.

Lesser, R., (1987). Cognitive neuropsychological influences on aphasia therapy. *Aphasiology, 1*, 189–200.

Lesser, R., & Perkins, L. (1999). *Cognitive neuropsychology and conversation analysis in aphasia*. London: Whurr Publishers.

Lew, H. L, Poole, J. H., Guillory, S. G., Salerno, R. M, Leskin, G., & Sigford, B. (2006). Persistent problems after traumatic brain injury: The need for long-term follow-up and coordinated care. *Journal of Rehabilitation Research & Development, 43*, vii–x.

Liles, B. Z. & Coelho, C. A. (1988). Cohesion analyses. In L. R. Cherney, B. B. Shadden, & C. A. Coelho (Eds.), *Analyzing discourse in communicatively impaired adults* (pp. 65–84). Gaithersburg, MD: Aspen Publishers.

Luria, A. R. (1964). Factors and forms of aphasia. In A. V. S. de Reuck & M. O'Connor (Eds.), *Ciba Foundation Symposium on disorders of language* (pp. 143–161). London, UK: J. & A. Churchill Ltd.

Manasco, M. H. (2014). *Introduction to neurogenic communication disorders.* Burlington, MA: Jones & Bartlett Learning.

March, E., Wales, R., & Pattison, P. (2003). Language use in normal ageing and dementia of the Alzheimer type. *Clinical Psychologist, 7*, 44–49.

McDonald, S. (1993). Pragmatic language skills after closed head injury: Ability to meet the informational needs of the listener. *Brain and Language, 44*, 28–46.

Moran, C. A., Nippold, M. A., & Gillon, G. T. (2006). Working memory and proverb comprehension in adolescents with traumatic brain injury: A preliminary investigation, *Brain injury, 20*, 417–423.

Murdoch, B. E. (1988). Language disorders in dementia as aphasia syndromes. *Aphasiology, 2*, 181–185.

Murdoch, B. E. (1990). *Acquired speech and language disorders: A neuroanatomical and functional neurological approach.* London: Chapman and Hall.

Murdoch, B. E. & Theodoros, D. G. (2001). *Traumatic brain injury: Associated speech, language, and swallowing disorders.* San Diego, CA: Delmar Singular Publishing Group.

Myers, P. S. (1999). *Right hemisphere damage: Disorders of communication and cognition.* San Diego, CA: Singular Publishing Group, Inc.

Myers, P. S. & Blake, M. L. (2008). Communication disorders associated with right-hemisphere damage. In R. Chapey (Ed.), *Language intervention strategies in aphasia and related neurogenic communication disorders* (pp. 963–987). Baltimore, MD: Lippincott Williams and Wilkins.

Myers, P. S. & Brookshire, R. H. (1996). Effect of visual and inferential variables on scene description by right-hemisphere-damaged and non-brain-damage adults. *Journal of Speech and Hearing Research, 39*, 870–880.

National Aphasia Association. (2021). Aphasia fact sheet. www.aphasia.org/aphasia-resources/aphasia-factsheet/),

National Institute on Deafness and Other Communication Disorders (NIDCD). (1997). Fact Sheet: Aphasia (NIH Pub. No. 97–4257). Bethesda, MD: NIDCD.

National Institute on Deafness and Other Communication Disorders (NIDCD). (2017). Aphasia (NIH Pub. No. 97–4257). Bethesda, MD: NIDCD. www.nidcd.nih.gov/health/aphasia

National Stroke Association. (2008). www.stroke.org

Obler, L. K., & Albert, M. L. (1981). Language in the elderly aphasic and in the dementing patient. In M. T. Sarno (Ed.), *Acquired aphasia* (pp. 385–398). New York: Academic Press Inc.

Papathanasiou, I. Coppens, P., & Davidson, B. (2022). Aphasia and related neurogenic communication disorders: Basic concepts, management, and use of technology. In I. Papathanasiou & P. Coppens (Eds.), *Aphasia and related neurogenic communication disorders* (pp. 3–14). Burlington, MA: Jones & Bartlett Learning.

Reinvang, I. (1984). The natural history of aphasia. *Advances in Neurology, 42*, 13–22.

Riddoch, M. J., & Humphreys, G. W. (1987). Perceptual action system in unilateral neglect. In M. Jeannerod (Ed.), *Neurophysiological and neuropsychological aspects of spatial neglect* (pp. 151–181). Amsterdam: Elsevier.

Ripich, D. N., & Terrell, B. Y. (1988). Patterns of discourse cohesion and coherence in Alzheimer's disease. *Journal of Speech and Hearing Disorders, 53*, 8–15.

Rivers, D. L. & Love, R. J. (1980). Language performance on visual processing tasks in right hemisphere lesion cases. *Brain and Language, 10*, 348–366.

Robb, M. (2015). Editorial. *Speech, Language, and Hearing, 18*(3), 125.

Rochon, E., Saffran, E. M., Berndt, R. S., & Schwartz, M. F. (2000). Quantitative analysis of aphasic sentence production: Further development and new data. *Brain and Language, 72*, 193–218.

Roman, M., Brownell, H. H., Potter, H. H., Seibold, M. S., & Gardner, H. (1987). Script knowledge in right hemisphere–damaged and normal elderly adults. *Brain and Language, 31*, 151–170.

Saffran, E. M., Berndt, R. S., & Schwartz, M. F. (1989). The quantitative analysis of agrammatic production: Procedure and data. *Brain and Language, 37*, 440–479.

Schwartz, M. F., Marin, O. S. M., & Saffran, E. M. (1979). Dissociation of language function in dementia: A case study. *Brain and Language, 7*, 277–306.

Semenza, C., Borgo, F., Mondini, S., Pasini, M., & Sgaramella, T. (2000). Proper names in the early stages of Alzheimer's disease. *Brain and Cognition, 43*, 384–387.

Simmons-Mackie, N. & Kagan, A. (2007). Application of the ICF in aphasia. *Seminars in Speech and Language, 28*, 244–253.

Snow, P. C., Douglas, J. M., & Ponsford, J. L. (1999). Narrative discourse following severe traumatic brain injury: A longitudinal follow up. *Aphasiology, 13*, 529–551.

Stemmer, B., Giroux, F., Joanette, Y. (1994). Production and evaluation of requests by right hemisphere brain-damaged individuals. *Brain and Language, 47*, 1–31.

Swinburn, K., Porter, G., & Howard, D. (2004). *Comprehensive Aphasia Test*. Hove, UK: Psychology Press.

Taber, K. H., Warden, D. L., & Hurley, R. A. (2006). Blast-related traumatic brain injury: What is known? *The Journal of Neuropsychiatry and Clinical Neurosciences, 18*, 141–145.

Tomoeda, C. K. & Bayles, K. A. (1993). Longitudinal effects of Alzheime disease on discourse production. Alzheimer Disease and Associated Disorders, 7, 223–236.

Tompkins, C. A. (1995). *Right hemisphere communication disorders: Theory and management*. San Diego, CA: Singular.

Tompkins, C. A., Klepousniotou, E., & Scott, A. G. (2011). Nature and assessment of right hemisphere disorders. In I. Papathanasiou, P. Coppens, & C. Potagas (Eds.), *Aphasia and related neurogenic communication disorders* (pp. 297–343). Burlington, MA: Jones & Bartlett Learning.

Trupe, E. & Hillis, A. (1985). Paucity vs. verbosity: Another analysis of right hemisphere communication deficits. *Clinical Aphasiology, 15*, 83–92.

Tucker, D., Watson, R., & Heilman, K. (1977). Discrimination and evocation of affectively intoned speech in patients with right parietal disease. *Neurology, 27*, 947–950.

Turkstra, L. S. & Holland, A. (1998). Assessment of syntax after adolescent brain injury: Effects of memory on test performance. *Journal of Speech, Language, and Hearing Research, 41*, 137–149.

Ulatowska, H. K., Chapman, S. B., Highley, A. P. & Prince, J. (1998). Discourse in healthy old-elderly adults: A longitudinal study. *Aphasiology, 12*, 619–633.

Ulatowska, H. K., North, A. J., & Macaluso-Haynes, S. (1981). Production of narrative and procedural discourse in aphasia. *Brain and Language, 13*, 345–371.

Ulatowska, H. K. & Olness, G. S. (2007). Pragmatics in discourse performance: Insights from aphasiology. *Seminars in Speech and Language, 28*, 148–158.

Veterans Health Initiative. (2010). *Traumatic brain injury*. Birmingham, AL: Department of Veterans Affairs.

Wade, D. T., Hewer, R. L., David, R. M., & Menderby, P. M. (1986). Aphasia after stroke: Natural history and associated deficits. *Journal of Neurology, Neurosurgery & Psychiatry, 49,* 11–16.

Weintraub, S., Mesulam, M. & Kramer, L. (1981). Disturbances in prosody: A right hemisphere contribution to language. *Archives of Neurology, 38,* 742–744.

Wepman, J. M., Bock, R. D., Jones, L. V., & Van Pelt, D. (1956). Psycholinguistic study of the concept of anomia. *Journal of Speech and Hearing Disorders, 21,* 468–477.

Wernicke. C. (1874). *Der aphasische symptomenkomplex.* Breslau, Germany: Cohn & Weigart.

Wilson, S. M., Eriksson, D. K., Schneck, S. M., Lucanie, J.M. (2018). A quick aphasia battery for efficient, reliable, and multidimensional assessment of language function. *PLoS One, 13*(2), e0192773.

World Health Organization (WHO). (2001). *International classification of functioning, disability and health (ICF).* Geneva, Switzerland: World Health Organization.

Worrall, L., & Foster, A. (2020). Does intensity matter in aphasia rehabilitation? *Lancet, 389*(10078), 1494–1495.

Worrall, L., Simmons-Mackie, N., Wallace, S. J., Rose, T., Brady, M. C., Kong, A. P. H., Murray, L., & Hallowell, B. (2016). Let's call it "aphasia": Rationales for eliminating the term "dysphasia". *International Journal of Stroke, 11*(8), 848–851.

Ylvisaker, M., & Szekeres, S. F. (1989). Metacognitive and executive impairments in head-injured children and adults. *Topics in Language Disorders, 9,* 34–49.

Ylvisaker, M., Szekeres, S. F., & Feeney, T. (2008). Communication disorders associated with traumatic brain injury. In R. Chapey (Ed.), *Language intervention strategies in aphasia and related neurogenic communication disorders* (pp. 879–962). Baltimore, MD: Lippincott Williams and Wilkins.

Youse, K. M. & Coelho, C. A. (1995). Working memory and discourse production abilities following closed-head injury. *Brain Injury, 19,* 1001–1009.

Appendix 1.1

Case History Form / Intake Questionnaire (for Aphasia)

Preparation:

- Review any referral information or related documentation ahead of time and take note of the sections in this form/questionnaire you want to explore during the interview.
- Arrange for comfortable seating and lighting. Ensure there will be minimal distraction that may affect the client.
- Interview the client alone. Arrange for the caregiver or accompanying person to join the interview, if applicable.
- Record the interview on audio or video.

Introduction:

- Introduce yourself. Explain to the client your assessment plan and how long it will take.
- Example: "Hello Mr./Mrs. _____. My name is _____. I am the clinician in charge who will conduct the assessment today. I would like to start by reviewing the case history and asking you some questions. After we finish talking, I will work with you. Today's assessment should take about _____ minutes."

A) General Information:

Name: _____ I.D. #: _____

Address: _____

Home/cell phone: _____ E-mail: _____

Date of interview: _____ Date of birth: _____

Age: _____ Gender: _____

1. What was the highest grade level you completed in school? _____

2. Is English your first language? Yes or No
   - What other languages do you speak? _____

3. Did you have any premorbid learning or behavioral problems? Yes or No
   - If yes, please describe _____

4. Did you need any special assistance premorbidly? Yes or No
   - If yes, please describe _____

B) Family/Psychosocial Information:

1. What is your marital status?
   Single ____ Married ____ Divorced ____ Separated ____ Widowed ____

2. Do you live alone? Yes or No
   • If no, whom do you live with? (Name and relationship)
   _____

3. Who is your primary caregiver? (Name and relationship)
   _____

4. Current support system

Name	Age	Relationship

5. What was your premorbid leisure interest and community involvement?
   Hobby _____   Social/civic group _____
   Recreation _____   Volunteer work _____
   Music or movie _____   Others _____

6. What is your current leisure interest and community involvement?
   Hobby _____   Social/civic group _____
   Recreation _____   Volunteer work _____
   Music or movie _____   Others _____
   Same as or similar to question 5 above _____

7. Did you have a use/abuse pattern?
   Alcohol ____   Tobacco____   Illegal drugs ____

8. Emergency contact: (Name and phone) _____

C) Medical Information:

1. What is the nature of your illness? Stroke or Accident or Other
   _____
   • Date of incident: _____

2. Were you unconscious? Yes or No or Not sure
   • If yes, how long? _____

3. Were you paralyzed? Yes or No or Not sure
   • If yes, where? _____

4. Were you right or left handed before the incident? _____

5. Did you have swallowing issues as a result? Yes or No
   • If yes, please describe _____

6. Do you have any longstanding health conditions/problems? Yes or No
   • If yes, please describe _____

7. What are the current medications and dosages you are currently taking?

Medication	Dosage	Frequency

8. Are you on a special diet? Yes or No
   • If yes, please describe _____

9. Do you have any allergies? Yes or No
   • If yes, please describe _____

10. Do you wear glasses? Yes or No

11. Do you wear hearing aids? Yes or No
    • If yes, how long? _____

12. Are you ambulatory? Yes or No
    • If no, how far can you go independently? _____

13. Do you use a wheelchair? Yes or No
    • If yes, please describe the type _____

14. Do you need assistance with the restroom? Yes or No

Primary Care Physician
Physician name: _____   Facility: _____
Address: _____
Phone: _____   Email/Fax: _____

Speech-and-Language Assessment/Therapy
Clinician name: _____   Facility: _____
Address: _____
Phone: _____   Email/Fax: _____
Dates attended: _____
Focus of previous speech–and–language training: _____
_____

Psychology/Counseling/Social Work
Clinician name: _____   Facility: _____
Address: _____
Phone: _____   Email/Fax: _____
Dates attended: _____

Physical Therapy
Clinician name: _____   Facility: _____
Address: _____
Phone: _____   Email/Fax: _____
Dates attended: _____

Occupational Therapy
Clinician name: _____   Facility: _____
Address: _____
Phone: _____   Email/Fax: _____
Dates attended: _____

Other Health Care
Clinician name: _____   Facility: _____
Address: _____
Phone: _____   Email/Fax: _____
Dates attended: _____

D) Language/Communication Skills

To assist us in establishing functional communication goals, please complete the following questions:

1. Rank which ways you are most successful in conveying your message, with 1 being the most successful and 5 being the least successful. You may use N/A for "not applicable".
    Speaking ____   Writing ____   Gesturing ____ Facial Expressions ____
    Drawing ____   Others ____ (please describe:_____)

2. Please check all that apply:
    a. Speaks in   single words ____
                     phrases ____
                     sentences ____
    b. Formulates questions ____
    c. Carries on conversations ____
    d. Understands   single words ____
                       yes/no questions ____
                       wh-questions ____
                       conversations ____
    e. Reads   single words ____
                 newspaper ____
                 novels ____
    f. Writes   name ____
                  single words ____
                  sentences ____

3. List situations where you are most successful in communicating.

4. List situations where you are least successful in communicating.

5. What do you hope to gain from therapy?

6. What activities do you want to be able to do? (For example: go to movies, do a sport, or dine in a restaurant with friends)

E) Employment History:

Job title/Duties	Company and location	Dates
		From to
		From to
		From to
		From to

1. Were you employed at the time of your stroke/accident/illness? Yes or No
2. Are you on a leave of absence? Yes or No
   - If yes, how long? _____
3. Are you retired? Yes or No
   - If yes, how long? _____
4. Are you retired due to your stroke/accident/illness? Yes or No

---

Wrap-up:
- "It looks like I have most of the information I wanted from you. Do you have any questions for me at this point?"
- "Thank you for the information you provided. It is helpful in my assessment. We will now proceed to the next part of the assessment to better understand your problem. When we are done, we will discuss our findings."

Appendix 1.2

Case History Form / Intake Questionnaire (for TBI or RHD)

Preparation:

- Review any referral information or related documentation ahead of time and take note of the sections in this form/questionnaire you want to explore during the interview.
- Arrange for comfortable seating and lighting. Ensure there will be minimal distraction that may affect the client.
- Interview the client alone. Arrange for the caregiver or accompanying person to join the interview, if applicable.
- Record the interview on audio or video.

Introduction:

- Introduce yourself. Explain to the client your assessment plan and how long it will take.
- Example: "Hello Mr./Mrs. _____. My name is _____. I am the clinician in charge who will conduct the assessment today. I would like to start by reviewing the case history and asking you some questions. After we finish talking, I will work with you. Today's assessment should take about _____ minutes."

A) General Information:

Name: _____   I.D. #: _____
Address: _____
Home/cell phone: _____   E-mail: _____
Date of interview: _____   Date of birth: _____
Age: _____   Gender: _____

1. What was the highest grade level you completed in school? _____

2. Is English your first language? Yes or No
   - What other languages do you speak? _____

3. Have you had a guardian assigned by the courts to make decisions for you? Yes or No
   - If yes: (Name and relationship) _____

4. Did you have any premorbid learning or behavioral problems? Yes or No
    - If yes, please describe _____
5. Did you need any special assistance premorbidly? Yes or No
    - If yes, please describe _____

B) Family/Psychosocial Information:

1. What is your marital status?
    Single ____ Married ____ Divorced ____ Separated ____ Widowed ____
2. Do you live alone? Yes or No
    - If no, whom do you live with? (Name and relationship)
    _____
3. Who is your primary caregiver? (Name and relationship)
    _____
4. Current support system

Name	Age	Relationship

5. What was your premorbid leisure interest and community involvement?
    Hobby _____ Social/civic group _____
    Recreation _____ Volunteer work _____
    Music or movie _____ Others _____
6. What is your current leisure interest and community involvement?
    Hobby _____ Social/civic group _____
    Recreation _____ Volunteer work _____
    Music or movie _____ Others _____
    Same as or similar to question 5 above _____
7. Did you have a use/abuse pattern?
    Alcohol ____   Tobacco____   Illegal drugs ____
8. Emergency contact: (Name and phone) _____

C) Medical Information:

1. What is the nature of your accident? Motor vehicle accident or Fall or
    Other _____
    - Date of incident: _____

2. Did you lose consciousness? Yes or No or Not sure
   • If yes, how long? _____

3. Were you in a coma? Yes or No or Not sure
   • If yes, how long? _____

4. Did you have post-traumatic amnesia? Yes or No or Not sure
   • If yes, how long? _____

5. Were you hospitalized for the accident? Yes or No
   • If yes, where? (Including any facilities transferred to) _____
   • How long were you in the hospital? _____
   • Discharge date: _____

6. What is the chief complaint? _____

7. Do you have any sensory deficits?
   Vision ____   Hearing ____   Smell ____   Taste ____
   Temperature ____   Touch ____   Proprioception ____

8. Were you right or left handed before the incident? _____

9. Did you have swallowing issues as a result? Yes or No
   • If yes, please describe _____

10. Did you have cognitive changes as a result? Yes or No
    • If yes, please describe _____

11. Did you have communicative changes as a result? Yes or No
    • If yes, please describe _____

12. Did you have behavioral changes as a result? Yes or No
    • If yes, please describe _____

13. Did you have seizure activities as a result? Yes or No
    • If yes, please describe _____

14. Did you have changes in appetite and weight as a result? Yes or No
    • If yes, please describe _____

15. Did you have changes in sleep habits as a result? Yes or No
    • If yes, please describe _____

16. Do you have any longstanding health conditions/problems? Yes or No
    • If yes, please describe _____

17. What are the current medications and dosages you are currently taking?

Medication	Dosage	Frequency

18. Are you on a special diet? Yes or No
    • If yes, please describe _____

19. Do you have any allergies? Yes or No
    - If yes, please describe _____

20. Do you wear glasses? Yes or No

21. Do you wear hearing aids? Yes or No
    - If yes, how long? _____

22. Are you ambulatory? Yes or No
    - If no, how far can you go independently? _____

23. Do you use a wheelchair? Yes or No
    - If yes, please describe the type _____

24. Do you need assistance with the restroom? Yes or No

Primary Care Physician

Physician name: _____   Facility: _____
Address: _____
Phone: _____   Email/Fax: _____

Speech-and-Language Assessment/Therapy

Clinician name: _____   Facility: _____
Address: _____
Phone: _____   Email/Fax: _____
Dates attended: _____
Focus of previous speech-and-language training: _____
_____

Psychology/Counseling/Social Work

Clinician name: _____   Facility: _____
Address: _____
Phone: _____   Email/Fax: _____
Dates attended: _____

Physical Therapy

Clinician name: _____   Facility: _____
Address: _____
Phone: _____   Email/Fax: _____
Dates attended: _____

Occupational Therapy

Clinician name: _____   Facility: _____
Address: _____
Phone: _____   Email/Fax: _____
Dates attended: _____

Other Health Care

Clinician name: _____   Facility: _____
Address: _____
Phone: _____   Email/Fax: _____
Dates attended: _____

D) Language/Communication Skills

To assist us in establishing functional communication goals, please complete the following questions:

1. Rank which ways you are most successful in conveying your message, with 1 being the most successful and 5 being the least successful. You may use N/A for "not applicable".
   Speaking ____ Writing ____ Gesturing ____ Facial Expressions ____
   Drawing ____ Others ____ (please describe:_____)

2. Please check all that apply:
   a. Speaks in   single words ____
                   phrases ____
                   sentences ____
   b. Formulates questions ____
   c. Carries on conversations ____
   d. Understands   single words ____
                     yes/no questions ____
                     wh-questions ____
                     conversations ____
   e. Reads   single words ____
               newspaper ____
               novels ____
   f. Writes   name ____
                single words ____
                sentences ____

3. List situations where you are most successful in communicating.
   _____

4. List situations where you are least successful in communicating.
   _____

5. What do you hope to gain from therapy?
   _____

6. What activities do you want to be able to do? (For example: go to movies, do a sport, or dine in a restaurant with friends)
   _____

E) Employment History:

Job title/Duties	Company and location	Dates
		From to
		From to
		From to
		From to

1. Were you employed at the time of your accident? Yes or No
2. Are you on a leave of absence? Yes or No
   - If yes, how long? _____
3. Are you retired? Yes or No
   - If yes, how long? _____
4. Are you retired due to your accident? Yes or No

Wrap-up:

- "It looks like I have most of the information I wanted from you. Do you have any questions for me at this point?"
- "Thank you for the information you provided. It is helpful in my assessment. We will now proceed to the next part of the assessment to better understand your problem. When we are done, we will discuss our findings."

Appendix 1.3

Case History Form / Intake Questionnaire (for Dementia)

Preparation:

- Review any referral information or related documentation ahead of time and take note of the sections in this form/questionnaire you want to explore during the interview.
- Arrange for comfortable seating and lighting. Ensure there will be minimal distraction that may affect the client.
- Interview the client alone. Arrange for the caregiver or accompanying person to join the interview, if applicable.
- When the client fails to provide an answer, it may be necessary to pose the same question by rewording it to the caregiver or accompanying person.
- Record the interview on audio or video.

Introduction:

- Introduce yourself. Explain to the client your assessment plan and how long it will take.
- Example: "Hello Mr./Mrs. _____. My name is _____. I am the clinician in charge who will conduct the assessment today. I would like to start by reviewing the case history and asking you some questions. After we finish talking, I will work with you. Today's assessment should take about _____ minutes."

A) General Information:

Name: _____   I.D. #: _____
Address: _____
Home/cell phone: _____   E-mail: _____
Date of interview: _____   Date of birth: _____
Age: _____   Gender: _____

1. What was the highest grade level you completed in school? _____
2. Is English your first language? Yes or No
    - What other languages do you speak? _____
3. Have you had a guardian assigned by the courts to make decisions for you? Yes or No
    - If yes: (Name and relationship) _____

4. Did you have any premorbid language, learning or behavioral problems?
    Yes or No
    - If yes, please describe _____

5. Did you need anyspecial assistance? Yes or No
    - If yes, please describe _____

B) Family/Psychosocial Information:

1. What is your marital status?
    Single ____   Married ____   Divorced ____
    Separated ____   Widowed ____

2. Do you live alone? Yes or No
    - If no, whom do you live with? (Name and relationship)

    _____

3. Who is your primary caregiver? (Name and relationship)

    _____

4. Current support system

Name	Age	Relationship

5. Before the diagnosis of dementia, what was your leisure interest and
    community involvement?
    Hobby _____   Social/civic group _____
    Recreation _____   Volunteer work _____
    Music or movie _____   Others _____

6. What is your current leisure interest and community involvement?
    Hobby _____   Social/civic group _____
    Recreation _____   Volunteer work _____
    Music or movie _____   Others _____
    Same as or similar to question 5 above _____

7. Did you have use/abuse pattern?
    Alcohol ____   Tobacco ____   Illegal drugs ____

8. Emergency contact: (Name and phone) _____

C) Medical Information:

1. Do you have concerns regarding your memory? Yes or No or Not sure
   - If yes, what is your main concern? _____

2. How would you describe your memory problem? _____

3. When did you first notice that your memory was different? _____

4. Has your memory changed over time? Yes or No or Not sure
   - If yes, how? _____

5. Are there times when your memory is better or worse? For example, is it better in the morning than in the evening? Yes or No or Not sure
   - If yes, what time is better? _____

6. Have you seen your family doctor about your memory? Yes or No
   - If yes, who and where? (Including any facilities visited) _____
     _____
   - What were the findings and/or recommendations? _____
     _____

7. Did your family doctor refer you to a specialist? Yes or No or Not sure
   - If yes, who and where? (Including any facilities visited) _____
     _____
   - What were the findings and/or recommendations? _____
     _____

8. Besides a memory problem, are you concerned with any of the following aspects?
   Speech ____ Daily activities ____ Behavior ____ Personality ____
   Job ____ Social interactions ____ Others____ (please describe:____)

9. Did you have changes in sleep habits? Yes or No
   - If yes, please describe _____

10. Do you have any longstanding health conditions/problems? Yes or No
    - If yes, please describe _____

11. What are the current medications and dosages you are currently taking?

Medication	Dosage	Frequency

12. Do you wear glasses? Yes or No

13. Do you wear hearing aids? Yes or No
    - If yes, how long? _____

14. Do you use a wheelchair? Yes or No
    - If yes, please describe the type _____

15. Do you need assistance with the restroom? Yes or No

Primary Care Physician

Physician name: _____   Facility: _____

Address: _____

Phone: _____   Email/Fax: _____

Speech-and-Language Assessment/Therapy

Clinician name: _____   Facility: _____

Address: _____

Phone: _____   Email/Fax: _____

Dates attended: _____

Focus of previous speech-and-language training: _____
_____

Psychology/Counseling/Social Work

Clinician name: _____   Facility: _____

Address: _____

Phone: _____   Email/Fax: _____

Dates attended: _____

Physical Therapy

Clinician name: _____   Facility: _____

Address: _____

Phone: _____   Email/Fax: _____

Dates attended: _____

Occupational Therapy

Clinician name: _____   Facility: _____

Address: _____

Phone: _____   Email/Fax: _____

Dates attended: _____

Other Health Care

Clinician name: _____   Facility: _____

Address: _____

Phone: _____   Email/Fax: _____

Dates attended: _____

D) Language/Communication Skills

To assist us in establishing functional communication goals, please complete the following questions:

1. Rank which ways you are most successful in conveying your message, with 1 being the most successful and 5 being the least successful. You may use N/A for "not applicable".
    Speaking ___   Writing ___   Gesturing ___   Facial Expressions ___
    Drawing ___   Others ___ (please describe:_____)

2. Please check all that apply:
   a. Speaks in   single words ___
                   phrases ___
                   sentences ___
   b. Formulates questions ___
   c. Carries on conversations ___
   d. Understands   single words ___
                    yes/no questions ___
                    wh-questions ___
                    conversations ___
   e. Reads   single words ___
               newspaper ___
               novels ___
   f. Writes   name ___
               single words ___
               sentences ___

3. List situations where you are most successful in communicating.
   _____

4. List situations where you are least successful in communicating.
   _____

5. What do you hope to gain from therapy?
   _____

6. What activities do you want to be able to do? (For example: go to movies, do a sport, or dine in a restaurant with friends)
   _____

E) Employment History:

Job title/Duties	Company and location	Dates
		From to
		From to
		From to
		From to

1. Were you employed at the time of your diagnosis? Yes or No
2. Are you retired? Yes or No
   • If yes, how long? _____

Wrap-up:

- "It looks like I have most of the information I wanted from you. Do you have any questions for me at this point?"
- "Thank you for the information you provided. It is helpful in my assessment. We will now proceed to the next part of the assessment to better understand your problem. When we are done, we will discuss our findings."

Chapter 2

Elicitation Procedures of Discourse Samples

Chapter Objectives

The reader will be able to:

1. define a discourse
2. identify the various types of discourse production and describe their characteristics
3. identify the clinical features of discourse deficits
4. describe and explain the clinical significance of measuring discourse production
5. describe the principles of discourse elicitation for speakers with aphasia and related language disorders
6. describe the use of various pictorial stimuli to collect narrative samples
7. apply different methodologies in collecting narrative samples for the purpose of clinical evaluation as well as for the purpose of conducting research about oral discourse
8. explain the possible reasons for lower reliability on discourse elicitation and analysis.

What Is Discourse?

A discourse is generally defined as "a language unit whose organization supersedes any single word or sentence" (Olness, 2006, p.176) or "a unit of language above and beyond the sentence [level]" (Schiffrin, 2006, p.169). A discourse has also been defined as an instance of language use in which the classification of types is based on the grammatical and lexical choices as well as the distribution of content and theme of a message (Crystal, 1985). It is composed of a series of sentences connected for conveying a message (Cherney, 1998) and can be the most elaborative linguistic activity (Ska et al., 2004). Clark (1994) described another approach to studying discourse and suggested there are two main categories of discourse: (1) spontaneous oral narrative, in which speakers usually produce an extemporaneous discourse

DOI: 10.4324/9781003254775-2

without detailed planning beforehand, such as conversations, and (2) carefully crafted written discourse, which usually involves one's planned writing, rewriting, and editing, such as novels or newspaper articles. In this chapter, our discussion will focus on oral discourse.

Clinical Significance of Discourse Production

Discourse produced by speakers with aphasia or related cognitive–communication disorders contains rich and valuable information for researchers to understand the manifestation of specific language disorders (Booth & Perkins, 1999). A careful quantification of discourse performance can also provide clinicians with useful information to plan specific treatment components for their clients (Kong, 2009). More specifically, clinicians are particularly interested in the aspects of discourse structure and discourse function. The structure of a discourse is often related to the sounds, syllables, words, phrases, clauses, and sentences used in an oral text. The function aspect, on the other hand, concerns how the discourse is used for a particular purpose for communication (such as informational, expressive, or social) (Schiffrin, 1994).

In the past two decades, cross-sectional studies on aphasia (e.g., Armstrong, 2000; Olness et al., 2010), traumatic brain injury – more specifically closed head injury (e.g., Coelho et al., 1995; Duff et al., 2012; Le, Coelho et al., 2011, Le et al., 2012), and dementia (e.g., Ash et al., 2006; Ehrlich et al. 1997) have provided clinically important evidence regarding discourse impairment associated with these neurological conditions. These findings have critical clinical implications not only to a more sensitive and reliable assessment of verbal discourse production among speakers with disordered narratives, but also a clearer direction to clinicians' planning of language remediation.

Objective measurement of discourse production as a part of a comprehensive assessment has been promoted in the past two decades and has become more popular as a routine of clinical language evaluation in Western countries (e.g., American Speech-Language-Hearing Association, 2004; Armstrong et al., 2006; Capilouto et al., 2006; Royal College of Speech & Language Therapists, 2005). As a result of increased accessibility to published guidelines and protocols of some clinically feasible discourse analyses, clinicians are more prepared (and feel more comfortable) to include this assessment as part of their daily practice. Subsequently, discourse deficits evident in day-to-day interpersonal interactions can now be identified within everyday clinical settings. In addition, more fine-tuned and appropriate targets of language therapy can be provided to speakers with acquired neurogenic communication disorders beyond the sentence level. More critically, at the same time, the effectiveness of these interventions can be better evaluated because some of these discourse analytic systems can be used as a form of outcome measure.

Discourse production is of particular interest to researchers in the field of communication sciences and disorders (or speech pathology), linguistics, neuro-linguistics, psychology, cognitive psychology, gerontology, and other health-related professions. While there is a high prevalence of communication difficulties at the discourse level among individuals with acquired neurogenic language disorders, the degree of the actual difficulty can only be objectively quantified when one uses detailed discourse analyses. Any alternations in the performance of discourse production demonstrated by a speaker can also reliably reflect a meaningful change in response to language treatment (Wright, 2011), especially for intervention targeting post-sentence level performance (see Chapter 7 for more details about discourse intervention). Even for physicians who generally do not pay special attention to objective oral discourse analysis, research has suggested that transcripts of patient-doctor conversations could reveal patients' use of verbal or non-verbal strategies during communication breakdown, which could further inform physicians about the social well-being of their patients. This would, in turn, allow more sensitive treatment and consultation that can address the needs of patients (Elwyn & Gwyn, 1999).

Characteristics of Discourse Breakdown

Successful construction of an oral discourse involves formulation of a communicative intent, organization of a message, and accounting for listeners' (or communication partners') perspective. The process also requires efficient and effective coordination between resources of working memory and attention in the auditory, visual, and/or verbal domains. Causes of discourse breakdown may include impairment in forming a thought (e.g., Gerson et al., 1977), deficits or impoverishment of language abilities or incompetence of communication abilities or skills (e.g., Olness, 2006), breakdown in formulating a complete linguistic output (e.g., Kong, 2009; Kong et al., 2016), and reduction of cognitive skills supporting language production (e.g., Ahmed et al., 2013; Ash et al., 2011). Note that the actual discourse symptoms of a patient may manifest at various linguistic levels with reference to their **etiology**.

Application of techniques in research studies for eliciting aphasic discourse and research findings of the symptoms found in speakers with aphasia have been used to expand our knowledge regarding the problematic processes underlying language deficits associated with other cognitive-communication disorders. For example, while the classical discourse symptoms and linguistic disorders in aphasia are different from those observed in dementia, it has been reported that related linguistic deficits existed in these two populations (Au et al., 1988). Nevertheless, some common clinical signs of impaired abilities in producing oral discourse include:

- reduced information content or total **propositions**
- increased incidence of errors, such as paraphasias or neologisms

- higher proportion of lexical deficits and higher usage of non-specific lexical items
- decreased efficiency to convey ideas, expressed in terms of the amount of verbal output or time needed for expressing a particular piece of information
- lower degree of grammatical accuracy and increased frequency of syntactic breakdown or errors, such as omission or misuse of function words, inflections, and grammatical morphemes or markers
- lower degree of grammatical complexity, such as reduced amount of embedding, subordination, or lower number of arguments attached to verbs
- restricted abilities to use language to convey feelings, give opinions, and express emotions
- increased frequency of using unconventional forms of language to convey meaning
- reduced use of cohesive devices, such as pronouns or synonyms, that reduces the overall continuity of output
- reduced overall coherence of an oral output.

Types, Examples, Strengths and Limitations of Existing Elicitation Methods

Three characteristics of oral discourse are highly dependent to the tasks used for eliciting language sample. They include (1) the overall quality, amount, and density of content; (2) the complexity of narrative structure; and (3) the quantity of discourse proposition. Many linguistic processes, such as vocabulary diversity or language features as small and specific as aspects of sentence structure, are sensitive to the task of elicitation (Armstrong, 2000; Armstrong and el., 2011; Fergadiotis & Wright, 2011).

There are two broad categories of discourse genres, including monologues and interactive dialogues. Analyses of monologic discourse, such as descriptive narratives, procedural discourse, and expository discourse (Cherney, 1998), allow one to reveal the microstructural and macrostructural impairments demonstrated by a speaker. Potential relationships between discourse symptoms (or skills) and cognitive functions underlying language production can also be captured. On the other hand, interactive dialogue, usually in the form of conversational discourse, allows one to understand the pragmatic aspects of discourse production because of the alternating roles one plays as a speaker and listener to exchange ideas, thoughts, and feelings (Wilkinson et al., 2003). In other words, instead of focusing on the linguistic or grammatical structures of sentences in a text, analysis of a conversation genre can highlight the sociological uses of language (Hodges et al., 2008).

The elicitation tasks listed below are a selection of some frequently used methods to obtain language samples from individuals with aphasia and related cognitive-communication disorders. These techniques vary in terms of their use of different stimulus types, the cognitive demands of each task, and how the content in stimuli is controlled for different evaluation purposes. In a recent report, Stark (2019) identified differences in discourse produced during different elicitation tasks, and concluded that different genres tax the language system in different ways. It was further concluded that clinicians should employ more than one single discourse task and select the most sensitive discourse tasks when attempting to assess specific language abilities and outcomes in their clients. Details regarding the testing purposes, appropriateness for disorder types, administration procedures and concerns, and information and factors relevant to sample analyses are given as follows.

Descriptive Discourse

Descriptive discourse entails the attribution of features and concepts of a stimulus. Depending on the complexity of the discourse, as pre-determined by the content within a stimulus (e.g., number of key items in a picture), there may be descriptions about a set of events that can, but not necessarily, be presented in a specific sequential order. Single or sequential pictures that are in the form of black and white line drawings, color drawings, or photos are typically used as materials for speech elicitation.

Traditional aphasia assessment batteries typically use single picture stimuli to elicit spontaneous oral narrative from an examinee. For example, the Western Aphasia Battery (Kertesz, 1982) uses a single black and white line drawing depicting a picnic scene to elicit a discourse sample for subsequent evaluation of its information content and degree of fluency and grammatical completeness. Another example is the Cookie Theft picture (Goodglass & Kaplan, 1972; Goodglass et al., 2001) from the Boston Diagnostic Aphasia Examination. It is the most widely used stimulus in the field of speech pathology for investigation of spoken production by speakers with aphasia (e.g., Menn et al., 1994; Nicholas & Brookshire, 1993), individuals with Alzheimer's disease (e.g. Giles et al., 1996; Kavé & Levy, 2003) or brain injuries (e.g. Thompkins & Rose, 1994), as well as unimpaired elderly individuals (e.g. Cooper, 1990). It has also been used to examine language production in non-adult speakers. For example, Chapman and Schwartz (1998) have used the Cookie Theft picture to examine the production deficits of English-speaking children and adolescents with Down's syndrome. Wilson and Proctor (2002) also asked adolescents with closed head injury to provide written narratives to the Cookie Theft picture; the written discourses produced were then compared to those by unimpaired adolescents. Although this picture stimulus has been widely used to assess language in the field of speech pathology (since it was first introduced about half a century ago), Berube et al. (2019) have highlighted some of its intrinsic problems, such as it being outdated in appearance, and its relatively limited target objects and actions of characters, which inhibits collection of a more extensive descriptive sample. Hence, an updated and more "politically correct" version of the same picture that depicts additional events was proposed (see Box 2.1 for details about the updates). Berube et al. (2019) concluded that the updated Cookie Theft picture was more useful and reliable for collecting information about impaired connected speech.

Box 2.1 Traditional Versus Updated Cookie Theft Picture

	The traditional 1972 version	The updated 2019 version
Scene	• A hectic scene of a kitchen in the 70s	• A hectic scene of a modern kitchen and another scene of the lawn outside the kitchen window
Appearance	• Black and white line drawing	• Colored drawing
Characteristics	• Contains a variety of actions and illustrates activities that one can easily interpret and integrate • Speakers tend to make comments about the stereotypical roles of characters, e.g., a woman washing dishes and looking after the children	• Addresses some of the weaknesses of the traditional picture and retains its strengths • Depicts events that better suit gender roles in modern society, e.g., a man washing the dishes and looking after the children • Contains items that are more evenly distributed between the left and right side of the drawing, making it a more sensitive tool to test contra-lesional hemi-spatial neglect in both left and right hemisphere strokes • Another version portraying a mixed-race family is also available, making it more appropriate for the current time – this also allows one to assess if racial and ethnic diversity influences the description content
Events depicted	Original events: • boy stealing cookies and falling off the stool • girl asking for a cookie • woman washing dishes and daydreaming • sink overflowing	Retained events: • boy stealing cookies and falling off the stool • girl asking for a cookie • sink overflowing Revised events: • man washing dishes and daydreaming Additional events: • dog eating cookies from the floor • cat chasing birds in the lawn • mother mowing over flowers while talking on her cell phone

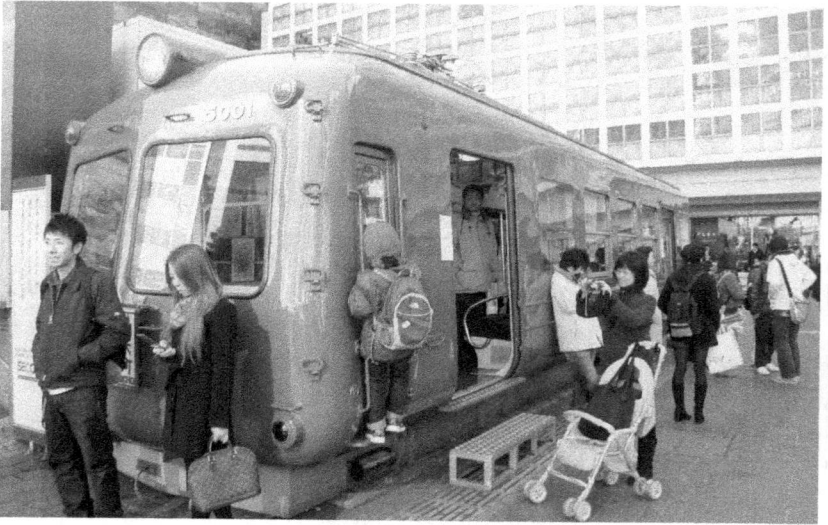

Figure 2.1 An example of a photo stimulus for eliciting descriptive discourse
Source: © Anthony Pak-Hin Kong, Ph.D.

As highlighted by Mueller et al. (2018), describing pictures is a constrained task that relies more on semantic knowledge and retrieval skills within the cognitive demands of a communication context, and poses less demand on a speaker's episodic memory. An example of a photo stimulus for eliciting descriptive discourse is shown in Figure 2.1. There are multiple characters in the photo that may seem to be engaged in different actions unrelated to each other. For example, on the left side of the photo, a couple is standing in front of a train. The man is smiling and standing with his hands inside the pockets of his jacket, while the woman is holding a cell phone and possibly making a call, sending, or reading a text message. Next to the couple is a child who is climbing on the train door. The boy's mother, standing next to a stroller, is holding a camera and taking a picture. There is also a man standing inside the train and a crowd behind the mother. One can appreciate how much information is present in the stimulus after carefully examining the photo. Multiple non–overlapping object items and actions depicted in the photo will allow an examiner to readily identify the potential word-finding behaviors and problems in constructing certain syntactic structures demonstrated by an examinee. Furthermore, to fully understand the photo, one needs to pay attention to the obvious features (such as the actions, facial expressions, and body language of the characters), to the overall setting (such as the fact that it cannot be a train station because the back of the train is a building), as well as to the more subtle cues (such as the absurdity embedded in the photo, including that the stroller seems to be too small for the boy or that a man is standing inside a non-moving train).

Unlike the use of a single picture stimulus, it has been reported that the use of sequential pictures to elicit verbal description from speakers with aphasia is better suited to sentence level analyses (Capilouto & Wright, 2009; Potechin et al. 1987). The major advantage was that language samples elicited are generally longer with a higher total word count. Furthermore, the samples tend to consist of descriptions on a related sequence of activities; this is in contrast to the tendency to list content items (i.e., predominant production of single nouns or verbs and single phrases) without the consideration of the underlying relationships among characters or items in a single picture stimulus. Narratives for sequential picture stimuli also tend to be more lexically diverse than those for single picture stimuli (Capilouto & Wright, 2009). The Broca's transcript in Table 2.1, elicited using the "Cat Rescue" picture (Figure 2.2), is a good example of this labelling behavior. In particular, unlike the speaker with anomic aphasia who was able to use sentences to provide more spontaneous description of the relations among different characters in the picture, the non-fluent speaker was mainly attempting to relay the main characters of the picture through naming individual items (and using a non-verbal means of pointing and gestures) to complete the task. (More details about the capturing of non-linguistic behaviors accompanying oral discourse can be found in Chapter 6.)

An example of the sequential picture stimuli from Kong (2016) is given in Figure 2.3. The propositions or key content depicted by the drawings were validated based on the performance of unimpaired speakers consisting of different age ranges and education levels. Table 2.2 displays the transcripts of a male examinee with early dementia and a control speaker. It is noticeable that both sets of discourse contain more "story-like" statements related to the pictures. However, one should also note that, content-wise, a longer sample elicited by a picture sequence does not necessarily contain more information than a shorter sample elicited by a single picture stimulus (Potechin et al., 1987). What primarily determines the richness of the output is a speaker's ability to interpret the picture content and to formulate a message to convey what the stimulus represents or depicts.

Common instructions clinicians may use include "Tell me everything you see happening in this picture/these pictures" or "Can you tell me what is going on in the picture(s)?" Clinicians should ask examinees to pay attention to all aspects of the stimuli and, if necessary, move the stimulus items to the examinees' intact visual field. Sometimes, it may be needed to encourage examinees to try to talk in sentences or to try to tell a story based on the stimuli with a beginning, a middle, and an end. For example, the use of the instruction "Make up your own story about what happened, with a beginning, middle, and an end" was reported to be able to improve the conveying of the temporal-causal interrelationship depicted in single pictures among

Table 2.1 Language samples of descriptive discourse in response to the "Cat Rescue" picture

Speaker	Language samples
A 71.2-year-old male speaker with anomic aphasia	+ *[Investigator <INV>: Take a look at everything that's going on in the picture and tell me a story about what you see happening with a beginning, a middle, and an end.]* + Mm [speaker sighs] mm [long pause] + well [speaker sighs] ... + Uh I see he's got a cat [speaker points to cat] in the tree and a [speaker points to bird] and a bird in tree. + [speaker shrugs] + Okay. + [speaker points to girl] and she's [speaker points to cat] [speaker points to girl] trying to get him down. + She is trying to get the cat down. + Uh, he climbs up [speaker taps on man] on the, the mother (father) or the (m)ale climbs up in top of the tree. + The, but the dog comes over and barks him [speaker taps on man] and [speaker points to ladder] knocks his, uh, luh, knocks his, uh, knocks his uh [long pause] whatever it is, knocks [speaker points to ladder] his his, uh, ladder down. + Then the... and and [speaker points to girl] she's still trying to get the cat down so... [speaker points to man] and he's yelling at the, at the dog. + So the firemen [speaker taps on fire ladder] come with uh a ladder. + I guess it, that'll be about the end of it [speaker points to firetruck]. + *[INV: Okay.]*
A 74.5-year-old female speaker with Broca's aphasia	+ [speaker points to tricycle] the bike... + [speaker points to girl] girl... + [speaker points to cat] cat ...[speaker mimics the action of moving] + [speaker points to dog] + the man and ... [speaker points to man] [speaker points to tree] tree + [speaker points to firetruck] [speaker points to man] [speaker looks up] hm... + [speaker points to firetruck] + [speaker points to bird] singing... + Yes.

Note: Remarks of the use of extra-linguistic behaviors are given in [square parentheses]. The investigator's verbal prompts are italicized. Correct targets the speaker originally intended to use are given in (parentheses).

Source: Kong (2016)

speakers with aphasia (Olness, 2006) and to increase the key content of a descriptive discourse among unimpaired typical speakers (Capilouto & Wright, 2009; Wright et al., 2006).

From the perspective of clinical evaluation, using single versus sequential pictures permits an examiner to control the content of the picture

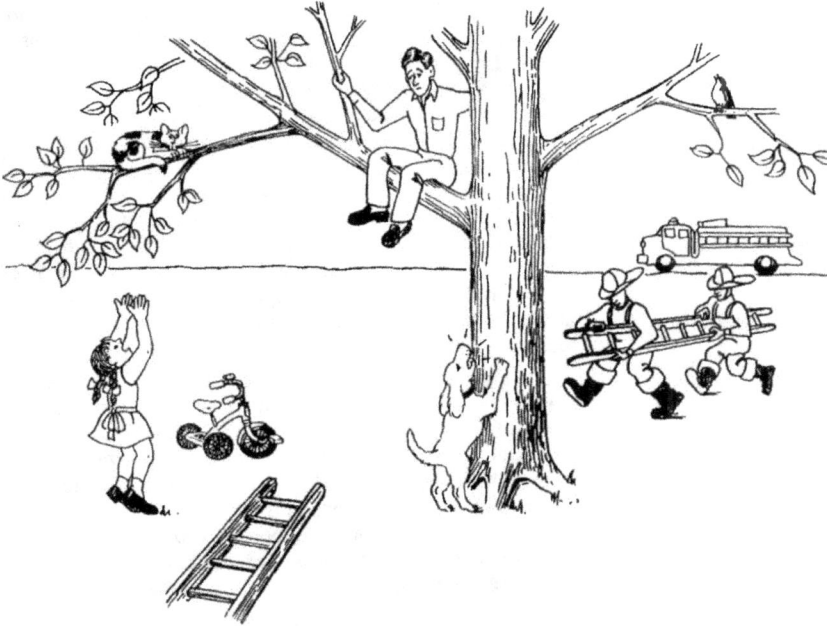

Figure 2.2 "Cat Rescue" picture in Nicholas and Brookshire (1993)
Source: http://talkbank.org/AphasiaBank/protocol/pictures/cat.jpg

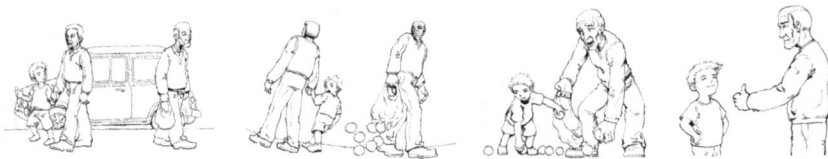

Figure 2.3 Sequential main concept pictures (set 4) from Kong (2016). This set of pictures contains three characters, including an old man, a boy, and the boy's father. The depicted story begins by the old man carrying a grocery bag and walking in the opposite direction to the father and his son. All of a sudden, the oranges from the old man's bag fall on the ground. The boy notices the incident and turns around to help the old man. The story ends with the old man praising the boy.
Source: © Anthony Pak-Hin Kong, Ph.D.

Table 2.2 Language samples of descriptive discourse in response to a set of sequential pictures

Speaker	Language samples
A 77-year-old male speaker with early dementia	+ Well, that poor guy that's carrying his bag of groceries. I don't think that he's very happy. Here's a little kid that's happy. This guy (is) not very happy either and that guy's really not happy. I think he's got old arthritis in his head. Okay. Little kid ready to go. This is an old car. Wow. Okay. He's lost all of his oranges. This guy did. Could be tomatoes, could be potatoes, oranges, baseballs. [speaker laughs]
	+ [Investigator <INV>): Okay.]
	+ It could. Look at all the round ones, ya know got a big hole in his [short pause] uh sack, you don't really know you're looking at round things. It might be small, um those things when guys set up their little, um like, little bowling balls but they're not ya know. And they throw them down out in the backyard. The same way with this. This must be some kind of fruit or something because grandpa's picking them up putting them in the bag. They did a good job so the grandpa gave him a thumbs up.
A male control speaker matched in age, education level, and gender	+ Uh what's going on? I guess there's a car in the background. Either one of these uh persons came out of the car. There's a man with a package, uh, on his right sh right hand. He's carrying a bag. I guess it's got groceries in it or something. And there's a man walking with his son or little boy the opposite way, walking in front of the car. And the second one is the man that's walking away from the car with the bag has the bag break. And whatever was in the bag, oranges, apples, whatever they are, fell out. And the little boy hears the commotion, I guess. He turned around and looked at it. He was still walking away with the other man. And it shows the little boy helping the man pick up the oranges or apples, whatever they are, whatever fruit they are. And putting it in the bag to help the old guy out. The old guy, looks like, he's ah he's kinda old. He looks haggard, he looks worse than I do. The other picture is, I guess, the man thanking the boy. He's got his left thumb up, left hand with the thumb up saying, I guess, thank you to the little boy for helping him.

Note: Remarks of the use of extra-linguistic behaviors are given in [square parentheses]. The investigator's verbal prompts are italicized. Correct targets the speaker originally intended to use are given in (parentheses).

Source: Kong (2016)

stimuli as well as the complexity of how the information is expressed by an examinee. For example, it has been reported that a sequential picture set containing more characters had a tendency to elicit more verbal content because of the higher number of inter-relationships among characters (Kong,

2009). The sequence of how content is mentioned by a speaker is also less constrained, as compared to other methods in this section (see procedural discourse or story telling). When using sequential pictorial sets that contain detached materials, clinicians should also pay attention to whether the standard procedures of examination require the examinee or examiner to arrange the picture order before the oral description begins. Prior to the start of description, the examinee should be informed that, instead of just a stack of single pictures, these pictures are in a sequence that depicts a meaningful act or event in order, or a story. After presenting the pictures in the correct order, it will be more desirable that the examiner points to each piece of depicted proposition to make sure that the examinee is aware of the content to be described (Kong, 2009, 2011).

One common question asked by clinicians is whether the selection of black and white versus color drawings to elicit spontaneous descriptive discourse matters. In fact, it is of interest to researchers as well as clinicians regarding the role color plays in potentially influencing the quality and quantity of samples. One may assume that the details of a line drawing, irrespective of it being single or sequential pictures, may be obscured because of the absence of color. However, contrary to the hypothesis that the presence of color would improve discourse measures, such as proportion of main events (or the key propositions) of a picture, **lexical diversity**, lexical errors, and total word count, it has been reported that using black and white sequential pictures resulted in a higher quantity of words in the description (Capilouto & Wright, 2008). The increase in proportion of content relayed was also found to approach the significance level in their study. On the other hand, Brown and Thiessen (2018) have illustrated that pictures lacking color could cause people with aphasia problems with the interpretation of intended objects or information embedded within the stimuli. This was echoed by Heuer (2016) who emphasized that colored picture materials could encourage easier and faster comprehension of depicted information, in both speakers with aphasia and neurologically healthy adults, and subsequently more comprehensive and naturalistic language production.

What should be highlighted here is the suggestion of paying attention to the age of examinees when determining the "best" pictorial stimuli (Capilouto & Wright, 2008) because different age groups may respond to color differently. Along this line of thinking, it is believed that other factors that are also worth considering include, but are not limited to, visuospatial processing skills (Dessalegn et al., 2013) and cultural differences in using color terms (Iijima et al., 1982). For instance, Mazumdar et al. (2020) have suggested that culturally appropriate color photographs are viable picture stimuli to elicit grammatically complex language samples spontaneously produced by neurologically healthy adults in a picture description task. Future investigations on the effects of these factors on discourse production can potentially provide more guidelines for clinicians to select the most appropriate test items for clinical evaluation.

Procedural Discourse

Procedural discourse usually centers on events that are contingent one on another. It may include explanations of a series of steps or actions to perform a task (e.g., describing the daily routine of getting ready for work) or presentation of a series of procedures to achieve a goal (e.g., instructions of how to fix a broken window or preparing a turkey for a Thanksgiving meal). In some cases, there is a chronologically ordered series of events that are conceptually related and violation of the event order is problematic (e.g., procedures of changing a flat tire on a bike or steps for checking in for an international flight at the airport).

Unlike a picture description task, use of pictorial stimuli for elicitation of a procedural discourse is optional. If necessary, clinicians may provide cues such as written words, pictures or photos of target items related to the anticipated content, or clips of pre-recorded video showing the actual event or sequence to provide assistance to the examinee. Examples of transcripts of describing the procedures to prepare a peanut butter and jelly sandwich, from the same two speakers with aphasia in Table 2.1, can be found in Table 2.3. The output from the speaker with anomic aphasia appears to be more informative and somewhat more complete. Unlike the Broca's speaker who needed prompts from the examiner using visual cues of photos to show the major ingredients, the anomic speaker was able to spontaneously describe the key steps to make this sandwich, even though at the end he mentioned he cooked a lot but seldom prepared this sandwich in particular. Iconic gestures to mimic actions or steps to prepare the sandwich were employed by the non-fluent speaker to compensate for her expressive difficulties. Chapter 6 has more detailed descriptions of analyzing non-verbal behaviors in a discourse tasks.

Instructions similar to those used for eliciting a descriptive discourse can be used in this task. However, if applicable, reminding an examinee to take time and to internalize the order or the steps involved in the whole event before providing the oral description may sometimes facilitate the quantity and overall quality of the verbal sequence. If the examiner attempts to focus on the verbal responses, he or she should try to encourage the examinee to refrain from using non-verbal means of expression, such as pointing, gestures, finger tracing, or writing, as much as possible.

Expository Discourse

Story-telling and retelling are the two most commonly used tasks to elicit expository discourse from speakers with neurogenic communication

Table 2.3 Language samples of procedural discourse – describing how to prepare a peanut butter and jelly sandwich

Speaker	Language samples
A 71.2-year-old male speaker with anomic aphasia	+ *[Investigator <INV>:Tell me how you would make a peanut butter and jelly sandwich.]* + Take two pieces of bread. + Peanut butter on [gesture of spreading] one side, jelly on the other side. + Slap (th)em together [hands clap] + *[INV chuckles]* + I cook a lot. + *[INV: Do you?]* + Yeah I… No not peanut butter and jelly but that's the way you do it.
A 74.5-year-old female speaker with Broca's aphasia	+ *[Investigator <INV>: Here's what I'm gonna ask you, to tell me how you would make a peanut butter and jelly sandwich.]* + … (no response) + *[INV: Here are the things that you would need.]* + [speaker points to bread] + [speaker points to peanut butter] [speaker points to jelly] Spreads bread. + [speaker mimics action of covering bread] + [speaker raises fist] Yes

Note: Remarks of the use of extra-linguistic behaviors are given in [square parentheses]. The investigator's verbal prompts are italicized. Correct targets the speaker originally intended to use are given in (parentheses).

Source: Kong (2016)

disorders. A story typically includes a setting (such as the characters and story context), interrelated episodes of the story (including the events, responses, and consequences), and an end (such as a moral or summary of the story). More complicated stories, which usually involve more characters, should contain more episodes. This type of discourse is very informative to a listener in terms of how the fact(s) or interpretation(s) of a topic is delivered through and draws upon higher-level thinking skills (such as comparison and contrast, cause and effect, as well as generalization). From a clinical perspective, expository discourse provides an optimal linguistic content that allows a systematic examination of the cohesion and coherence of language.

Auditory-oral retelling and story-telling elicited using videos or cartoons (e.g., Cherepski & Drummond, 1987) mainly differ in terms of the tapping of cognitive functions sub-serving language. The former involves auditory and verbal short-term memory on the part of the examinees because it requires them to carefully listen to the story and to retain details and sequence of information presented. Story-telling using visual stimuli, on the other hand, will rely on the examinees' visuospatial processing skills (to carefully scan and read the stimuli pictures), and visual short-term memory (to carefully remember the details of the stimuli pictures without a pre-set structure of the story). The content of a story, such as particular lexical items in relation to the story content, as well as the complexity of expressing these propositions should be controlled for as much as possible, based on factors such as length (or episodes) of a story or emotional content of story stimuli (Bottenberg et al., 1987). As compared to a picture description task, speakers who are telling or re-citing a story tend to produce a significantly higher proportion of main events and significantly more past-tense verbs (Capilouto & Wright, 2009). Language samples of the Cinderella story from two speakers with aphasia in Table 2.4 illustrate the higher proportion of these action words in the past tense (such as "hired," "happened," "went," "met," "was," and "had"), as compared to transcripts shown in Table 2.1 and Boxes 1.1 to 1.5.

Depending on the language skills (or deficits) of a story-teller, a story can be conveyed through words, vocal intonation, gestures, facial expressions, and body movements (Mallan, 1997). Pragmatic skills of an examinee, such as how well he or she can maintain eye contact and adapt the telling of the story to specific listeners, is another underlying dimension of producing expository discourse. Detailed and objective quantification of the above skills can inform clinical practitioners of the relevant issues on how language is used, which are crucial for language remediation.

Asking an examinee to tell or retell a common well-known story, such as Cinderella or Aesop's Fables, or plots of a favorite movie or television drama are common methods to elicit required speech samples during a language assessment session. Sufficient amount of discourse output for research-oriented analyses has been suggested to be at least 150 words that represent the narrative core of one's attempts to tell the story (Saffran et al., 1989). This "narrative core" should not include output such as neologisms, direct responses to a specific question from the examiner, or comments made on the narrative or the task (more detailed discussion on content-based discourse analyses is given in Chapter 3). When it comes to clinical implementation, clinicians should also apply similar criteria to elicit a speech sample, such that corresponding quantification measures suggested in the literature can be readily used for clinical evaluation. Consistent with the elicitation methods of procedural discourse, use of a picture book of the story is encouraged if the examinee needs reminders of the content of the story, but written text in the story book should be covered or removed to avoid direct reading aloud of the story. The examinee should be asked to tell the story in their own words after the picture stimuli are removed and the examiner should avoid asking specific questions about the story. With only the use of general verbal prompts or **reinforcement** (such as "Good, please go on" or "What happens next?"), interruptions from the examiner should be kept to a minimum. The same principle on encouraging one to internalize the

Table 2.4 Language samples of expository discourse – telling the Cinderella story

Speaker	Language samples
A 71.2-year-old male speaker with anomic aphasia	+ *[Investigator <INV>: Have you heard of the story of Cinderella?]* + Yes, I remember some of it. Some of it a while back. + *[INV: I just want you to look through the book to remind yourself of some of the details of how Cinderella goes. Then I'm going to take the book away and ask you to tell me the story.]* + Okay I don't know. [speaker chuckles] We'll see. + *[INV chuckles].* + We'll see. She was a maid I think, and has a mother, uh has a daughter, not th(e)... she she's she's a maid and she has uh she's the... The woman there was the, her, hired hired the her hired her and two girls [fingers showing two] were behind her. + Uh [long pause] a mother and two daughters. Okay? + Uh [long pause] uh [long pause] I, I don'know. + Uh she eventually goes to the wedding ball or something like that, wedding ball. And she had a what's his name, has a shoe that w... went with her. I don't know how that worked though. The shoe was a glass boot (slipper) glass [long pause] glass shi sh glass boot (slipper). I'm sorry. The boot it's not a boot but glass. And um [short pause] uh and she met that guy, the good lookin(g) young man that he (she) liked. And she went home from the ball I think. That was about it you know. + *[INV: What happened next?]* + [speaker sighs] [head shaking no] I don't know really. I just don't know, I'm sorry. + *[INV: okay]* + I'm sorry. + *[INV: No no that's fine]* + Yeah.
A 74.5-year-old female speaker with Broca's aphasia	+ *[Investigator <INV>: Tell me as much of the story of Cinderella as you can.]* + I don't [long pause] + *[INV: Did Cinderella go to a ball?]* + no. [gesture mimicking travelling] + ball. + *[INV: Did she meet the prince?]* + [head nodding yes] yes. + *[INV: And then what happened?]* + What to do what happens was have... Oh and go away tomorrow. + And... and (w)hat happened was it [speaker exhales] and what happened was [gesturing the action of picking up] he... + What happened? And what happens was he (she) was goin(g) to the ball. + And what happens was he (she) goes to the ball... go(es) to the ball. And we one [speaker sighs] and goes to the ball. + *[INV: Ready to move on to something else?]* + Yes.

Note: Remarks of the use of extra-linguistic behaviors are given in [square parentheses]. The investigator's verbal prompts are italicized. Correct targets the speaker originally intended to use are given in (parentheses).

Source: Kong (2016)

episodes of a story and not to rush in finishing the story suggested for elicitation of a procedural discourse is also applicable here.

Another method to elicit an expository speech is by asking an examinee
to describe an important event. Clinicians can instruct an examinee to talk
about an event that is important in his or her life, which can be about anything. According to Renvall et al. (2013a, 2013b), persons with aphasia tend
to focus on the here and now in their spoken output and are restricted to
conversation topics concerning individuals socially close to them. In this
"Important Event" narrative task, if the examinee demonstrates difficulties
coming up with a particular event, a simple prompt such as "Perhaps talk
about a memorable event" or "This event can take place a while ago or
recently. It can be happy or sad. Try your best to think of an important or
memorable event" can be provided (Law et al., 2018). Box 2.2 summarizes a
list of topics that have been found to be common in spoken output elicited
from both unimpaired speakers and those with aphasia.

Box 2.2 Topics of "An Important Event" Reported to Be Common in Individuals With Aphasia and Neurologically Unimpaired Speakers

Topic category (following Stuart et al., 1994)	Examples (in descending order of frequency of popularity)
Time frame	• Past events • Childhood memories • Weekly activities • Childbirth • Holidays • Celebratory occasions • Social events • Humorous events
Persons/things	• Children or grandchildren • Marriage • Friends and neighbors • Family • Work or colleagues • Photographs
Happening	• Food and drinks • Travel • Recreation activities • Health issues or illness • Hobbies or interests • Pet • Accident • Opinion on life

Topic category (following Stuart et al., 1994)	Examples (in descending order of frequency of popularity)
	• Death
	• Significant other's activities
	• Weather
	• Garden
	• Plans for the day
	• Car and driving
	• Television
	• Hospitals or nursing homes
	• Overseas countries
	• Sport
	• Home furnishings
	• Plans for meals
	• Music
	• Household maintenance
	• Job or occupation
	• Parts of a country
	• Household chores
	• Church or religious days
	• Transport or traffic
	• Lottery or raffles
	• Local suburbs
	• Books or magazines
	• News or current affairs
	• Government or politics
	• Finances
	• Computers

Source: Law et al. (2018); Renvall et al. (2013b)

Conversational Discourse

When someone is engaged in a conversation with a communication partner, his or her roles as a listener or as a speaker change from time to time within the verbal interaction. In addition, there are always some underlying rules or rituals (that may be culturally specific) that both **interlocutors** of the verbal exchange need to follow. This is related to the pragmatics of language. For example, people who are conversing should talk to each other, face each other, and should not speak simultaneously. Most people will start a conversation by greeting one another, followed by taking turns to speak without interrupting each other too often. At the end, the conversation ends appropriately with the interlocutors finishing what they want to say and saying goodbye to each other. Any violation of the above process is an indicator of pragmatic problems.

Conversation samples of two individuals with aphasia are given in Table 2.5. With reference to the transcripts, one can easily notice the communication breakdown for both speakers during a conversation task. The fluent speaker demonstrates a higher amount of oral content, whereas the non-fluent speaker seems to rely more on non-verbal means to keep the conversation going. Both **conversation dyads** show adequate conversation relation, which is related to the relevancy of the examinees' contribution, as well as manner, which is related to the clarity of the examinee's contribution. More detailed description on conversation analyses is given in the next chapter.

Depending on the content and purpose of a conversation, as well as the communication partner(s) involved, examination of conversational discourse and behaviors will provide clinicians with a lot of important and clinically useful information to determine the degree of language impairment among speakers with aphasia and related cognitive-communication disorders. More specifically, clinicians may get a better idea of how a person uses concepts of language in a specified communicative context or **speech act**. How well various communication functions are used, such as making a statement or request, asking a question, giving an order, showing gratitude, or offering an apology, can also be assessed (Wambaugh et al., 1991).

Although golden standards regarding the most appropriate conversation sample size have not been established in the literature, an investigation of the relationship between conversation duration and selected measures on conversational discourse analysis was reported by Boles and Bombard (1998). In particular, it was suggested that the use of conversation samples of five to ten minutes is sufficient for studying repair behaviors, speaking rate, and utterance length of disordered conversations in aphasia. In particular, it was reported that ten-minute samples adequately represented the "parent" conversations from which they were derived when measuring conversation repair behaviors in six out of eight cases of the study. For measuring speaking efficiency, such as length of utterance and speaking rate, conversation samples of five minutes was adequate for all the eight cases. Clinically, this amount of time should be sufficient for clinicians to obtain relevant case history from a new client and any family member(s) and to establish report with them during the initial assessment. At the same time, clinicians will be able to make some initial estimation of the linguistic strengths and weaknesses of the client, which can further guide the selection of relevant areas requiring further assessment.

When obtaining a conversational discourse from individuals with brain injuries, the personal and emotional relevance of topic(s) chosen will have a significant effect on the amount and quality of the language produced. Therefore, careful selection of a conversational topic is encouraged because different topics may influence how interlocutors convey ideas. More importantly, the topic selected can affect what a speaker may assume about the

Table 2.5 Language samples of conversation

Speaker	Language samples
A 71.2-year-old male speaker with anomic aphasia	+ [Investigator <INV>:*Thinking back, can you tell me about something important that happened to you in your life? Something that meant a lot to you. It could be happy or sad. From any time, from when you were a child or more recently.*]
	+ Well hmm... well I guess going to Georgia State University [speaker points to behind] and got a Ph.D. was most fun to do. Then I moved to, finished it and came down to Florida. And I felt real good about that. Yeah.
	+ [INV: *mhm? Can you tell me about what that was like... um going to Georgia State?*]
	+ Oh in nineteen seventy, nineteen sixty, (s)ixty [short pause] eight to seventy two... Nineteen seventy two about four years.
	+ [INV: *mhm.*]
	+ I worked on the... uh I worked on the school. I was a instructor. Uh not an instructor not teaching courses but [one arm flails] dealing with students.
	+ [INV: *mhm.*]
	+ You know, dealing with students. That was fun, you know... and uh we had a good time. Uh [speaker shrugs] and then I came to Georgia... to Georgia State University, but, you know, um... [head shaking no] I don't know what to say really.
	+ [INV: *okay.*]
A 74.5-year-old female speaker with Broca's aphasia	+ [Investigator <INV>:*What were you doing before you had your stroke? Were you working?*]
	+ [head shaking no] No, I... I...
	+ [long pause]
	+ [INV: *Were you retired?*]
	+ [head nodding yes] Yes.
	+ [INV: *What did you do before you retired? What kind of work did you do?*]
	+ [arm mimicking sweeping and moving]
	+ [INV: *Was it somethin(g) you enjoyed?*]
	+ [head nodding yes] Yes. You... I, I want to tell you but I can't.
	+ [INV: *Okay, well, one of the things I'm wondering is can you figure out a way to show me something that you did at work?*]
	+ [speaker mimics typing]
	+ [INV: *Is that a computer?*]
	+ [head nodding yes] Yes.
	+ [INV: *You worked on a computer*]
	+ [speaker presses on table]
	+ [INV: *uhhuh*]
	+ [speaker traces a line]
	+ [INV: *And did you do programming?*]
	+ [head nodding yes] Yes and no and...

Note: Remarks of the use of extra-linguistic behaviors are given in [square parentheses]. The investigator's verbal prompts are italicized. Correct targets the speaker originally intended to use are given in (parentheses).

Source: Kong (2016)

(shared) knowledge of the listener (Nolasco & Arthur, 1987). In addition, speech acts within a conversational discourse can vary with the topic of conversation (Wambaugh et al., 1991). For example, while referential topics (e.g., directing someone to finish a task) tend to contain more speech acts with request functions, there are more descriptive speech acts in a conversation on planning an activity (e.g., planning a family trip or activities for a vacation). Communication partners also play an important role in the overall quantity and quality of speech output. Partners of higher familiarity to the speakers, such as family members or significant others versus a speech–and-language pathologist the patient meets for the first time, may affect the selection of referents that are conversed. Linguistic options used to engage in a conversation, or more specifically to code references, can also be different (Boles, 1997).

With reference to the premises that conversational discourse is the most prevalently used type of discourse in humans, one major advantage concerning the ecologic validity of conversation is that it should better reflect the "real-life situations" in which a speaker with acquired language impairment communicates. This is, in fact, one of the major rationales for why conversation analysis (CA) is an important assessment procedure for speakers with traumatic brain injuries (Lê, Mozeiko, & Coelho, 2011; Liles et al., 1989). However, unlike the above-mentioned monologic discourse, control of topic and/or content of a conversation can be challenging. Comparison across patients in terms of the amount or accuracy of content, as well as the use of conversational strategies, is less straightforward, since controlling the content of discourse elicited and introducing the conversational topic(s) to elicit the same amount of output for subsequent analyses can be tricky. For example, examiners can readily identify the elements of targeted output in a descriptive discourse or story-telling task, which can serve as the standard for comparison across examinees. The same approach of examinations using conversational transcripts can be methodologically difficult. Examiners also cannot truly "compare" and quantitatively evaluate the elicited interaction across conversational dyads since equivalent targets are not available in the first place.

Voicemail Elicitation Task

Recently, a novel standardized computerized language sampling procedure in a role-play task called "voicemail elicitation task" (Meulenbroek & Cherney, 2019) was introduced. It was developed with a specific purpose to measure **politeness markers** in people with moderate or severe traumatic brain injury, who typically have difficulties in dialogues essential to professional or work communication. Specifically, there are four role-play voicemail scenarios in this voicemail elicitation task. Each scenario, presented individually via a computer, mimics a context to provide a voicemail audio recording and elicits two common workplace speech acts, including the spoken communication behaviors of "informing" and "requesting." Moreover, the four voicemail role plays target four different work-related recipients based on status and familiarity level: subordinate, friend, colleague, and supervisor (see details in Box 2.3).

Box 2.3 Examples of Voicemail Elicitation Task

Instructions: "*We are going to do a role-play activity on this computer. In order to do this task, you will read situations on the computer screen and then leave voicemail messages using this telephone receiver. You have a pen and paper to take notes*" (Meulenbroek & Cherney, 2019).

Condition	Role-play scenario	To elicit speech act of "informing"	To elicit speech act of "requesting"
Subordinate	"William reports to you for a project at work you are in charge of. You notice that he has not been following the dress code recently. The weather outside has warmed up and he has started wearing shorts every other day."	To remind a subordinate that shorts are not allowed in the workplace	To ask him to follow the dress code rules
Friend	"Brandon has a birthday on Friday and you want to throw him a party. You will be busy setting up the party on Friday night and you need someone to pick up a sandwich platter from a local restaurant."	To tell a friend about the party you are planning	To ask him to pick up the sandwich platter
Colleague	"Your car just broke down and will be in the shop for the rest of the week. Now you need a ride to work. You recently got to know a co-worker named Stanley because you are working on a project together. Stanley mentioned he drives by your house his way to work."	To tell a co-worker about your car problem	To ask him for some help with getting to and from work for the next week

Condition	Role-play scenario	To elicit speech act of "informing"	To elicit speech act of "requesting"
Supervisor	"Your sister is getting married in Mexico in three months. Your job has a strict rule about requesting time off three months advance. You are close to the three-month deadline."	To tell your boss you are planning a vacation	To ask him/ her to start the required paperwork

Source: Meulenbroek et al. (2013)

Note that this task differs from other previously-mentioned elicitation methods in which an examinee is allowed to prepare written notes to be used throughout the process. However, the examinee cannot script a standard or prepared response to read aloud when producing the language sample. To assist with any memory problems, the full scenario instructions are also displayed continuously.

Considerations Common Across Elicitation Tasks

There are some general principles of collecting and recording spoken texts. The use of appropriate recording equipment for the right recording medium needed is critical. Depending on whether the purpose of discourse data collection is research- or clinically-related, one may want to carefully consider the selection of appropriate stimuli and task instructions for discourse elicitation. More specifically, an examiner should do the following:

- Carefully select and use picture stimuli or stories with content that is culturally appropriate for the local population being evaluated. Using materials with content that an examinee fails to recognize or cannot relate to is problematic. For example, the employment of the Cookie Theft picture in the Chinese population has been reported to be inappropriate (Kong & Law, 2003) because the kitchen scene was wrongly identified as a living room. Similarly, use of the Cinderella story in non-Western populations may sometimes lead to lower capability for speakers to produce target information, and, therefore, underestimation of an examinee's performance.
- Provide more explicit instructions when asking an examinee to provide oral discourse. It has been suggested that, upon a more explicit instruction, such as "Tell me what you see as if you are telling me a

story with a beginning, middle, and end," examinees tended to produce samples with richer contents that include more of the underlying relationships between characters and events (Capilouto & Wright, 2009; Olness, 2006).

- Consider the practicalities of recording and determine whether audio or video recordings, or both, are needed. For example, visual details captured by videos are important for analyses of use of co-verbal as well as non-verbal behaviors, such as gestures, facial expressions, or body movements. However, some examinees may feel uncomfortable performing a narrative task in front of a camera and therefore may be affected by the recording. Because video recordings include images, which are considered as readily available in identifying information of examinees, they pose a greater concern to most Institutional Review Boards (IRB) that review and monitor the running of research studies and/or Operating Boards that monitor daily clinical operations. For audio files, analog recording should be sufficient in most cases, especially if the main purpose of recording the examinee is to facilitate offline orthographic transcription of his or her output. However, use of digital equipment will be needed if subsequent analyses of the discourse involve acoustic measurement of data. Note that as compared to traditional paper-based documentation, storage of these digital video or audio files may require additional resources. How long these digital files are retained for clinical, educational, or research purposes should also be considered.

- Ensure sufficient amount of discourse data for subsequent analyses. Examiners are recommended to record a much longer sample than the minimum required for an assessment and/or description or discourse task (Crystal et al., 1989). Collecting discourse samples from an examinee on more than one occasion may enhance the degree of representativeness of his or her performance. Discourse produced by the same examinee in different communication contexts and/or with different communication partners may also better reflect his or her natural use of spontaneous language output.

- Avoid interruption and refrain from providing directive cues or prompts during a discourse task. The occasions of communication breakdown or word-finding difficulty during a conversation demonstrated by an examinee and how he or she compensates for the impairment contain rich clinical information about the nature of the language impairment. Examiners can evaluate what compensatory strategies are used by an examinee to overcome communication breakdown. Facilitative feedback or constructive behaviors demonstrated by different communication partners can also be recorded.

The type of discourse elicited and the length of the oral samples should be determined by the purpose for which the samples are needed. For example, methodologically, use of narrative discourse allows systematic and quantitative analyses not offered by conversational discourse. Examiners can easily identify the targeted elements or content from discourse output elicited through the use of stories or procedures. Comparison across examinees can be made readily with reference to the standard target elements of a particular discourse task (Liles et al., 1989). In contrast, conversation is more open ended. Control and manipulation of context and target content within a conversational task can, therefore, be more difficult. However, use of **illocutionary acts** can be readily examined using conversational language, as compared to monologic discourse.

Reliability Issues in Discourse Transcription and Analysis

The observation, recording, analysis, and interpretation of how people use discourse to communicate rely on some form of transcription (Müller & Guendouzi, 2006). Unlike scoring performance at the word level, such as object or action naming, which is often straightforward and likely to get higher consistency across and within raters, preparation of a discourse transcript and its subsequent analysis always involves one's personal judgment and can potentially lead to some degree of subjectivity and, therefore, discrepancy of inter-rater and/or intra-rater agreement. This is because the process of translating spoken data to an orthographic medium involves the making of multiple decisions along the way. However, the degree of how many decisions are made by an examiner in preparing and processing a transcript and how reliable these decisions are will depend on factors such as the type of the discourse tasks, experience of preparing transcription and conducting text-based discourse analyses on the part of the raters, and the nature of the actual analyses.

A common procedure to check for consistency within or across raters in the discourse analytic process is by calculating the point-to-point agreement. Obtaining this information is particularly critical for ensuring that quantification of discourse samples by multiple examiners does not vary too much. This percentage agreement can be used for measures involving frequency counts, such as coding of parts-of-speech, sentence structures, or cohesive devices as well as number of words or utterances. A random sample of 5% to 10% of the total raw data can be selected for reassessment by the same or independent rater to obtain the intra-rater and inter-rater reliability, respectively. After that, the agreement can be computed by the formula below (Hula et al., 2003; Kong, 2009; Nicholas & Brookshire, 1995):

$$\frac{\text{Total agreements}}{\left(\text{Total agreements} + \text{Total disagreements}\right)} \times 100$$

In terms of stability of discourse analysis over time, shorter connected speech samples have been found to be more problematic in speakers with language disorders. In other words, short transcripts are highly unstable across sessions, i.e., low test-retest reliability (Brookshire & Nicholas, 1994). Measures of discourse production (such as words per minute, correct information units per minute, or percentage of correct information units) demonstrated a higher degree of test-retest stability when the sample length increased. Concerning representativeness, discourse samples composed of a wider range of discourse tasks are more representative of the examinee's everyday performance on connected speech.

Text-Based Versus Transcription-Less Analysis

Because of the time required for accurate transcription and objective analyses of discourse production, inclusion of detailed discourse quantification has been out of reach for most practicing clinicians. However, a transcription-less approach to analyze discourse can make this component of language evaluation more accessible to clinicians (Armstrong et al., 2006).

The principle of conducting a transcription-less approach of discourse analysis involves an examiner's careful, slow, and repeated listening to an audio file and/or watching a video file of a pre-recorded discourse recording (Armstrong et al., 2007). Similar to the conventional text-based analyses, a rater generally needs to refer to the raw data (i.e., sound or video files) multiple times before a final "judgement" is made. This "judgement" can be in the form of a rating or score that reflects the speaker's performance. A number of investigations have also been conducted to evaluate the intra-rater and inter-rater reliability of this transcription-less method. For example, the potential of using a transcription-less analytic procedure of aphasic discourse was explored by Armstrong et al. (2007), who were able to establish a high degree of concurrent validity for the concept production measures, adopted from the **main concept** measures in Nicholas and Brookshire (1995), between the agreements of transcription-based analyses and their transcription-less analyses. It was, therefore, suggested that the transcription-less analyses were promising in capturing a range of discourse features among speakers with aphasia. In addition, the use of gestures in people with right hemisphere damage was investigated by Brady and Mackenzie (2001), who profiled gesture employment directly from video-recordings. Intra-rater reliability was reported to range between 88% and 99%. Skills of turn-taking in speakers with dysarthria were also examined by Comrie et al. (2001). Analysis of videos of conversational samples yielded an average of 90% intra-rater agreement and 86.7% for inter-rater reliability over seven aspects of turn-taking. The major source of lower agreement was reported to be the frequency of within-turn pauses.

Although the approach of transcription-less discourse analysis seemed to be quite promising (e.g., Brady et al., 2005; Mackenzie & Armstrong, 2003), when it comes to analysis that is more difficult (such as the case of overlapping turns in a conversation sample), Comrie et al. (2001) admitted that conventional transcription-based analysis is still a more valid and reliable option.

Conclusions

The definition of a discourse and the significance of its measurement to inform clinicians on issues around clinical assessment and management were discussed in this chapter. Information on the practical considerations of the use of various discourse tasks and their specific elicitation methods was also provided. It is recommended that researchers and clinical practitioners should carefully evaluate the pros and cons of each assessment option and to determine the most adequate and appropriate one to highlight the nature of discourse deficits in their clientele. More detailed information on the traditional versus contemporary methods to quantify different types of discourse samples can be found in other chapters of this book.

References

Ahmed, S., Haigh, A. M. F., de Jager, C. A., & Garrard, P. (2013). Connected speech as a marker of disease progression in autopsy-proven Alzheimer's disease. *Brain, 136*, 3727–3737.

American Speech-Language-Hearing Association. (2004). Admission/Discharge criteria in speech-language pathology. *ASHA, 24*(suppl.), 65–70.

Armstrong, E. (2000). Aphasic discourse analysis: The story so far. *Aphasiology, 14*, 875–892.

Armstrong, L., Brady, M., Mackenzie, C., & Norrie, J. (2007). Transcription-less analysis of aphasic discourse: A clinician's dream or a possibility? *Aphasiology, 21*, 355–374.

Armstrong, L., Brady, M., & Norrie, J. (2006, May 29–June 2). Evaluating a transcription-less approach to the analysis of aphasic discourse [Paper presentation]. Thirty-sixth annual Clinical Aphasiology Conference, Ghent, Belgium.

Armstrong, E., Ciccone, N., Godecke, E., & Kok, B. (2011). Monologues and dialogues in aphasia: Some initial comparisons. *Aphasiology, 25*, 1347–1371.

Ash, S., McMillan, C., Gross, R. G., Cook, P., Morgan, B., Boller, A., Dreyfuss, M., Siderowf, A., & Grossman, M. (2011). The organization of narrative discourse in Lewy body spectrum disorder. *Brain and Language, 199*, 30–41.

Ash, S., Moore, P., Antani, S., McCawley, G., Work, M., & Grossman, M. (2006). Trying to tell a tale: Discourse impairments in progressive aphasia and frontotemporal dementia. *Neurology, 66*, 1405–1413.

Au, R., Albert, M. L., & Obler, L. K. (1988). The relation of aphasia to dementia. *Aphasiology, 2*, 167–173.

Berube, S., Nonnemacher, J., Demsky, C., Glenn, S., Saxena, S., Wright, A., Tippett, D. C., & Hillis, A. E. (2019). Stealing cookies in the twenty-first century: Measures of spoken narrative in healthy versus speakers with aphasia. *American Journal of Speech-Language Pathology, 28*(1S), 321–329.

Boles, L. (1997). Conversational analysis as a dependent measure in communication therapy with four individuals with aphasia. *Asia Pacific Journal of Speech, Language and Hearing, 2*, 43–61.

Boles, L., & Bombard, T. (1998). Conversational discourse analysis: Appropriate and useful sample sizes. *Aphasiology, 12*, 547–560.

Booth, S., & Perkins, L. (1999). The use of conversation analysis to guide individualized advice to carers and evaluate change in aphasia: A case study. *Aphasiology, 13*, 283–303.

Bottenberg, D., Lemme, M., & Hedberg, N. (1987, May 31–June 4). Effect of story content on narrative discourse of aphasic adults [Paper presentation]. Seventeenth annual Clinical Aphasiology Conference, Lake of the Ozarks, MO, United States.

Brady, M., Armstrong, L., & Mackenzie, C. (2005). Further evidence on topic use following right hemisphere brain damage: Procedural and descriptive discourse. *Aphasiology, 19*, 731–47.

Brady, M., & Mackenzie, C. (2001). Gesture use following right hemisphere brain damage. *International Journal of Language and Communication Disorders, 36* (suppl.), 35–40.

Brady, M., Mackenzie, C., & Armstrong, L. (2003). Topic use following right hemisphere brain damage during three semi-structured conversational discourse samples. *Aphasiology, 17*, 881–904.

Brookshire, R. H. & Nicholas, L. E. (1994). Test-retest stability of measures of connected speech in aphasia. *Clinical Aphasiology, 22*, 119–133.

Brown, J., & Thiessen, A. (2018). Using images with individuals with aphasia: Current research and clinical trends. *American Journal of Speech–Language Pathology, 27*, 504–515.

Capilouto, G. J. & Wright, H. H. (2008, May 27–June 1). The impact of stimulus on narrative discourse production [Paper presentation]. Thirty-eighth annual Clinical Aphasiology Conference, Jackson Hole, WY, United States.

Capilouto, G. J. & Wright, H. H. (2009). Manipulating task instructions to change narrative discourse performance. *Aphasiology, 23*, 1295–1308.

Capilouto, G. J., Wright, H. H., & Wagovich, S. A. (2006). Reliability of main event measurement in the discourse of individuals with aphasia. *Aphasiology, 20*, 205–216.

Chapman, R. S., & Schwartz, S. E. (1998). Language skills of children and adolescents with Down syndrome: II. Production deficits. *Journal of Speech, Language and Hearing Research, 41*, 861–873.

Cherepski, M., & Drummond, S. (1987). Linguistic description in nonfluent dysphasia: Utilization of pictograms. *Brain and Language, 30*, 285–304.

Cherney, L. R. (1998). Pragmatics and discourses: An introduction. In L. R. Cherney, B. B. Shadden, & C. A. Coelho (Eds.), *Analyzing discourse in communicatively impaired adults* (pp. 1–7). Gaithersburg, MD: Aspen Publishers Inc.

Clark, H. (1994). Discourse in production. In M. A. Gernsbacher (Ed.), *Handbook of psycholinguistics* (pp. 985–1021). London: Academic Press.

Coelho, C. A., Liles, B. Z., & Duffy, R. J. (1995). Impairments of discourse abilities and executive functions in traumatically brain-injured adults. *Brain Injury, 9*, 471–477.

Comrie, P., Mackenzie, C., & McCall, J. (2001). The influence of acquired dysarthria on conversational turn taking. *Clinical Linguistics and Phonetics, 15*, 383–398.

Cooper, P. V. (1990). Discourse production and normal aging: Performance on oral picture description tasks. *Journal of Gerontology, 45*, 210–214.

Crystal, D. (1985). *A dictionary of linguistics and phonetics.* New York: Basil Blackwell.

Crystal, D., Fletcher, P., & Garman, M. (1989). *Grammatical analysis of language disability.* London: Whurr.

Dessalegn, B., Landau, B., & Rapp, B. (2013). Consequences of severe visual-spatial deficits for reading acquisition: Evidence from Williams syndrome. *Neurocase, 19*, 328–347.

Duff, M. C., Mutlu, M., Byom, L. & Turkstra, L. S. (2012). Beyond utterances: Distributed cognition as a framework for studying discourse in adults with acquired brain injury. *Seminars in Speech and Language, 33*, 44–54.

Ehrlich, J. S., Obler, L. K., & Clark, L. (1997). Ideational and semantic contributions to narrative production in adults with dementia of Alzheimer's type. *Journal of Communication Disorders, 30*, 79–99.

Elwyn, G. & Gwyn, R. (1999). Stories we hear and stories we tell: Analysing talk in clinical practice. *British Medical Journal, 318*, 186–188.

Fergadiotis, G. & Wright, H. H. (2011). Lexical diversity for adults with and without aphasia across discourse elicitation tasks. *Aphasiology, 25*, 1414–1430.

Gerson, S. N., Benson, D. F., & Frazier, S. H. (1977). Diagnosis: Schizophrenia versus posterior aphasia. *The American Journal of Psychiatry, 134*, 966–969.

Giles, E., Patterson, K., & Hodges, J. R. (1996). Performance on the Boston Cookie Theft Picture Description task in patients with Alzheimer's disease: Missing information. *Aphasiology, 10*, 395–408.

Goodglass, H., & Kaplan, E. (1972). *The Boston Diagnostic Aphasia Examination.* Philadelphia: Lea & Febiger.

Goodglass, H., Kaplan, E., & Barresi, B. (2001). *The Boston Diagnostic Aphasia Examination: Stimulus cards, short form.* Philadelphia, PA: Lippincott Williams & Wilkins.

Heuer, S. (2016). The influence of image characteristics on image recognition: A comparison of photographs and line drawings. *Aphasiology, 30*, 943–961.

Hodges, B. D., Kuper, A., & Reeves, S. (2008). Discourse analysis. *British Medical Journal, 337*, 570–572.

Hula, W. D., McNeil, M. R., Doyle, P. J., Rubinsky, H. J., & Fossett, T. R. D. (2003). The inter-rater reliability of the story retell procedure. *Aphasiology, 17*, 523–528.

Iijima, T., Wenning, W., & Zollinger, H. (1982). Cultural factors of color naming in Japanese: Naming tests with Japanese children in Japan and Europe. *Anthropological Linguistics, 24*, 245–262.

Kavé, G., & Levy, Y. (2003). Morphology in picture descriptions provided by persons with Alzheimer's disease. *Journal of Speech, Language, and Hearing Research, 46*, 341–352.

Kertesz, A, (1982). *The Western Aphasia Battery.* New York: Grune & Stratton.

Kong, A. P. H. (2009). The use of main concept analysis to measure discourse production in Cantonese-speaking persons with aphasia: A preliminary report. *Journal of Communication Disorders, 42*, 442–464.

Kong, A. P. H. (2011). The main concept analysis in Cantonese aphasic oral discourse: External validation and monitoring chronic aphasia. *Journal of Speech, Language, and Hearing Research, 54*, 148–159.

Kong, A. P. H. (2016). *The Main Concept Analysis (MCA) for oral discourse production.* Hong Kong: The Commercial Press (H.K.) Limited.

Kong, A. P. H. & Law, S. P. (2003). A Cantonese linguistic communication measure. *Asia Pacific Journal of Speech, Language and Hearing, 8*, 229–234.

Kong, A. P. H., Whiteside, J., & Bargmann, P. (2016). The Main Concept Analysis: Validation and sensitivity in differentiating discourse produced by unimpaired English speakers from individuals with aphasia and dementia of Alzheimer type. *Logopedics Phoniatrics Vocology, 41*(3), 129–141.

Law, S. P., Kong, A. P., & Lai, C. (2018). An analysis of topics and vocabulary in Chinese oral narratives by normal speakers and speakers with fluent aphasia. *Clinical linguistics & phonetics, 32*(1), 88–99.

Lê, K., Coelho, C., Mozeiko, J., Krueger, F., & Grafman, J. (2011). Measuring goodness of story narratives: Implications for traumatic brain injury. *Aphasiology, 25*, 748–760.

Lê, K., Coelho, C., Mozeiko, J., Krueger, F., & Grafman, J. (2012). Predicting story goodness performance from cognitive measures following traumatic brain injury. *American Journal of Speech-Language Pathology, 21*, S115–S125.

Lê, K., Mozeiko, J., & Coelho, C. (2011). Discourse analyses: Characterising cognitive-communication disorders following TBI. *The ASHA Leader, 16*(2), 18–21.

Liles, B. Z., Coelho, C. A., Duffy, R. J., & Zalagens, M. R. (1989). Effects of elicitation procedures on the narratives of normal and closed head-injured adults. *Journal of Speech and Hearing Disorders, 54*, 356–366.

Mallan, K. (1997). Storytelling in the school curriculum. *Educational Practice and Theory, 19*, 75–82.

Mazumdar, B., Donovan, N. J., & Sultana, A. (2020). Comparing language samples of Bangla speakers using a colour photograph and a black-and-white line drawing. *International journal of language & communication disorders, 55*(5), 793–805.

Menn, L., Ramsberger, G., & Helm-Estabrooks, N. (1994). A linguistic communication measures for aphasic narratives. *Aphasiology, 8*, 343–359.

Meulenbroek, P., & Cherney, L. R. (2019). The voicemail elicitation task: Functional workplace language assessment for persons with traumatic brain injury. *Journal of Speech, Language, and Hearing Research, 62*(9), 3367–3380.

Meulenbroek, P. A., Togher, L., & Turkstra, L. (2013, May 28–June 2). Functional workplace communication elicitation for persons with traumatic brain injury [Paper presentation]. Forty-third annual Clinical Aphasiology Conference, Tuscon, AZ, United States.

Mueller, K. D., Hermann, B., Mecollari, J., & Turkstra, L. S. (2018). Connected speech and language in mild cognitive impairment and Alzheimer's disease: A review of picture description tasks. *Journal of Clinical and Experimental Neuropsychology, 40*(9), 917–939.

Müller, N. & Guendouzi, J. A. (2006). Transcribing at the discourse level. In N. Müller (Ed.), *Multilayered transcription* (pp.113–134). San Diego, CA: Plural Publishing.

Nicholas, L. D., & Brookshire, R. H. (1993). A system for quantifying the informativeness and efficiency of the connected speech of adults with aphasia. *Journal of Speech and Hearing Research, 36*, 338–350.

Nicholas, L. E., & Brookshire, R .H. (1995). Presence, completeness, and accuracy of main concepts in the connected speech of non-brain-damaged adults and adults with aphasia. *Journal of Speech and Hearing Research, 38*, 145–156.

Nolasco, R. & Arthur, L. (1987). *Conversation.* New York, NY: Oxford University Press.

Olness, G. S. (2006). Genre, verb, and coherence in picture-elicited discourse of adults with aphasia. *Aphasiology, 20*, 175–187.

Olness, G. S., Matteson, S. E., & Stewart, C. T. (2010). "Let me tell you the point": How speakers with aphasia assign prominence to information in narratives. *Aphasiology, 24,* 697–708.

Potechin, G. G., Nicholas, L. E., & Brookshire, R. H. (1987). Effects of picture stimuli on discourse production. *Aphasiology, 17,* 216–220.

Renvall, K., Nickels, L., & Davidson, B. (2013a). Functionally relevant items in the treatment of aphasia (part I): Challenges for current practice. *Aphasiology, 27*(6), 636–650.

Renvall, K., Nickels, L., & Davidson, B. (2013b). Functionally relevant items in the treatment of aphasia (part II): Further perspectives and specific tools. *Aphasiology, 27*(6), 651–677.

Royal College of Speech & Language Therapists. (2005). *RCSLT Clinical Guidelines.* Bicester, Oxon: Speechmark Publishing.

Saffran, E. M., Berndt, R. S., & Schwartz, M. F. (1989). The quantitative analysis of agrammatic production: Procedure and data. *Brain and Language, 37,* 440–479.

Schiffrin, D. (1994). *Approaches to discourse.* Oxford: Blackwell.

Schiffrin, D. (2006). Discourse. In R. W. Fasold & J. Connor-Linton (Eds.), *An introduction to language and linguistics* (pp. 169–203). Cambridge, UK: Cambridge University Press.

Ska, B., Duong, A., & Joanette, Y. (2004). Discourse impairments. In R. D. Kent (Ed.), *The MIT encyclopedia of communication disorders* (pp. 302–304). Cambridge, MA: The MIT Press.

Stark B. C. (2019). A comparison of three discourse elicitation methods in aphasia and age-matched adults: Implications for language assessment and outcome. *American Journal of Speech-Language Pathology, 28*(3), 1067–1083.

Stuart, S., Vanderhoof-Bilyeu, D., & Beukelman, D. (1994). Differences in topic reference of elderly men and women. *Journal of Medical Speech-Language Pathology, 2,* 89–104.

Thompkins, C. A., & Rose, C. G. R. (1994). Working memory and inference revision in brain-damaged and normally aging adults. *Journal of Speech and Hearing Research. 37(4),* 896–912.

Wambaugh, J. L., Thompson, C. K., Doyle, P. J., & Camarata, S. (1991). Conversational discourse of aphasic and normal adults: An analysis of communicative functions. In Clinical Aphasiology Conference (Ed.), *Clinical Aphasiology Conference* (pp. 343–353). Santa Fe, NM: Pro-Ed.

Wilkinson, R., Beeke, S., & Maxim, J. (2003). Adapting to conversation: On the use of linguistic resources by speakers with fluent aphasia in the construction of turns at talk. In C. Goodwin (Ed.), *Conversation and brain damage* (pp. C59–89). New York, NY: Oxford University Press.

Wilson, B. M., & Proctor, A. (2002). Written discourse of adolescents with closed head injury. *Brain injury, 16*(11), 1011–1024.

Wright, H. H. (2011). Discourse in aphasia: An introduction to current research and future directions. *Aphasiology, 25,* 1283–1285.

Wright, H., Capilouto, G., Carrico, J., & Siever, C. (2006, May 29–June 2). Impact of manipulating task instructions on narrative discourse performance [Paper presentation]. Thirty-sixth annual Clinical Aphasiology Conference, Ghent, Belgium.

Chapter 3

Clinical Assessment of Disordered Discourse

Chapter Objectives

The reader will be able to:

1. describe the principles and methods of subjectively assessing disordered discourse using rating scales
2. compare and contrast the general principles of various clinically oriented, linguistically-based discourse analytic systems for aphasia and related language disorders
3. discuss the general principles of propositional- or content-based discourse analytic systems for aphasia and related language disorders
4. discuss the general principles of conversation analysis for discourse in aphasia and related language disorders
5. explain the pros and cons for conducting various types of clinical discourse assessments
6. apply selectively one or more approaches of clinical discourse assessment.

Historical Background of Clinical Discourse Analysis

Various approaches of clinical assessment of disordered discourse have been proposed to facilitate the evaluation of aphasia beyond the single word or sentence levels. According to Spreen and Risser (2003), early investigations of aphasic language production conducted between the 1930s and 1950s had mainly focused on screening procedures and the development of clinical batteries for diagnostic purposes. It was not until the 1960s that researchers started to investigate open-ended free speech by measuring different linguistic parameters. Many of these clinically oriented tools were intended to assist clinicians in quantifying aphasic production by native English speakers. Their results might serve as an initial assessment of a speaker's linguistic abilities, which might then lead to more in-depth and detailed evaluation of aphasia. A small number of these systems have also been used to investigate the progressive changes of disordered narratives across time, such as the

DOI: 10.4324/9781003254775-3

positive change in aphasia recovery or regression over the course of different stages in dementia. More specifically, open ended or spontaneous language samples have been analyzed in terms of their rate, prosody, length of production, pronunciation, degree of grammatical correctness, and distribution of errors. The above pioneering work became the basis for the later development of other discourse quantitative systems.

In this chapter, we first discuss the approach of using subjective rating scales to assess disordered discourse. We then explore some linguistic-based and content-based analyses, with illustrations of what these various methodologies are based on and how they can be applied clinically. For some of these analyses, we will also discuss how extensions of a tool can be used to assess a more specific disorder population. Finally, the approach of conversation analysis and its components for evaluation will be discussed. The pros and cons for each of the above approaches will be briefly discussed, so that readers can better understand their clinical importance, diagnostic values, as well as potential challenges.

Subjective Ratings

A number of clinically oriented standardized tools have been developed for a quick evaluation of the general performance of individuals with aphasia. These tools have in common a series of criterion-referenced tasks that yield scores on the dimensions of auditory comprehension, verbal and/or non-verbal expression, and alternative means of communication present in speakers with aphasia, such as reading, writing, and gestures (e.g., Enderby et al, 1987; West et al., 1998). Among various existing published standardized assessment batteries, the Western Aphasia Battery (WAB; Kertesz, 2006), Minnesota Test for Differential Diagnosis of Aphasia (MTDDA; Schuell, 1965), and the Boston Diagnostic Aphasia Examination (BDAE; Goodglass & Kaplan, 1983) are commonly used in the diagnosis of aphasia because they are well validated with clinical rating scales on one or more aspects of language performance.

Standardized Aphasia Assessment Batteries

To illustrate, the WAB utilizes conversational questions and a picture description task to elicit spontaneous language output from an examinee. The output can be rated from a scale of 0 (the poorest) to 10 (the best) based on the number of questions an examinee can respond to correctly and the amount of propositions provided in the description sample (see Table 3.1). A fluency rating scale (0 to 10) that briefly addresses the degree of word-finding difficulty, presence of paraphasias and jargons, length of utterances, and sentence structure is also available in the WAB, as well as its bedside form (see Table 3.2). A simpler clinical rating from the MTDDA, focusing on the

Table 3.1 Rating scale on scoring information content of spontaneous speech in Western Aphasia Battery-Revised (WAB-R)

Level	Description
0	No information.
1	Incomplete responses only.
2	Correct responses to any one (out of six) conversational question.
3	Correct responses to any two (out of six) conversational questions.
4	Correct responses to any three (out of six) conversational questions.
5	Correct responses to any three (out of six) conversational questions plus some response to the picture description task.
6	Correct responses to any four (out of six) conversational questions plus some response to the picture description task.
7	Correct responses to any four (out of six) conversational questions and a mention of at least six things in the picture.
8	Correct responses to any five (out of six) conversational questions and an incomplete description of the picture.
9	Correct responses to all six conversational questions and an almost complete description of the picture; at least ten people, objects, or action should be named. Circumlocution may be present.
10	Correct responses to all six conversational questions and a reasonably complete description of the picture. Sentences of normal length and complexity, referring to most of the items and activities.

Source: Adapted from Kertesz (2006).

Table 3.2 Rating scale on scoring fluency of spontaneous speech in Western Aphasia Battery (Bedside)-Revised

Level	Description
0	No words or short, meaningless utterances.
1	Recurrent, **stereotypic utterances** with meaningful intonation.
2	Single words, often paraphasias, effortful and hesitant.
3	Mostly unintelligible, low-volume mumbling; some single words.
4	Agrammatic, effortful; verb-noun phrases, but only one or two propositional sentences.
5	Halting, paraphasic, but more complete sentence; significant word-finding difficulties.
6	Logopenic but normal syntax; few, if any, paraphasias; significant word-finding difficulties.
7	Fluent phonemic jargon, semblance to English syntax and phonology.
8	Circumlocutory, fluent speech with semantic paraphasias and word-finding difficulties.
9	Some hesitations and word-finding difficulties.
10	Normal speech.

Source: Kertesz (2006).

Table 3.3 Rating scale on expressive speech in Minnesota Test for Differential Diagnosis of Aphasia (MTDDA)

Level	Description
6	No functional speech.
5	Expresses needs and wishes in limited or defective manner.
4	Ready communication with single words and short phrases.
3	Some conversational speech but marked difficulty in expressing long or complex ideas.
2	Conversational speech, with mild difficulty finding words or expressing ideas.
1	Converses easily with occasional difficulty.
0	No observable impairment.

Source: Schuell (1965).

quality of speech content on a scale between 6 (the poorest) and 0 (the best), is also displayed in Table 3.3. On the other hand, based on the performance of free conversation, picture description, and telling of Aesop's Fables, the BDAE contains scales that are more detailed and quantifiable for an examiner to establish a profile of linguistic characteristics encompassing features such as the following:

- Phrase length: From a scale of 1 – "one word," 4 – "four words," to 7 – "seven words."
- Grammatical form: From a scale of 1 – "no syntactic word group," 4 – "simplified or incomplete forms with omission of grammatical morphemes," to 7 – "normal range of syntax with normal use of grammatical words."
- Intrusion of paraphasic errors: From a scale of 1 – "present in every utterance," 4 – "one to two instances per minute of conversation," to 7 – "absent."
- Anomia: From a scale of 1 – "fluent but empty speech," 4 – "informational words proportional to fluency," to 7 – "output contains primarily content words."
- Degree of repetition: From a scale of 1 – "0 to 20 percentile score," 4 – "50 percentile score," to 7 – "90 to 100 percentile score."

Functional Communication Measures (FCMs) by American Speech-Language-Hearing Association

Another example of the subjective use of clinical ratings is the Functional Communication Measures (FCMs) developed by the American Speech-Language-Hearing Association (ASHA, 2002, 2013) which contains a total of 15 disorder-specific, seven-point rating scales, ranging from Level

1(the least functional) to Level 7 (the most functional). The development of the FCMs is part of ASHA's National Outcome Measurement System (NOMS) data collection and reporting tool and it can be applied clinically to describe the different aspects of an examinee's functional communication (and swallowing) abilities over the course of speech-and-language pathology intervention. Based on the treatment plan of an examinee, suitable FCMs are chosen and scored by a certified speech-and-language pathologist on admission and again at discharge to reflect the amount of change. The FCM on spoken language expression is shown in Table 3.4.

Table 3.4 American Speech-Language-Hearing Association's Functional Communication Measure (FCM) on spoken language expression

Level	Description
1	The individual attempts to speak, but verbalizations are not meaningful to familiar or unfamiliar communication partners at any time.
2	The individual attempts to speak, although few attempts are accurate or appropriate. The communication partner must assume responsibility for structuring the communication exchange, and with consistent and maximal cueing, the individual can only occasionally produce automatic and/or imitative words and phrases that are rarely meaningful in context.
3	The communication partner must assume responsibility for structuring the communication exchange, and with consistent and moderate cueing, the individual can produce words and phrases that are appropriate and meaningful in context.
4	The individual is successfully able to initiate communication using spoken language in simple, structured conversations in routine daily activities with familiar communication partners. The individual usually requires moderate cueing, but is able to demonstrate use of simple sentences (i.e., semantics, syntax, and morphology) and rarely uses complex sentences/messages.
5	The individual is successfully able to initiate communication using spoken language in structured conversations with both familiar and unfamiliar communication partners. The individual occasionally requires minimal cueing to frame more complex sentences in messages. The individual occasionally self-cues when encountering difficulty.
6	The individual is successfully able to communicate in most activities, but some limitations in spoken language are still apparent in vocational, **avocational**, and social activities. The individual rarely requires minimal cueing to frame complex sentences. The individual usually self-cues when encountering difficulty.
7	The individual's ability to successfully and independently participate in vocational, avocational, and social activities is not limited by spoken language skills. Independent functioning may occasionally include use of self-cueing.

Note: This FCM should not be used for individuals using an augmentative/alternative communication system.

Source: National Outcomes Measurement System (NOMS): Adults Speech-Language Pathology User's Guide (American Speech-Language-Hearing Association, 2013).

Pros and Cons of Subjective Ratings

One major advantage of using the above-mentioned checklists or rating scales is that they can be readily administered within a clinical setting for a quick and easy evaluation of disordered narrative. This is particularly popular for daily practice for two reasons: (1) detailed and quantitative analysis of spontaneous discourse in speakers with neurogenic communication disorders is not a straightforward task, and (2) it is a very time-consuming process to conduct an oral discourse analysis from the start of collecting a language sample and having it properly transcribed to the time the sample is objectively analyzed. Hence, this approach becomes suitable for clinicians who need a quick diagnosis of language impairment, which is often treated as a supplement to standardized testing or to provide additional direction for further assessment of the discourse difficulties demonstrated by a patient. The validity of using this approach of subjective ratings is often challenged by the lack of systematic and detailed guidelines on its clinical application. Moreover, potential problems of judgment consistency across raters exist. This is especially the case for clinicians who have different degrees of clinical experience of working with a particular disorder population. The application is more problematic, perhaps, when there are discrepancies in the interpretation of rating descriptors across raters. An intra-rater reliability issue within the same examiner over time is another possible inevitable limitation due to the subjectivity involved in providing a clinical rating. In fact, conducting a reliable subjective evaluation of oral discourse always requires a high level of clinical skills because an examiner must be sensitive to the various discourse characteristics in the context of narrative production frameworks. According to Murray and Chapey (2001), collection of samples using other tasks apart from those in the above-mentioned aphasia batteries may improve the reliability and validity in assessing connected speech (see Chapter 2 on procedures about other discourse elicitation tasks). Nevertheless, one should note that although systematic quantitative discourse analyses (see Chapter 4) can provide information on specific language skill areas, some of them do not always reflect how the improvement of a skill translates into improved performance in functional day-to-day activities, such as in the case of ASHA's FCMs.

Linguistically-Based Analyses

As psycholinguistic analysis of aphasic output is complex and analytic procedures are not readily understood by clinicians who lack prior linguistic training, it remains unrealistic to expect clinicians to conduct a full-scale quantitative analysis of disordered language samples in everyday clinical settings. In light of this notion, a number of researchers have proposed discourse analytic systems that are brief but linguistically-focused as well as quick and easily learned. Specifically, these systems are characterized by (1) their capability to reflect aspects of language performance that have been found to differ among speakers with language impairments (e.g., efficiency of transmitting information content) as well as between disordered speakers and unimpaired individuals (e.g., performances at the lexical and syntactic levels), (2) the relatively little linguistic background required on the part of the examiners to learn to use the system, and (3) the use of discourse measures that can be obtained through quick and straightforward computation. Examples of some popular tools used by clinicians, or speech-and-language pathologists to be specific, are outlined below.

The Yorkston and Beukelman Quantification Method

Yorkston and Beukelman (1980) introduced a systematic and clinically oriented scoring framework to analyze the description of the Cookie Theft picture of the BDAE. This analytic system is referred to as the "Yorkston and Beukelman quantification method" because it was considered innovative back when it was first reported and has become a classical method of clinical discourse assessment. In particular, the procedures of analysis focused on two main areas of aphasic connected speech production: the amount and the efficiency of information conveyed. The former could be measured by comparing target words produced by the examinee with a list of content units, which were defined as information expressed to describe a key element of the picture. These content units included nouns, such as "the boy," "the girl," "the mother," "cookie," "water," or "sick," and action words such as "to steal," "to wash," "to fall," or "to daydream." As for the efficiency of communication, it was indicated by speaking rate (syllables per minute) and the rate at which content units were uttered (content units per minute). These indices were reported to be able to differentiate between speakers with low-moderate and mild aphasia as well as between speakers with high-moderate aphasia and unimpaired individuals. In a later study by Craig et al. (1993), which replicated the Yorkston and Beukelman study in 1980, a larger number of participants with aphasia were recruited. Among the 103 individuals with aphasia encompassing a range of impairment severity (i.e., mild, moderate, and severe grades of aphasia), it was found that the three severity groups differed significantly from each other with regard to all measures, except for the syllable rate measure between those with mild and moderate degrees of aphasia. It was concluded that this technique adequately acted as a "systematic and highly efficient way to quantify connected speech... and is strongly recommended as ... a clinical method for documenting change(s) in the expressive language of adults with aphasia" (p. 162).

Core Lexicon Analysis

To quantify word-retrieval ability at the discourse level, the method of measuring **core lexicons** (or lexical items that play a critical and significant role in constructing a semantically coherent narrative) has been proposed (MacWhinney et al., 2010). This approach of core lexicon analysis can help determine if words (such as nouns and verbs, or an aggregated list of core lexicons) most frequently present in oral production of cognitively healthy adults are adequately and appropriately used by speakers with discourse deficits. Typically, task-specific lists of core lexicons are first generated based on the performance of a group of representative unimpaired speakers to provide a reference to understand if and how different clinical populations deviate from the norms. For example, MacWhinney et al. (2010) have extracted the ten most frequent nouns and verbs (i.e., the core lexicons) from 25 healthy participants, and found that speakers with aphasia showed a reduced degree of lexical diversity and a greater proportion of light verbs than their control counterparts.

Motivated by the fact that selective impairments of content versus function words have been reported across aphasia subtypes, Dalton and Richardson (2015) believe that it is ecologically important to develop separate core lexicon lists by word class. With reference to normative language samples from 92 cognitively healthy adults, the authors built a core lexicon list including function words. Apart from a superior production of more core lexical items by the healthy group (than speakers with aphasia), it was found that participants with fluent aphasia performed better than the non-fluent group. Kim et al. (2021) have recently published an exploratory study to develop "core function word lists" to evaluate function word use in discourse and to examine how well the lists can help identify aphasia. Each of these lists contains the top 25 commonly used function words extracted from narrative language samples from healthy adults of seven age groups: 20s, 30s, 40s, 50s, 60s, 70s and 80s. Their results replicated the conclusions by Dalton and Richardson (2015); more importantly, their findings revealed significant correlations between function word production and aphasia severity (as reflected by the Aphasia Quotient of the Western Aphasia Battery).

In short, one major advantage of core lexicon measures lies on its clinical feasibility. In most cases, clinicians will only need to use a checklist of core lexicon items and apply a simple binary scoring system to check the presence (or absence) of these targets in an examinee's discourse output. Not only can this greatly reduce the valuable in- or off-session time needed for completing an analysis, clinicians can also reliably perform scoring without undertaking special or required training like they do for other traditional narrative-based analyses. Real time scoring within a clinical session or completing a scoring with pre-recorded audio or video files without orthographic transcripts is also possible (Dalton et al., 2020). Kim and Wright

---

Box 3.1 Advantages and Disadvantages of Clinical Measures of Word Retrieval in Connected Speech

Advantages	Disadvantages
✓ Convenient for clinical application	✗ Unable to fully measure subtle difficulties in word retrieval
✓ Easy to measure a speaker's word retrieval failure and to reflect general fluency	✗ Not easy to identify word choice errors
✓ Useful to reveal a speaker's vocabulary knowledge and lexical diversity in discourse	✗ Unclear if use of unique words reflects a speaker's failure or success in word retrieval
✓ Possible to use word retrieve performance to help predict everyday language	✗ Unclear if underlying cognitive processes of word retrieval differ across discourse tasks

Source: Modified from Kavé and Goral (2017)

(2020) have recommended this new approach of analysis for its clinical usability, practicality, and good time efficiency to assess and manage aphasia, and offered additional suggestions for clinical application and implementation. Box 3.1 outlines the advantages and disadvantages of measuring word retrieval in connected speech.

Correct Information Units (CIUs)

By adopting the principle and scoring method of the Yorkston and Beukelman (1980) study, Nicholas and Brookshire (1993) introduced another system to examine the accuracy and efficiency of aphasic connected speech elicited through the description of single pictures, a picture sequence, and a report of personal and procedural information. Unlike the original scoring method in Yorkston and Beukelman, in which the quantification of the amount of information was specific (and therefore limited) to the Cookie Theft picture, a rule-based method to quantify the information conveyed by a speaker was proposed. Specifically, the system utilized the following five measures to analyze samples from 20 speakers with aphasia and their control counterparts:

1. The total number of words.
2. The total number of "correct information units" (CIUs), defined as "words that are intelligible in context, accurate in relation to the picture(s) or topic, and relevant to the informative about the content of the picture(s) or the topic" (p.348). Note that this definition was quite

similar to that of content units described by Yorkston and Beukelman (1980).

3. Rate of word production in minute.
4. The number of CIUs produced per minute.
5. The ratio of CIUs to the total number of words (percentage of CIUs).

All the measures were found to reveal statistically significant differences between the non-brain-damaged and speakers with aphasia. Furthermore, measures 3, 4, and 5 were reported to be higher in sensitivity and able to discriminate between speaker groups better than the other two measures.

Shewan Spontaneous Language Analysis (SSLA)

A more comprehensive quantification system was introduced by Shewan (1988a), namely the Shewan Spontaneous Language Analysis (SSLA). In this analysis, language samples were elicited through a picture description task using the picture stimulus from the standardized version of the Western Aphasia Battery (Shewan & Kertesz, 1980). The samples were then analyzed using 12 SSLA variables that are meant to evaluate the semantic, phonological, and syntactic components of oral discourse:

1. Number of utterances: A measure of the total number of utterances spoken by an examinee.
2. Time: The total speaking time in minutes for the sample, measured by counting the start at the first syllable and the end at the last syllable.
3. Rate: The total number of syllables spoken per minute.
4. Length: Percentage of short utterances, calculated by dividing the number of utterances that contained five or fewer words by the total number of utterances spoken.
5. Melody: A 7-point melody rating scale on the rhythm of speech, the stress patterns employed, and the intonation contours expressed. This scale was similar to the melody rating in the BDAE.
6. Articulation: A 7-point articulation rating scale on the articulatory accuracy of speech with consideration of the presence of imprecise speech, verbal dyspraxia, articulatory errors, and/or phonological disturbance. This scale was similar to the articulatory agility rating in the BDAE.
7. Complex sentences: Percentage of complex utterances with at least one independent clause and one or more dependent clauses, calculated by dividing the number of complex utterances by the total number of utterances in the sample.
8. Errors: Percentage of syntactic and morphological errors relative to the total number of utterances spoken.
9. Content units: Total number of grouping of information expressed by the examinee, similar to the definition of "content unit" in Yorkston and Beukelman (1980).

10. Paraphasias: Percentage of paraphasias (in place of correct content) relative to the total number of utterances in the sample.
11. Repetition: Percentage of repeated words or phrases relative to the total number of utterances in the sample.
12. Communication Efficiency: calculated by dividing the total number of content units by the time of the language sample in minutes.

The author concluded that ten of the variables were reported to reveal significant differences between the aphasic and unimpaired speaker groups with "Content units," "Rate," and "Number of utterances" being the top three discriminating variables in the system. According to Shewan (1988a), the analysis of connected speech may help judge the general communicative ability of speakers with aphasia.

The SSLA was then used to monitor changes in expressive language during recovery as a function of severity (Shewan, 1988b). The study tested 47 participants with different degrees of aphasia, from mild to severe, who had suffered from a single unilateral **cerebrovascular accident**. Two language samples were obtained from all participants through the same picture description task. The first sample was taken between two and four weeks post onset; the second was taken within the period of three to twelve months after the collection of the first sample. The two sets of language samples were then compared using the SSLA variables. The results indicated that eight of the variables were useful in tracing the recovery of language function as they showed positive changes towards the normal level of the older unimpaired participants from Shewan's (1988a) study, including "Content units," "Number of utterances," "Errors," "Time," "Rate," "Melody," "Articulation," and "Communication efficiency." However, a potential issue in the study was the possible practice effect of the repeated measurement of the SSLA. It was crucial to see whether changes in the SSLA variables would occur between the two speech samples of the controls elicited on the two occasions. Shewan (1988b) also attempted to use the system to distinguish aphasia syndromes and severity. It was found that both the type and the degree of aphasia impairment significantly affected the aphasic group's performance on a subset of variables measuring quantity ("Length"), propositions ("Content units"), efficiency ("Rate" and "Communication efficiency"), and error production ("Errors" and "Paraphasias") in the speech output. The speakers with anomic aphasia were found to produce the highest amount of errors, followed by those with conduction and Wernicke's aphasia. The speakers with global and Broca's aphasia, on the other hand, produced the fewest errors, but they were also the most impaired as measured by the remaining variables. Except for the index of "Paraphasias" in which there was a lack of significant difference among the aphasic types, the global and Broca's participants differed significantly from the other three types of aphasia. Concerning the aphasia severity, as expected, it was found that the participants with severe aphasia were significantly more impaired than the moderate and mild groups with regard to the measures of "Rate," "Content units," "Paraphasias," and "Communication efficiency." Interestingly, the mildly and moderately impaired individuals used significantly more utterances that were short, and produced significantly more errors than the severe group. These results seemed to suggest a lack of direct relationship between the quality of errors committed and the degree of aphasia severity.

Linguistic Communication Measure (LCM) and Its Extended Versions

Another quick method of analyzing aphasic narratives is presented by Menn et al. (1994), which is referred to as the Linguistic Communication Measure (LCM). This tool was designed with the clear purpose of supplementing, rather than replacing, standard aphasia batteries. Using the Cookie Theft picture of the BDAE as the stimulus, its aim was to reflect progress or deterioration in oral narratives over time among speakers with aphasia. It contains a small number of indices, the computation of which required minimal clinical experience and linguistic training to quantify the following linguistic aspects of verbal output:

1. Amount of information conveyed – "Number of content units," with the same definition as in Yorkston and Beukelman (1980).
2. Extent of word-finding difficulty and emptiness of speech – "Index of Lexical Efficiency (ILE)," defined as the ratio of correct content units to the total number of words produced.
3. Occurrence of morphological errors and omissions – "Index of Grammatical Support (IGS)," which was the average number of correctly used supporting words and grammatical elements (such as grammatical endings and contractions) per content unit.

According to Menn et al. (1994), the computation of these LCM indices was relatively quick and easy. Although these performance indices were not intended to differentiate between aphasia syndromes, it was argued that they reflected clinically important differences among individuals with aphasia (which was related to the use of correct grammatical morphemes) that were missing in the Yorkston and Beukelman quantification method. To investigate the use of the LCM for monitoring changes in patients with aphasia over time, Menn et al. (1994) followed three fluent and three non-fluent speakers' performances on describing the same picture stimulus. The speakers were required to regularly provide oral samples during a period of recovery ranging from two months to seven years. It was found that over time, the performances of these participants either approached the normal means or became more stable towards the end, as reflected by the number of content units and the ILE. However, it should be noted that the measure of grammatical support was also only supposed to be a brief description of speakers' syntactic ability, not a detailed description as in Saffran et al. (1989) and Rochon et al. (2000) (see details in Chapter 4). Nevertheless, the strength of the LCM lies in the fact that the collection of speech samples is relatively quick and its analytic procedures are simple and straightforward enough to be used in general clinical situations.

Kong and Law (2004) have put forth the Cantonese Linguistic Communication Measure (CLCM) for use by speech-and-language pathologists to conduct clinical discourse analysis among native Cantonese Chinese speakers in Hong Kong. It was developed based on the original LCM with some of the indices devised based on the SSLA. Similar to the original tool, the CLCM was designed to be a quick, objective, and simple evaluation that would require little linguistic background of the user. Computation of the indices continued to be easy and straightforward. As such, it ensured a short rater training period and good intra-rater and inter-rater reliabilities. Four pictures, depicting scenes of a picnic, a kitchen, a living room, and a restaurant were developed. Language samples were elicited through a picture description task, which were then orthographically transcribed and analyzed in terms of the following seven indices:

1. Number of **informative words** (IW): An informative word was defined as a key lexical item of the picture stimuli, similar to the definition of "content units" in Yorkston and Beukelman (1980), and was counted only when it was used accurately in the oral output. In the case where the speaker attempted to self-correct an informative word, only the final version of the production would be used for scoring. That is, when a speaker wrongly self-corrected his or her word(s), only the final version of the production would be counted (as an error), without any credit being given to the previously produced correct informative word. On the other hand, when a speaker correctly self-corrected the word, the final version of the production would be counted as an informative word. All previous incorrect productions when he or she was struggling for the corresponding informative word were counted as errors.

2. Index of Lexical Efficiency (ILE): The ratio of total number of words to number of informative words.

3. Index of Communication Efficiency (ICE): Calculated by dividing the number of informative words by the duration of the recording in minutes, similar to the "rate" index in the SSLA.

4. Index of Grammatical Support (IGS): Modified from the original IGS in the LCM; calculated by dividing the total number of correctly used grammatical morphemes by the total number of words. Instead of counting the gross number of closed class items in the language sample,

only those that had appropriately modified the correct informative words in the sample were counted toward this index.

5. Index of Elaboration (IEl): The ratio of correctly used stem morphemes (or open class morphemes) to informative words.

6. Index of Error (IEr): Obtained by dividing the total number of jargons, neologisms, phonemic paraphasias, and semantic paraphasias produced by the number of informative words.

7. Index of Lexical Richness (ILR): The language sample elicited from each of the four pictures was trimmed to 40 words. The **type-token ratio (TTR)** (see Chapter 4) for the total 160 words from the four stimulus pictures was then computed.

Kong and Law (2004) have shown that native unimpaired speakers of Cantonese and adults with aphasia in Hong Kong differed significantly on all the indices when tested on a single occasion. Kong and Law (2009a) subsequently performed a multivariate analysis of language samples from 34 adults with fluent aphasia, 26 with non-fluent aphasia, and 60 unimpaired speakers. The CLCM indices, when used together, were able to differentiate among the three speaker groups. A discriminant function analysis was also carried out to classify speaker groups and to predict group membership for individual participants. A specificity of 100% in classifying normal and a sensitivity of 85% in classifying speakers with aphasia were obtained. While the IEr was the most discriminative between unimpaired speakers and adults with aphasia, the IGS and ICE were found to be most useful to distinguish those with fluent from non-fluent aphasia. A follow-up study by Kong and Law (2009b) has also provided further evidence of the CLCM's capability to monitor changes of language production over time. Specifically, changes of narrative production in five adults with aphasia in the period of spontaneous recovery (SR group) and four who underwent anomia therapies (Tx group) were monitored. Language samples elicited from the same picture description task were collected among the SR participants at regular intervals within the first six months post-onset and among the Tx participants before and after treatment. The results showed that the CLCM indices could reflect changes of language production in both the SR and Tx participants over time. More critically, the changes of index values were consistent with the expectations of performance during early stages after stroke for the SR participants and treatment outcomes of the Tx participants, indicating the sensitivity of the CLCM for adults with aphasia who can at least produce short utterances and sentences during recovery.

More recently, Kong and Yeh (2019) have translated and adapted a Mandarin version of the LCM for the local population in Taiwan (i.e., TM-LCM). Informative words that were geographically sensitive to Taiwanese were first established from neurologically intact native speakers recruited in

Taiwan. Based on the performance of 36 control participants and 10 individuals with aphasia, the TM–LCM was found to be able to highlight and distinguish impaired spoken output in aphasia. Specifically, discourse performance, as reflected by TM–LCM indices, was found to associate with aphasia severity. Similar to other versions of the LCM, calculation of TM–LCM indices continued to be reliable and clinically feasible.

Hilger et al. (2014) have also introduced an extended version of the LCM, namely the Linguistic Communication Measure – Speech Sounds (LCM-SS). It was utilized to report a detailed multidimensional analysis of connected speech, elicited through the description of the Cookie Theft picture, gathered over the course of 27 months in a participant with logopenic variant **primary progressive aphasia (PPA)**. The development of the LCM-SS was motivated by the lack of a sensitive tool in the literature to reflect the observed gradual deterioration of speech sounds within the production of a discourse that was exhibited by this participant with logopenic PPA. In particular, while other clinical linguistic systems could capture the speaker's lexical, syntactic, pragmatic, and/or morphological abilities, they did not respond well to the increasing speech sound difficulties (such as phonetic and phonological errors and stutter-like onsets in an oral discourse). In light of the limitations of existing quantification systems, the following counts and indices were newly added to the LCM-SS:

1. Counting of morphosyntactic errors: All morphosyntactic errors in the complete language sample were identified and tallied. Errors of morphology included all incorrect bound grammatical morphemes (i.e., word endings and prefixes). Syntactic errors included incorrect forms of words (e.g., "you have going" which should be "you have gone" or "you are going"), words that were missing (e.g., "She gave it me" which should be "She gave it to me"), changes in tense and aspect within a phrasal unit, and word order violations as reflected by a word group that was not spoken in the correct and grammatical order.

2. Counting of semantic errors: This involved a frequency count of all semantic errors in the complete sample, such as semantic paraphasias and wrong gender terms. Attempts at a word that was not eventually produced correctly, even if the speaker recognized the attempts were incorrect (e.g., "Skip? No. Trip? No. Anyway …" in reference to a boy falling off a stool), were also included in the count.

3. Counting of sound errors: All sound errors were identified and tallied, including phonological **paraphasia**, neologisms, jargon segments, words that are broken off (e.g., "cook jar" for "cookie jar"), and words produced incorrectly that were eventually corrected.

4. Counting of repetitions: All full and partial word and phrasal repetitions in the complete sample were identified and tallied. For full word repetitions, each instance of the repeated word was counted. For partial

word repetitions, each word that contained a partial word was counted. If a non-word was repeated, this error was counted as both a sound and a repetition error. Each phrasal repetition was counted as a single unit (e.g., "the boy is, he is" contained one phrasal repetition, although the exact words were not used the second time).

5. Index of grammatical errors (IGramE): ratio of the total morphosyntactic errors within content units (CU) to the total number of CU.
6. Index of semantic errors (ISemE): ratio of the total number of semantic (verbal) paraphasias within CUs to the total number of CUs.
7. Index of sound errors (ISouE): the sum of total sound errors and number of words with repetitions was divided by the number of CUs.

The last three indices were found to be sensitive to indicate the level of morphosyntactic impairment, semantic impairment, and level of sound production impairment during narration, respectively.

Functional Measures of Word Retrieval at the Narrative Level

Another quick and simple framework of the functional measure of word retrieval was introduced by Mayer and Murray (2003) who included a set of procedures for eliciting conversational samples and composite descriptions of picture sequences, as well as steps for analyzing samples. To ensure the collection of at least 300 words for each speaker, pictures that depicted a series of events, each of which included multiple characters and activities were used in this study. The final transcript from multiple tasks was combined, and the first 300 words were used for subsequent scoring. In case a speaker produced a total output of fewer than 300 words, the entire transcript was scored. The measures used for sequence analyses were:

1. number of accurately used nouns
2. number of accurately used verbs
3. number of error nouns
4. number of error verbs
5. percentage of noun retrieval attempts that were successful (%WR nouns)
6. percentage of verb retrieval attempts that were successful (%WR verbs)
7. percentage of substantive verbs (%SV)
8. percentage of corrected errors (%CERR).

Based on the results of seven individuals with mild aphasia and another seven with moderate aphasia, it was found that the speakers tended to better retrieve and self-correct errors (i.e., higher %WR and %CERR) in connected speech as compared to single-word naming tasks. The measures of %WR and %SV was also found to be able to detect verb retrieval deficits in aphasia, with a higher sensitivity for the mild aphasic group. The authors concluded that the above functional measures were simple and easily quantifiable with high clinical feasibility.

Pros and Cons of Linguistically-Based Analyses

It is fair to say that, overall, the above linguistically-based analyses were designed to be clinically oriented with more focused and specific measures and were developed to assist an examiner to clinically quantify disordered discourse production. Often, clinicians may use the results of one or more of these analytic systems to serve as an initial estimation of a speaker's linguistic abilities, which then lead to more in-depth evaluation of the discourse performance. Some of these quantification frameworks have also been proved to reflect the progressive changes of narratives among individuals with aphasia over time. A recent comparison study by Kong and Wong (2018) has concluded that linguistically-based measures worked the best to detect discourse impairments in aphasia and were the most powerful to characterize impaired performance of spoken aphasic discourse. For examples, linguistic measures focusing on the quantity and efficiency of production were particularly useful to estimate the fluency status of aphasia. The linguistic approach of discourse analysis also best correlated with and predicted aphasia severity.

Clinically, having an objective, easily administrable, and reliable tool for everyday assessment and monitoring of changes in language ability in speakers with disordered narratives can offer practitioners important diagnostic information (Gao & Benson, 1990). A particular clients' performance as reflected by these tools will provide clinicians with directions for devising a suitable intervention plan. Furthermore, communication about the client's progress across different clinical settings or among professionals can also be greatly enhanced. A few recent systematic reviews and/or meta-analyses of disordered spoken discourse suggest the growth in research and clinical application of discourse analysis. An example of these reviews is the summary by Bryant et al. (2016) that focused on methodological applications of linguistic discourse analysis in aphasia. Although this linguistic approach of evaluation has received credits for its clinical usability, one should note that some users may challenge that the measurement cannot adequately or fully reflect discourse production by the disordered population in real-world settings.

Content-Based Analyses

A content-based analysis is another clinical approach that employs some rule-based procedures to score key episodes or scenarios expressed in a connected speech; it has been extensively reported in the literature. Unlike the linguistically-based analyses outlined above that focus on specific linguistic components of a discourse, this approach emphasizes the quantification of amount of proposition or information content (i.e., degree of informativeness) in an examinee's discourse output. According to Van Dijk (1980), key concepts within a narrative are the fundamental building components of discourse macrostructure. Organized sequences of key concepts thus form the skeletal outline of a discourse. Some common content-based analyses of discourse suitable for clinical application are outlined below.

Main Concept Analysis and Its Extended Versions

Nicholas and Brookshire (1995) reported the use of a scoring method that measured the amount of main information conveyed about a topic and compared the performance between 20 English speaking individuals with aphasia and 20 non-brain-damaged adults. Connected speech samples were elicited from each participant using four single pictures (including the Cookie Theft picture from the BDAE, the "picnic" picture from the WAB, and two others in which each depicted a story-like situation with a central focus and interactions among pictured elements), two sets of sequential pictures (each of which contained six panels to form a story), two conversations related to participants' personal information ("Tell me what you usually do on Sundays" and "Tell me where you live and describe it to me"), and two procedural descriptions ("Tell me how you would go about doing dishes by hand" and "Tell me how you would go about writing and sending a letter"). The amount of main information within an output was reflected by the number of main concepts contained. In particular, a main concept was defined as "statements [that] provide an outline of the gist or essential information portrayed in the stimulus pictures or an outline of the essential steps in the procedures... and should contain one and only one main verb" (p. 148). Each elicited language sample was evaluated on whether all potential main concepts were present, and if so whether the essential information in each main concept mentioned was accurate and complete. For example, for the main concept of "The girl is asking for a cookie" within the Cookie Theft picture, the main verb is "to ask for" and pieces of essential information include "girl" and "cookie". Each main concept identified was then classified as one of the following four categories:

1. Accurate and Complete (AC): All essential information in a main concept was accurate and complete. Essential information did not have to be spoken in a standard grammatical form or standard word order, as long as deviations would not lead to miscomprehension of the essential meaning of the main concept. In addition, the production did not have to be correctly articulated to be considered accurate, as long as it was intelligible to a listener (i.e., the listener would understand the target

words in the context of what the speaker was saying). With reference to the above-mentioned example, acceptable AC main concepts include "The sister would like to get a cookie from her brother" or "She was asking for a cookie from him" as long as the pronoun "she" was indicating the "girl" instead of the "mother".

2.   Accurate but Incomplete (AI): One or more pieces of essential information in the main concept were missing, but all given essential information was accurate. For example, acceptable AI main concepts may include "The girl asked for something" (where the essential information of "cookie" is missing) or "She would like to get a cookie" (in case it is not clear whether the pronoun "she" is referring to the "girl").

3.   Inaccurate (IN): One or more pieces of essential information in the main concept given were inaccurate. Examples included paraphasias of action words or nouns, neologisms, and jargons or irrelevant lexical items that did not match with the content of the picture stimuli. More specifically, all of the following examples contain one or more errors in the output: "The boy is asking for a cookie," "The girl would like to get an ice-cream," and "The girl is giving a cookie and a plate."

4.   Absent (AB): None of the essential information in a target main concept was given, i.e., the speaker did not provide any essential information that appeared to be an attempt to communicate a particular main concept.

It was found that the non-brain-damaged group produced significantly more AC main concepts and significantly fewer AI, IN, and AB main concepts than the speakers with aphasia. Moreover, out of the four categories, the AI and IN were found to be more discriminating between the two speaker groups than the AC and AB. The results also revealed that the number of AB and AC main concepts was strongly correlated to the estimated severity of aphasia. The average point-to-point inter-rater and intra-rater reliability was 86% and 90% for the four scores, with the categories AC and IN achieving the highest level of agreement. A mean correlation coefficient of 0.77 for the four scores in test-retest reliability also indicated acceptably stable performance of description on two occasions seven to ten days apart. It was concluded that the measures of main concept production could reflect the overall communication success and could supplement existing measures of communicative informativeness and efficiency.

Adapting from the Nicholas and Brookshire study (1995), Kong (2009) developed the Main Concept Analysis (MCA), to measure the connected speech from 30 Cantonese speakers, including ten fluent and ten non-fluent persons with aphasia as well as ten healthy participants. The study involved the development of four novel sets of sequential pictures that were culturally appropriate for both the Western and Eastern populations, including the Chinese Cantonese speakers in Hong Kong, to elicit language samples.

Specifically, each picture set contains four detached, single, black-and-white line drawings with dimensions of 15 cm by 21 cm. While two of the sets contained only one character, the other two sets contained three characters and, therefore, should potentially contain more numbers of main concepts (than the first two sets) with reference to the inter-relationships among characters:

- Picture set 1 ("Cooking in a kitchen") depicts an old lady who is preparing a meal in a kitchen and accidently cuts her finger.
- Picture set 2 ("Waking up late for work") shows a man waking up late and rushing to go to work.
- Picture set 3 ("Buying ice cream") depicts a mother and her daughter visiting an ice cream shop and their interactions with the staff there.
- Picture set 4 ("Helping an old man") illustrates a boy walking with his father and helping an old man to pick up his grocery items that have fallen on the ground (see Figure 2.3).

The lexical items contained in the pictures were carefully controlled in a way that the same key item did not appear in more than one picture set. The method of analyzing the oral discourse directly adopted the four index measures (AC, AI, IN, and AB) from Nicholas and Brookshire (1995) with an addition of two new measures created by Kong:

1. The main concept score (MC): calculated by a formula ($3 \times AC + 2 \times AI + 1 \times IN$) to obtain a summary of the first four measures.
2. AC per minute: a ratio of AC to the total recording time in minutes to reflect the efficiency of a speaker's conveying of AC concepts.

Due to the linguistic differences between English and Chinese Cantonese, scoring rules of the MCA were altered. In particular, use of elliptical utterances (e.g. omissions of the subject or object of a sentence), right dislocation of nouns or pronouns in a sentence (VOS), and a word or phrase in the object position placed at the beginning of a sentence (OSV) were not correct in English but might be accepted in Cantonese. Therefore, with consideration of the characteristics of topic chain in Chinese grammar, an IN concept in English might be rated as AC or AI in Cantonese. Kong (2009) concluded that the unimpaired speakers had significantly higher scores on AC, AI, MC, and AC/minute but lower scores on IN and AB than the two aphasic groups. Moreover, aphasia severity, as reflected by the Cantonese version of the Western Aphasia Battery (CAB; Yiu, 1992), correlated significantly with most measures, except for AI and IN. Further work on the MCA was reported by Kong (2011) who recruited sixteen speakers with aphasia and established the external validation of the tool by examining the relationship between the MCA index scores and the CLCM (Kong & Law,

2004; see earlier discussion in this chapter) as well as subtests in the CAB. It was found that the main concept measures were highly correlated with the CLCM indices and CAB. More specifically, both AC and MC had positive relations with the total number of informative words as well as CAB scores on spontaneous speech (SS), naming subtest, and overall aphasia quotient (AQ). In addition, AC was found to positively correlate with the CLCM Index of Lexical Richness (ILR) but negatively correlate with the CLCM Index of Error (IEr). Finally, there was a positive relationship between AC/minute and CLCM Index of Communication Efficiency (ICE), between MC and CAB SS subtest, as well as between AC/minute and SS (Fluency) subtest. Subsequently, the MCA has been examined on its clinical applicability to the native Irish-English population with aphasia and controls living in Ireland (Kong et al., 2012), typical English speakers, individuals with aphasia and dementia in the United States (Kong at al., 2016), and people with and without aphasia who speak Taiwanese Mandarin residing in Taiwan (Kong & Yeh, 2015; Yeh & Kong, 2014). Newer adaptations of the MCA to populations from other geographic locations include native speakers of Spanish from four different dialect origins (Central American Caribbean, Andean-Pacific, Mexican, and Central-Southern Peninsular regions) (Kong, 2021), Japanese adults with aphasia and controls in Japan (Yazu et al., 2021), Flemish Dutch speakers and those with aphasia in Belgium (Criel et al., 2021), Mandarin speakers with traumatic brain injury in Mainland China (Gao et al., 2016), and Korean-speaking adults in South Korea (Kong, 2018). Consistent results were obtained in these studies which suggests the MCA continues to adequately discriminate disordered discourse from language output of healthy participants. More information about the assessment consideration of the culturally diverse population can be found in Chapter 8.

Numerous reports have added important evidence of the clinical feasibility and value of MCA in evaluating spoken discourse in aphasia. For example, to examine how well speakers with aphasia can conceptualize a sequence of concepts, select, and organize corresponding relevant information to produce in spoken discourse, Hameister and Nickels (2018) investigated the quantity of main concepts produced in a picture description task and focused on the sequence of occurrence of these concepts in the output. It was found that, compared with healthy speakers, individuals with aphasia produced significantly fewer main concepts (that could not be fully accounted for by their language production deficits) at the beginning of the oral descriptions. In addition, the aphasia group was characterized by a much higher proportion of marginally relevant information in the output and was more variable in their order of main concepts, suggesting impaired conceptualization. Deng et al. (2021) have also applied the MCA to score spoken discourse production (on two discourse tasks of single and sequential picture description) by native Mandarin Chinese speakers with anomic aphasia. Results similar to the original reports of the English-MCA and

Cantonese-MCA were replicated: compared with unimpaired individuals, speakers with anomic aphasia produced significantly fewer AC but more AI and AB main concepts, and subsequently lower overall main concept scores. In another recent study, the scoring principles and criteria of MCA have been applied to examine the impacts of language dominance on 83 young and unimpaired bilingual speakers of Spanish and English (Rivera et al., 2018). It was concluded that speakers' language proficiency correlated with their production of main concepts in spoken discourse; their word retrieval skills were also predictive of production of main concepts in both Spanish and English.

An example of the clinical administration of the MCA is given in Box 3.2. BJ was a 55-year-old, right-handed, Caucasian male speaker of English who pre-morbidly worked as a shop manager. He had sustained a left hemispheric cerebrovascular accident about 13 months before he received a formal evaluation of his language ability using the Western Aphasia Battery, in which he was diagnosed with anomic aphasia (with an aphasia quotient of 88.2 out of 100). Six days after the administration of the WAB, BJ was assessed on his narrative skills using the MCA which contained a more detailed quantification of his discourse language functions. The complete language sample is shown in Box 3.2, which contains the orthographical transcript of BJ's oral description of the fourth set of the MCA sequential pictures (see Figure 2.3). According to Kong et al. (2015), there are six target main concepts for this picture set, which are listed in the recording form. Note that there is only one target action word (bolded and underlined) in each main concept; pieces of essential information are underlined. BJ's transcript contains three accurate and complete (AC) concepts, i.e., concepts 1, 4, and 5. Note that in BJ's description of concept 1, "... are walking down the hall the street there...," mentioning of "the hall" which was then immediately self-corrected to "the street" should not compromise the scoring of AC. In contrast, his production in concept 2 was counted as an IN because of the semantic paraphasia "woman". His oral production on concept 3 and 6 is considered accurate but incomplete (AI). While the main action word "fall" is missing from the description of concept 3, the target action word "praise" was replaced by "thank" in concept 6. Concept 6 would have been scored AC if the speaker used a description such as "the older man gives him a thumb up." Notice that even though there is a grammatical error in concept 3, "The bag is tore opening and ...," it does not affect the MCA scoring because the MCA does not require information be spoken in standard grammatical from or standard word order, as long as the deviation does not lead to miscomprehension of the meaning of the main concept. With the total of three AC, two AI, and one IN concepts for this picture set, a total MCA score of 15 can be obtained. The total duration of the description was 30 seconds, which was then converted to 0.5 minutes. The final measure of AC per minute can then be computed, i.e., $3 \div 0.5 = 6$. A blank MCA scoring form is provided in

Box 3.2 An Illustration of the Main Concept Analysis (MCA)

Patient name:	B.J.	**Speech therapist:**	A.K.

Date of birth/Age: Nov 1966 /55   **Date of MCA testing:** Nov 16, 2022

Gender: M / F   **Date of WAB testing:** Nov 10, 2022

Onset of aphasia: Aug 23, 2021   **WAB AQ:** 88.2

Etiology: CVA   **Aphasia type:** anomic

Remarks: Fluent with occasional word finding difficulties and semantic paraphasias. No apparent motor speech disorders. Appropriate speech prosody.

Complete language sample:

The kid and his father are walking down the hall the street there. And there is a woman that is walking in the opposite direction and he's got a bag with something in it... And here is shows the fact that the bag is tore opening and it looks like it has maybe oranges and the kid sees it and turns around picks it up and helps the guy the older man pick it up... Then the older man thanks him.

Time = 0 min 30 sec = 0.50 minute

	AC	AI	IN	AB
1 The FATHER and the SON are WALKING on the street				
The kid and his father are walking down the hall the street there	1			
2 The OLD MAN is CARRYING a grocery bag				
a woman that is walking in the opposite direction and he's got a bag with something in it			1	
3 The ORANGES FALL on the floor				
The bag is tore opening and it looks like it has maybe oranges		1		
4 The BOY SEES the incident				
the kid sees it	1			
5 The BOY is HELPING the old man				
the kid sees it and turns around picks it up and helps the guy the older man pick it up	1			
6 The OLD MAN is PRAISING the BOY				
Then the older man thanks him		1		

	AC	AI	IN	AB
Index 1, 2, 3, 4 –	3	2	1	0
Index 5 – Main concept score (MC) = (3×**AC** + 2×**AI** + 1×**IN**)	14			
Index 6 – AC per minute =	6			

Appendix 3.1. If picture stimuli other than those in Kong (2009, 2011, 2016) are used, all main concepts with target action words and relevant essential information should be identified prior to their clinical application.

Richardson and Dalton (2016) reported a refined version of MCA to assess spoken discourse and utilized additional codes that address accuracy and completeness of a main concept to provide a more detailed measurement of the overall informativeness. Specifically, for a concept to be coded as "accurate," no essential elements within the concept can include incorrect information. On the other hand, for a concept to be coded as "complete," a speaker must have produced every essential element of the concept. Based on these principles, after determining whether all target main concepts of a discourse are present or not, each "present" concept would be given one of the four following codes:

1. Accurate and Complete (AC): Must contain all elements of the concept with no incorrect information.
2. Accurate but Incomplete (AI): Must contain no incorrect information, but one (or more) essential element is left out.
3. Inaccurate but Complete (IC): Typically contains at least one incorrect piece of information, but all essential elements of the concepts must be mentioned.
4. Inaccurate and Incomplete (II): A statement that clearly corresponds with a target concept, but includes at least one incorrect essential element and also misses at least one essential element.

A modified main concept score that is different from Kong (2009) was also proposed: $(3 \times AC + 2 \times AI + 2 \times IC + 1 \times II)$. This modification separated the previously combined "inaccurate" scores (IC and II) and gave more value to IC statements than the method in Kong (2009) or Nicholas and Brookshire (1995).

Based on transcripts of telling the Cinderella story and describing the procedures to make a peanut butter and jelly sandwich from 92 unimpaired speakers in English (stratified into four age groups: 20 to 39 years, 40 to 59 years, 60 to 79 years, and 80 years or older), Richardson and Dalton (2016) found that the two younger groups produced significantly more AC concepts on average than the two older groups. Hence, younger speakers achieved higher modified main concept scores. Although the same positive age effect was not found in transcripts of a picture sequence narrative (i.e., descriptions elicited using the sequential picture of "Broken Window" of the AphasiaBank protocol; MacWhinney et al., 2011), the authors have made the main concept checklists (specific to these three discourse tasks) available for clinicians and researchers to assess aphasic spoken discourse. To further contribute to the important development of objective discourse measures, Richardson and Dalton (2020) have recently replicated their 2016 study, and provided comparable main concept checklists that can be readily used to quantify two semi-spontaneous discourse tasks in the AphasiaBank protocol: a scene narrative of the "Cat Rescue" picture (see Figure 2.2) and another sequential picture narrative using the "Refused Umbrella" pictures.

The refined MCA has been reported to be able to identify speakers with aphasia who scored above the cut-off of WAB (Fromm et al., 2017) and to highlight discourse characteristics by aphasia types (Dalton & Richardson, 2019; Richardson, et al., 2021). Moreover, to explore the relationship between informativeness and macrostructure in aphasic discourse, Greenslade et al. (2020) and Richardson et al. (2021) reported a multilevel approach of discourse analysis that involved the application of "main concepts, sequencing, and story grammar" (MSSG). The authors concluded that MSSG could clinically distinguish between speakers with aphasia and healthy adults.

Main Event Analysis

Capilouto et al. (2006) have also modified the main concept measurement by Nicholas and Brookshire (1995) and investigated the ability to convey **"main events"** among eight adults with aphasia. With reference to the performance of describing two single pictures and two sets of sequential picture stimuli, the performance by the aphasic group was compared with eight healthy adults. In this study, a main event was defined as "an event that was of sufficient importance to the story as a whole and independent from the other events in the story" (p. 207). This definition differed from the main concepts of Nicholas and Brookshire (1995) in that a main event might contain more than one main verb. As claimed by the authors, this could allow the capturing of a speaker's ability to convey relationships between characters and events. At the same time, how well a speaker extracted critical ideas and inter-relationships from irrelevant details could be indirectly evaluated (Capilouto et al., 2005). A binary scoring system, which was arguably simpler than the calculation of main concepts, was used to calculate the proportion of main events produced by each participant. Only those main events that contained all necessary information were scored as "present;" otherwise, any other incomplete output would be scored as "absent." The results indicated that the aphasic group produced significantly fewer main events than their healthy counterparts, thus highlighting the usefulness of the main event measurement to characterize their impaired narrative discourse abilities. Test–retest reliability of the main events measured at 7–21 days apart was also calculated, with significant correlations of 0.88 and 0.73 for sequential picture and single picture stimuli, respectively.

Wright and Capilouto (2009) have further reported their application of the main event analysis to samples of picture descriptions and story-telling by 24 healthy older adults of English. A significant positive relationship between the proportion of main events in the transcripts of sequential picture description and percentage of information units was found. Moreover, proportion of main events in the single picture description correlated negatively with the overall type-token ratio (TTR; see Chapter 4). The authors provided an explanation that the participants' use of a limited range of, but specific, lexical items might have contributed to this observed pattern of increased level of informativeness but decreased amount of productive vocabulary. Nevertheless, together with the point-to-point inter- and intra-rater agreement of 86.4% and 95.3%, respectively, these findings were able to demonstrate the strength of this analytic method. A follow-up study conducted by this research group (Capilouto et al. 2016) applied the main event analysis to language samples (elicited by two single and two sequential pictures) from 240 healthy adults, separated into three age groups of young (20–39 years), middle-age (40–69 years), and older (70–89 years) speakers. It was found that, compared to the young and middle-age groups, the older participants relayed a significantly lower proportion of main events in their descriptions. One possible cause was the weakened working memory capacity demonstrated by the older adults. In addition, this trend of decreased production of main events by age was suggested to be contributed to by age-related decline in micro-linguistic processes, as evident by (a) lower degree of mean syntactic complexity in the older speakers and their significantly less complex utterances as compared to the young and middle-age groups, (b) for the young and middle-age group, significant correlations between total number of words and main event production, and (c) for the young group, significant correlations between lexical diversity and main event production.

A Frequency Analysis of Errors

Contrary to the method of tallying propositional content within an oral discourse, an approach focusing on counting and categorizing errors committed by speakers with aphasia was introduced by Ardila and Rosselli (1993). Specifically, language deviations in describing the Cookie Theft picture by 30 left hemispheric-damaged speakers with aphasia (who were sub-divided into five aphasic groups: Broca's, transcortical motor, conduction, Wernicke's, and anomic aphasia) were scored and analyzed. For each of the language deviations identified, it was scored as one of the following error types:

1. Literal paraphasias: Include (a) phonemic paraphasias, such as phoneme omissions, additions, displacements, and substitutions; and (b) articulatory paraphasias, which were usually perceived to be phonemic paraphasias.
2. Verbal paraphasias: Can be phonologically (i.e., formal paraphasias), morphologically, or semantically (e.g., words in the same semantic field, antonyms, superordinate, or proximity) related to the target. Unrelated verbal paraphasias are also included in this category.

3. Syntagmatic paraphasias.
4. Circumlocutions: Include description of an object (e.g., "a kind of food that is white or soft" for "bread") or an instrumental function (e.g., "it is for knowing the time" for "clock" or "watch").
5. Indefinite anaphors.
6. Neologisms.

Results on the classification of paraphasias based on the five aphasic groups suggested distinctive and syndrome-specific error patterns. For example, the Broca's group was characterized by a majority of literal paraphasias secondary to the speakers' phoneme omissions and substitutions. The conduction group had predominantly literal paraphasias in the output but the proportion of verbal semantic paraphasias was also high. Anomic speakers, on the other hand, only committed semantic verbal paraphasias in general. A mix of syntagmatic and formal verbal parpahasias were found in the transcortical motor group but some of the participants in this group did not commit any errors at all. The performance of Wernicke's speakers was the poorest among the five aphasia syndromes and contained massive errors of literal paraphasias and neologisms in addition to verbal and semantic paraphasias. The authors also applied the same error classification system to analyze these speakers' performance on the BDAE repetition and naming subtests. It was concluded that profiles of different of language impairment were similarly present among the five aphasic groups.

Word-Finding Behavior (WFB) With Reference to T-Units

Hunt (1964, 1965) developed a minimal **terminable unit (T-unit)** analysis, which has been used extensively to measure the overall syntactic complexity and degree of preserved grammatical correctness in both spoken and written samples of language. A T-unit of language was defined as a main (independent) clause plus all subordinate clauses and non-clausal structures (i.e., dependent modifiers of the main clause) that are attached to or embedded in it. It is the smallest word group that could be considered as a grammatical sentence, regardless of how it was punctuated. In the 1970s, analyses using T-units became an important measurement in sentence-combining research. The original design of this method was geared toward the examination of grammatical structures in written text by school-age children. According to Hunt (1964), given that the length of a T-unit paralleled the cognitive development in a child, T-unit analysis could act as a stable indicator of language development.

The use of T-units was standardized in the Test of Word Finding in Discourse (TWFD; German, 1991) which was proposed in the early 1990s for quantifying language samples by children. Specific guidelines on test administration (such as consideration of using standard picture stimuli for sample elicitation), scoring procedures, and result interpretation were proposed. The TWFD was applied for analyzing aphasic language of adults (Boyle, 2004, 2014). This was motivated by the lack of information in the aphasiology literature about the test-retest stability in word retrieval among speakers with aphasia, although session-to-session or day-to-day variability on informativeness and efficiency measures of aphasic connected speech has been well reported (e.g., Cameron et al., 2009; Nicholas & Brookshire, 1993). Since the TWFD was developed for children, the stimuli used in Set A in the study by Brookshire and Nicholas (1994) were utilized for eliciting the discourses. In addition, given that the original analytic system did not contain categories that were typically used to identify word-retrieval difficulty in aphasia (paraphasias or neologisms, to be specific), these two error classes were introduced in Boyle's studies. The first step of analysis involved counting of incidence of word-finding behavior (WFB), such as repetition, reformulation, empty/indefinite words, time fillers, and delays. Some other count measures modified for a more sensitive evaluation of acquired neurogenic disordered speech from adult speakers proposed by Boyle (2004) included the following:

1. Verbal paraphasia: A fluently produced phonemic substitution for a target, in a real word, with sound semblance to that target.
2. Phonemic paraphasia: A fluently produced non-word obviously related in sound to the target.
3. Initial sound: Partial production of the target or partial production of some attempt at the target, such as "wa" for "water" or "si" for "sister").
4. Comment: Statements made by a speaker about the task or the language process (e.g., "This is difficult" or "I can't think of the name").
5. Neologism: A non-word with no or only a remote (fewer than 50% of phonemes in common) relation to the target.

After calculating the total number of T-units and counting the number of different categories of word-finding difficulties, a global measure of word-finding impairment could be obtained by calculating the percentage of T-units that contained evidence of any type of word-finding behavior (%TWFB; German, 1991). Moreover, in order to compare different WFB categories of a speaker across sessions, the percentage of T-units containing each specific category of WFB can be calculated.

Pros and Cons of Content-Based Analyses

In summary, the systems mentioned in this section have an emphasis on the extraction of propositions (or errors) in an oral discourse and employ a rule-based approach to identify the key elements (or errors) contained in the output. The fact that an examiner does not need to pay specific attention to the linguistic integrity of a transcript makes this approach relatively easy for everyday clinical application. Relatively shorter time involved in the collection of discourse sample as well as straightforward and simple measure computation in data analysis also enhance the clinical feasibility over other systems mentioned in this chapter. Although most studies about discourse analysis have focused on reporting how individuals with chronic post-stroke aphasia demonstrate positive changes in discourse production, one should not neglect the improvements expected to be seen in some acute patients. For example, Brisebois et al. (2020) have recently applied measures on thematic informativeness to reflect improvements in picture description of 15 (out of 23) individuals with acute post-stroke aphasia (2 to 10 days post-onset). Apart from enhanced discourse content over time, the efficiency of thematic informativeness also improved. On the other hand, these content-based analyses may be limited in informing us about the direction of management because they do not inform clinicians on the specific micro- or macro-linguistic structure of the analyzed discourse. Practitioners may in some cases need to conduct additional evaluations when planning specific goals of discourse rehabilitation.

Conversation Analysis

Everyday talks involve the exchange of ideas and information between a speaker and his or her communication partner(s). Procedures in sampling and quantifying a conversational dyad are oriented toward the functional aspects of social interaction at the descriptive level of analysis. However, what makes clinical conversation analysis stand out from other formal clinical assessments is its dynamic interactions involving exchange of new (and old) information and management of turn taking. It also allows one to study how speakers with aphasia perform outside a contextualized testing environment, which tends to be more natural and interactive, and allows clinicians to determine a patient's language skills from a different perspective. Furthermore, how aphasia leads to difficulties with the unique features of conversation can be examined. Finally, how communication partners may enhance (or in some cases inhibit) the flow of a conversation can be evaluated. Below are a few well-known protocols for analyzing conversation.

Conversation Analysis Profile for People with Aphasia (CAPPA)

Several investigations on the measurement of conversational abilities among speakers with aphasia and the interactions between these individuals and their conversational partners have been reported (e.g., Boles, 1997; Boles & Bombard, 1998; Coelho et al., 1991; Coelho et al., 2002; Simmons-Mackie & Damico, 1996; Whitworth et al., 1997; Youse & Coelho, 2006). According to

Damico et al. (1999), conversation analyses reported between the 1960s and 1980s originally acted as a qualitative tool for describing social interactions among people of various nationalities. It was not until the early 1990s that this analytic framework was applied in clinical aphasiology for evaluation of the impact of aphasia on everyday conversations, as well as for determination of target interventions to be conducted in this group of speakers. A system of conversation analysis for aphasia was, therefore, proposed based on modifications from former studies in the 1960s. The system could focus on quantifying the communication abilities, social interactions, and pragmatics of individuals with aphasia during naturalistic verbal interactions, all of which were mainly achieved by:

1. counting the turn completions between individuals with aphasia and their conversational partner(s)
2. determining the successful and unsuccessful strategies demonstrated by individuals with aphasia
3. analyzing the manner of feedback given by partner(s)
4. determining the characteristics of feedback from partner(s) that could facilitate the overall conversations by individuals with aphasia.

For example, Whitworth et al. (1997) presented a Conversation Analysis Profile for People with Aphasia (CAPPA) using 26 questions to quantify aphasic speakers' initiation of conversations and turn taking (e.g., failure or delay in response), topic management (e.g., maintaining conversation topics), repair strategies (e.g., ability to repair errors with or without help from partners), and linguistic impairments (e.g., failure of word retrieval or production of jargons and paraphasias). Table 3.5 contains more detailed information on the conversational areas addressed in the CAPPA and their implications for clinical analysis of aphasia.

Boles (1997) presented a Conversational Discourse Analysis (CDA) to monitor the communication progress of four individuals with aphasia. The CDA contains variables that measured the quantity of verbal output (e.g., the total number of words per utterances and utterances per conversation) as well as communicative strategies demonstrated by speakers (e.g., self-repairs and requests for clarifications). According to Boles, conversation repair was defined as "an attempt to modify one's own or the other person's utterance for the purpose of clarification" (p.45). Understanding the use of repair strategies by speakers with impaired conversation skills could help clinicians modify therapeutic goals and objectives for training conversational dyads. Different categories of repair strategies suggested by Boles (1997) include the following:

1. Self-clarification: This includes self-correction, repetition of oneself, rephrasing oneself or paraphrasing oneself.

Table 3.5 Areas addressed in the Conversation Analysis Profile for People with Aphasia (CAPPA) and their clinical implications

Areas addressed	Clinical implications
Section 1: Linguistic abilities	
Failure in word retrieval	To inform the degree of struggle and give up during word finding
Production of circumlocutions	To inform the ability to use short and efficient output to get a message across
Production of uncorrected semantic paraphasias	To inform the use of wrong words or names for something without correcting
Production of phonemic paraphasias	To inform the degree of phonemic errors for a target
Production of apraxic errors	To inform the degree of struggle to get the sounds out in a word
Overuse of pronouns and proforms	To inform the degree of word-finding difficulty
Difficulty indicating yes and no reliably	To determine the functional use of affirmation and negation
Production of agrammatic speech	To determine the degree of agrammatism and dysfluency
Production of neologisms	To inform the degree of error in output
Production of jargon	To inform the degree of error in output
Failure in comprehension	To inform the degree of difficulties in understanding a conversational partner
Section 2: Repair	
Ability to initiate repair on conversational partner's turn	To determine the ability to indicate difficulty in following a conversation
Ability to initiate repairs on own errors	To estimate how well one can pick up a mistake in conversation and try to self-correct it
Ability to repair own errors after self-initiation without help	To determine the degree of self-awareness of own mistakes in conversation and ability to correct them without assistance
Ability to repair own turn when initiated by conversational partner	To determine ability to correct own mistakes in conversation upon assistance
Section 3: Initiation and turn taking	
Ability to initiate conversations	To determine the appropriateness of pragmatics
Failure to respond when selected as next speaker	To inform the sensitivity to turn sequences
Delay in responding when selected as next speaker	To determine the efficiency of verbal output and sensitivity to turn sequences
Production of long pauses in the middle of turns	To determine the efficiency of conversation

Table 3.5 Cont.

Areas addressed	Clinical implications
Violation of conversational partner's turns	To determine the appropriateness of pragmatics and to inform the sensitivity to turn sequences
Failure to hand over conversational floor	To determine the appropriateness of pragmatics and to inform the sensitivity to turn sequence
Reliance on minimal acknowledgements	To determine the ability to use external cues for verbal output
Section 4: Topic management	
Ability to initiate new topics	To inform the ability to provide new information with appropriate timing of conversation
Failure to orient conversational partner to new topics	To determine the sensitivity to a conversational partner's perspective
Ability to maintain topics	To determine the ability to stay on a topic
Repeated initiations of "favorite" topics	To determine the ability to initiate and provide self-related information

Source: Modified from Whitworth et al. (1997)

2. Other-repair using a cue: This involves a speaker being aware of the target utterance of the communication partner and his or her own attempts to induce that target. A "hint" is usually given to facilitate the repair process.
3. Other-repair using a model: This involves a speaker's simple use of a target utterance to communicate with the partner. This strategy is often used following the provision of a cue.
4. Other-repair using reflection: This involves a speaker's rephrasing or paraphrasing of what the communication partner has said. This strategy may be used specifically to induce a known target and/or simply as a kind of "bookmark" to keep the conversation flowing.
5. Other-repair by requesting for a clarification: This involves a speaker's request for a repetition or rephrasing from the communication partner when he or she has difficulties understanding the communication partner.
6. Other-repair using an undifferentiated request for clarification: This involves a speaker's request for a clarification from the communication partner using undifferentiated questions, such as "what?" or "huh?"

It was concluded that CDA could reveal useful pragmatic information that was less available or unavailable from other methods of discourse analyses, such as the ability to engage in social interaction. This system would also

inform clinicians how ready a patient is for receiving therapeutic intervention on conversation and if a conversation partner therapy is appropriate.
A follow-up study by Boles and Bombard (1998) concluded that a conversation sample of five to ten minutes was adequate for studying the conversation repair, speaking rate, and utterance length among individuals with
aphasia.

Conversational Appropriateness (CA)

To address the impaired communication skills among individuals with
closed head injuries during conversational exchange, Youse et al. (2011)
reported a comparison study to evaluate the application of two paradigms of
conversational discourse analyses and their effectiveness on reflecting these
speakers' conversational discourse deficits. They included the Conversational
Appropriateness (CA; Blank & Franklin, 1980; Coelho et al., 2002;
Coelho et al., 2005; Coelho et al., 2003) and a Modified Conversational
Appropriateness (Modified CA) paradigm. The analytic procedures in both
paradigms involved the evaluation of how appropriate a speaker is when
participating in a conversation. There are two distinct categories in the CA
to describe the interactions between the speaker (i.e., Speaker Initiation)
and the communication partner (i.e., Speaker Response) by defining each
person's contribution to the turn of speaking. Each conversational utterance
can be classified using five CA measures as follows:

1. Speaker Initiation:
   1a) Oblige: an utterance that contains an explicit and clear demand for
   a response.
   1b) Comment: an utterance that does not contain a demand for a
   response from the conversational partner.
2. Speaker Response:
   2a) Adequate response: a response that meets the initiator's verbalization. A response in a single word can also be acceptable here.
   2b) Adequate Plus response: a response that meets the initiator's verbalization and, at the same time, provides additional relevant information that has not been requested.
   2c) Inadequate response: a response that is inadequate, tangential, irrelevant, or insufficient (incomplete) and does not meet the initiator's
   verbalization.

The modified CA proposed by Youse et al. (2011) involved the expansion of
measures for both the categories of Speaker Initiation and Speaker Response.
With the assumption that this modified paradigm could better capture and
provide additional information about the nuances that have been known to

affect conversational performance in individuals with closed head injuries, the additional measures included the following:

1. Speaker Initiation:
   1c) Understanding: an utterance demonstrating that the communication partner is following along or understands what has been said. This may include non-linguistic (e.g., "okay," "uh huh," or "mmhmm") production.
   1d) Clarification: an utterance that demonstrates a need for repetition or clarification of information.
2. Speaker Response:
   2d) Adequate Minimum response: used when a single word response is not considered completely adequate (as in 2a). The response is usually an utterance that answers the initiator's verbalization but is limited to a single word.
   2e) No response: no response is provided following the initiator's verbalization.
   2f) Partially Unintelligible response: an utterance that contains some unintelligible information. However, enough information is still available such that the utterance can clearly be categorized.
   2g) Completely Unintelligible response: an utterance that is totally unintelligible and cannot be categorized.
   2h) Delayed response: an utterance that answers or addresses the initiator's verbalization but is delayed by at least four seconds. This kind of response is usually perceived as pragmatically awkward.

A set of conversation samples from one individual with closed head injury containing eight 10-minute verbal interactions, elicited over a period of three weeks of language treatment, was analyzed using both the CA and Modified CA. The results revealed that the modified scheme was more representational of the speaker's conversation deficits. The authors concluded that this scheme could provide therapists with additional details to be utilized when assessing and designing therapy goals for the clinical population of traumatic brain injury.

Pros and Cons of Conversation-Based Analyses

One critical advantage of applying conversation analysis to disordered oral output is that this framework provides clinicians with a good amount of information regarding how interaction works at the level of daily face-to-face interaction. The complex social actions involved in a conversation, such as how and when these social actions are used to convey messages, can also be clearly quantified. This will in turn lead to better planning of remediation for improvement of daily communication among those in need because the clinician can assess a speaker's use of oral discourse from a functional perspective. In other words, the results drawn from the above-mentioned conversation analyses allow clinicians to understand how social-pragmatic skills and conversational partners affect the face-to-face conversational ability among speakers with aphasia or related neurogenic communication disorders. They can also provide useful indications for setting intervention goals by reinforcing the existing strategies successfully used by these speakers, before introducing new strategies to improve communication among speakers with language impairments (and supporting strategies for their significant others, if needed).

However, the limitations of this approach include the difficulty in controlling conversation topics, content, and/or interaction contexts across (as well as within) examinees. The amount of oral content elicited through various topics may vary greatly, especially if we factor in the effect of personal interest or relevancy of a given topic to a speaker. Furthermore, the feedback from different conversational partners involved in a natural verbal interaction is a variable that one cannot easily control.

Conclusions

A number of clinically feasible approaches to discourse analyses were presented in this chapter, with discussion of their methodologies, strengths, and limitations. Clinical practitioners, especially speech-and-language pathologists, should carefully select one or more of these methods to assist their clinical work based on considerations such as the underlying rationale of conducting a discourse evaluation or the significant clinical symptoms demonstrated by a patient to be assessed. One may notice that the majority of research findings and implications presented in this chapter were based on investigations using the Cookie Theft picture. Readers may see this as an advantage because conclusions drawn from these studies can be readily compared. At the same time, one should not be limited to this single classic picture stimulus when it comes to eliciting discourse samples, primarily because the principles of most of the analytic frameworks discussed here can be generalized to other types of discourse genres (i.e., discourse tasks). Of course, consistency in applying the procedures of analyses is another important factor that requires attention by clinicians. More detailed information regarding research-oriented discourse analytic systems can be found in Chapter 4.

Due to the heterogeneous nature of measures and analytic methods reported in the literature of aphasic spoken discourse, a recent working group (Stark et al., 2021) has created recommendations for field-wide standards in methods, analysis, and reporting of spoken discourse outcomes. In the past decade, there was also a rapid and healthy growth of studies that have reported specific micro- (e.g., Fromm et al., 2017; Pritchard et al., 2018) and macro-linguistic (e.g., Greenslade et al., 2020; Hazamy & Obermeyer, 2020; Leaman & Edmonds, 2021) features of disordered discourse production. Readers are encouraged to refer to these updated investigations for additional insights into clinical application of discourse analysis.

References

American Speech-Language-Hearing Association. (2002). *National Outcomes Measurement System (NOMS): Adults Speech-Language Pathology User's Guide*. www. asha.org/NOMS

American Speech-Language-Hearing Association. (2013). *National Outcomes Measurement System (NOMS): Adults Speech-Language Pathology User's Guide*. www. asha.org/NOMS

Ardila, A., & Rosselli, M. (1993). Language deviations in aphasia: A frequency analysis. *Brain and Language, 44*, 165–180.

Blank, M., & Franklin, E. (1980). Dialogue with preschoolers: A cognitively-based system of assessment. *Applied Psycholinguistics, 1*, 127–150.

Boles, L. (1997). Conversational analysis as a dependent measure in communication therapy with four individuals with aphasia. *Asia Pacific Journal of Speech, Language and Hearing, 2*, 43–61.

Boles, L., & Bombard, T. (1998). Conversational discourse analysis: Appropriate and useful sample sizes. *Aphasiology, 12(7/8)*, 547–560.

Boyle, M. (2004). Semantic feature analysis treatment for anomia in two fluent aphasia syndromes. *American Journal of Speech Language Pathology, 13*, 236–249.

Boyle, M. (2014). Test-retest stability of word retrieval in aphasic discourse. *Journal of Speech, Language, and Hearing Research, 57*, 966–978.

Brisebois, A., Brambati, S. M., Désilets-Barnabé, M., Boucher, J., García, A. O., Rochon, E., Leonard, C., Desautels, A., & Marcotte, K. (2020). The importance of thematic informativeness in narrative discourse recovery in acute post-stroke aphasia. *Aphasiology, 34*(4), 472–491.

Brookshire, R. H., & Nicholas, L. E. (1994). Test-retest stability of measures of connected speech in aphasia. *Clinical Aphasiology, 22*, 119–133.

Bryant, L., Ferguson, A., & Spencer, E. (2016). Linguistic analysis of discourse in aphasia: A review of the literature. *Clinical Linguistics & Phonetics, 30*(7), 489–518.

Cameron, R., Wambaugh, J., & Mauszycki, S. (2009, May 26–30). *Quantifying the informativeness and efficiency of connected speech: An analysis of individual variability over time* [Poster presentation]. Thirty-ninth annual Clinical Aphasiology Conference, Keystone, CO, United States.

Capilouto, G. J., Wright, H. H., & Maddy, K. M. (2016). Microlinguistic processes that contribute to the ability to relay main events: influence of age. *Neuropsychology, Development, and Cognition. Section B, Aging, Neuropsychology and Cognition, 23*(4), 445–463.

Capilouto, G. J., Wright, H. H., & Wagovich, S. A. (2005). CIU and main event analyses of the structured discourse of older and younger adults. *Journal of Communication Disorders, 38*(6), 431–444.

Capilouto, G. J., Wright, H. H., & Wagovich, S. A. (2006). Reliability of main event measurement in the discourse of individuals with aphasia. *Aphasiology, 20*(2–4), 205–216.

Coelho, C. A., Liles, B. Z., & Dufft, R. J. (1991). Analysis of conversational discourse in head-injured adults. *Journal of Head Trauma Rehabilitation, 6,* 92–99.

Coelho, C., Ylvisaker, M., & Turkstra, L. S. (2005). Nonstandardized assessment approaches for individuals with traumatic brain injuries. *Seminars in Speech and Language, 26*(4), 223–241.

Coelho, C. A., Youse, K. M., & Le, K. N. (2002). Conversational discourse in closed-head-injured and non-brain-injured adults. *Aphasiology, 16,* 659–672.

Coelho, C. A., Youse, K. M., Le, K. N., & Feinn, R. (2003). Narrative and conversational discourse of adults with closed-head-injuries and non-brain-injured adults: A discriminant analysis. *Aphasiology, 17,* 499–510.

Craig, H. K., Hinckley, J. J., Winkelseth, M., Carry, L., Walley, J., Bardach, L., Higman, B., Hilfinger, P., Schall, C., & Sheimo, D. (1993). Quantifying connected speech samples of adults with chronic aphasia. *Aphasiology, 7*(2), 155–163.

Criel, Y., Deleu, M., De Groote, E., Bockstael, A., Kong, A. P. H., De Letter, M. (2021). The Dutch Main Concept Analysis: Translation and establishment of normative data. *American Journal of Speech-Language Pathology, 30*(4), 1750–1766. https://doi.org/10.1044/2021_AJSLP-20-00285

Dalton, S. G. H., Hubbard, H. I., & Richardson, J. D. (2020). Moving toward non-transcription based discourse analysis in stable and progressive aphasia. *Seminars in Speech and Language, 41*(1), 32–44.

Dalton, S. G., & Richardson, J. D. (2015). Core-lexicon and main-concept production during picture-sequence description in adults without brain damage and adults with aphasia. *American Journal of Speech-Language Pathology, 39,* 1125–1137.

Dalton, S. G. H., & Richardson, J. D. (2019). A large-scale comparison of main concept production between persons with aphasia and persons without brain injury. *American Journal of Speech-Language Pathology, 28*(1S), 293–320.

Damico, J. S., Oelschlaeger, M., & Simmons-Mackie, N. (1999). Qualitative methods in aphasia research: Conversation analysis. *Aphasiology, 13,* 667–679.

Deng, B, Lin, F., Lai, Q., Chen, Z., Zhou, L., & Jiang, Z. (2021). Applying Main Concept Analysis to discourse assessment in aphasia: Research on anomic aphasia based on normal controls. *Chinese Journal of Rehabilitation Medicine, 36*(4), 418–425.

Enderby, P., Wood, V., & Wade, D. (1987). *Frenchay aphasia screening test.* Windsor: NFER-NELSON Publishing Company Ltd.

Fromm, D., Forbes, M., Holland, A., Dalton, S. G., Richardson, J., & MacWhinney, B. (2017). Discourse characteristics in aphasia beyond the Western Aphasia Battery cutoff. *American Journal of Speech-Language Pathology, 26*(3), 762–768.

Gao, G., Kong, A., & Lau, K. (2016, Oct 16–18). *Production of main concepts by Mandarin-speakers with traumatic brain injury in China: A pilot study* [Poster presentation]. 54th Annual Academy of Aphasia Meeting, Llandudno, United Kingdom. http://doi.org/10.3389/conf.fpsyg.2016.68.00005

Gao, S. R. & Benson, D. F. (1990). Aphasia after stroke in native Chinese speakers. *Aphasiology, 4*(1), 31–43.

German, D. J. (1991). *Test of Word Finding in Discourse (TWFD): Administration, scoring, interpretation, and technical manual.* Austin, TX: Pro-Ed.

Goodglass, H., & Kaplan, E. (1983). *The assessment of aphasia and related disorders.* Philadelphia, PA: Lea & Febiger.

Greenslade, K. J., Stuart, J., Richardson, J. D., Dalton, S. G., & Ramage, A. E. (2020). Macrostructural analyses of Cinderella narratives in a large nonclinical sample. *American Journal of Speech-Language Pathology, 29*(4), 1923–1936.

Hameister, I., & Nickels, L. (2018). The cat in the tree – using picture descriptions to inform our understanding of conceptualisation in aphasia. *Language, Cognition and Neuroscience, 33*(10), 1296–1314.

Hazamy, A. A., & Obermeyer, J. (2020). Evaluating informative content and global coherence in fluent and non-fluent aphasia. *International Journal of Language & Communication Disorders, 55*(1), 110–120.

Hilger, A., Ramsberger, G., Gilley, P., Menn, L., & Kong, A. P. H. (2014). Analysing speech problems in a longitudinal case study of logopenic variant PPA. *Aphasiology, 28*(7), 840–861.

Hunt, K. (1964). *Differences in grammatical structures written at three grade levels, the structures to be analyzed by transformational methods: Report to the U. S. Office of Education, Cooperative Research Project.* Tallahassee, FL: National Council of Teachers of English (NCTE).

Hunt, K. (1965). *Grammatical structures written at three grade levels.* Champaign, IL: National Council of Teachers of English (NCTE).

Kavé, G., & Goral, M. (2017). Do age-related word retrieval difficulties appear (or disappear) in connected speech? *Aging, Neuropsychology and Cognition, 24*(5), 508–527.

Kertesz A. (2006) *Western Aphasia Battery-Revised.* San Antonio, TX: Harcourt Assessment, Inc.

Kim, H., Kintz, S., & Wright, H. H. (2021). Development of a measure of function word use in narrative discourse: Core lexicon analysis in aphasia. *International Journal of Language & Communication Disorders, 56*(1), 6–19.

Kim, H., & Wright, H. H. (2020). A tutorial on core lexicon: Development, use, and application. *Seminars in Speech and Language, 41*(10), 20–31.

Kong, A. P. H. (2009). The use of Main Concept Analysis to measure discourse production in Cantonese-speaking persons with aphasia: A preliminary report. *Journal of Communication Disorders, 42,* 442–464.

Kong, A. P. H. (2011). The Main Concept Analysis in Cantonese aphasic oral discourse: External validation and monitoring chronic aphasia. *Journal of Speech, Language, and Hearing Research, 54,* 148–159.

Kong, A. P. H. (2016). *The Main Concept Analysis (MCA) for oral discourse production.* Hong Kong: The Commercial Press (H.K.) Limited.

Kong, A. P. H. (2018). Main Concept Analysis (MCA) for acquired deficits of spoken narratives: Preliminary data on inter-rater agreement and potential application to the Korean-speaking population. *Clinical Archives of Communication Disorders, 3*(1), 14–21.

Kong, A. P. H. (2021). Dialectally-sensitive norms of the Spanish version of Main Concept Analysis (Span-MCA) for quantifying neurogenically impaired spoken discourse. *Revista de Investigación en Logopedia, 11*(2), e69932, 1–13.

Kong, A. P. H., & Law, S. P. (2004). A Cantonese linguistic communication measure for evaluating aphasic narrative production: normative and preliminary aphasic data. *Journal of Multilingual Communication Disorders, 2*(2), 124–146.

Kong, A. P. H., & Law, S. P. (2009a). Cantonese Linguistic Communication Measure (CLCM): A clinical tool for assessing aphasic narrative production. In S.P. Law, B.

Weekes, & A. Wong (Eds.), *Disorders of Speech and Language in Chinese* (pp. 255–272). Clevedon, UK: Multilingual Matters.

Kong, A. P. H., & Law, S. P. (2009b). A linguistic communication measure for monitoring changes in Chinese aphasic narrative production. *Clinical Linguistics and Phonetics, 23*(4), 255–269.

Kong, A. P. H., Ross, A., & Pettigrew, C. (2012). A Main-Concept Analysis for aphasic discourse in Irish-English speakers: Adaptation and preliminary report. *Journal of Clinical Speech and Language Studies, 19*, 19–43.

Kong, A. P. H., Whiteside, J., & Bargmann, P. (2016). The Main Concept Analysis: Validation and sensitivity in differentiating discourse produced by unimpaired English speakers from individuals with aphasia and dementia of Alzheimer type. *Logopedics Phoniatrics Vocology, 41*(3), 129–141.

Kong, A. P. H. & Wong, C. W.-Y. (2018). An integrative analysis of spontaneous storytelling discourse in aphasia: Relationship with listeners' rating and prediction of severity and fluency status of aphasia. *American Journal of Speech-Language Pathology, 27*, 1491–1505.

Kong, A. P. H. & Yeh, C. C. (2015). A Taiwanese Mandarin Main Concept Analysis (TM-MCA) for quantification of aphasic oral discourse. *International Journal of Language & Communication Disorders, 50*(5), 580–592.

Kong, A. P. H. & Yeh, C. C. (2019). A preliminary study of Mandarin Linguistic Communication Measure for the local population in Taiwan (TM-LCM): Clinical evaluation and linguistically-based quantification of aphasic oral discourse. *Journal of the Speech-Language-Hearing Association of Taiwan, 40*(2), 17–54.

Leaman, M. C., & Edmonds, L. A. (2021). Measuring global coherence in people with aphasia during unstructured conversation. *American Journal of Speech-Language Pathology, 30*(1S), 359–375.

MacWhinney, B., Fromm, D., Forbes, M., & Holland, A. (2011). AphasiaBank: Methods for studying discourse. *Aphasiology, 25*, 1286–1307.

MacWhinney, B., Fromm, D., Holland, A., Forbes, M., & Wright, H. (2010). Automated analysis of the Cinderella story. *Aphasiology, 24*, 856–868.

Mayer, J. F. & Murray, L. L. (2003). Functional measures of naming in aphasia: Word retrieval in confrontation naming versus connected speech. *Aphasiology, 17*, 481–497.

Menn, L., Ramsberger, G., & Helm-Estabrooks, N. (1994). A linguistic communication measure for aphasic narratives. *Aphasiology, 8*(4), 343–359.

Murray, L. L., & Chapey, R. (2001). Assessment of language disorders in adults. In R. Chapey (Ed.), *Language intervention strategies in aphasia and related neurogenic communication disorders* (pp. 55–126). Philadelphia: Lippincott Williams & Wilkins.

Nicholas, L. E., & Brookshire, R. H. (1993). A system for quantifying the informativeness and efficiency of the connected speech of adults with aphasia. *Journal of Speech and Hearing Research, 36*, 338–350.

Nicholas, L. E., & Brookshire, R. H. (1995). Presence, completeness, and accuracy of main concepts in the connected speech of non-brain-damaged adults and adults with aphasia. *Journal of Speech and Hearing Research, 38*, 145–156.

Pritchard, M., Hilari, K., Cocks, N., & Dipper, L. (2018). Psychometric properties of discourse measures in aphasia: Acceptability, reliability, and validity. *International Journal of Language & Communication Disorders, 53*(6), 1078–1093.

Richardson J. D., & Dalton S. G. (2016). Main concepts for three different discourse tasks in a large non-clinical sample. *Aphasiology*, 30(1), 45–73.

Richardson J. D., & Dalton S. G. (2020). Main concepts for two picture description tasks: An addition to Richardson & Dalton, 2016. *Aphasiology*, 34(1), 119–136.

Richardson, J. D., Dalton, S. G., Greenslade, K. J., Jacks, A., Haley, K. L., & Adams, J. (2021). Main concept, sequencing, and story grammar analyses of Cinderella narratives in a large sample of persons with aphasia. *Brain Sciences*, 11(1), 110.

Rivera, A., Hirst, J., & Edmonds, L. A. (2018). Evaluation of language predictors of main concept production in Spanish/English bilingual discourse using Nicholas and Brookshire stimuli. *American Journal of Speech-Language Pathology*, 27(1), 52–70.

Rochon, E., Saffran, E. M., Berndt, R. S., & Schwartz, M. F. (2000). Quantitative analysis of aphasic sentence production: Further development and new data. *Brain and Language*, 72, 193–218.

Saffran, E. M., Berndt, R. S., & Schwartz, M. F. (1989). The quantitative analysis of agrammatic production: Procedure and data. *Brain and Language*, 37, 440–479.

Schuell, H. (1965). *Minnesota Test for Differential Diagnosis of Aphasia*. Minneapolis, MN: University of Minnesota Press.

Shewan, C. M. (1988a). The Shewan Spontaneous Language Analysis (SSLA) system for aphasic adults: Description, reliability and validity. *Journal of Communication Disorder*, 21, 103–138.

Shewan, C. M. (1988b). Expressive language recovery in aphasia using the Shewan Spontaneous Language Analysis (SSLA) system. *Journal of Communication Disorder*, 21, 155–169.

Shewan, C. M., & Kertesz, A, (1980). Reliability and validity characteristics of the Western Aphasia Battery (WAB). *Journal of Speech and Hearing Disorders*, 45, 308–324.

Simmons-Mackie, N. N., & Damico, J. S. (1996). The contribution of discourse markers to communicative competence in aphasia. *American Journal of Speech-Language Pathology*, 5, 37–43.

Spreen, O., & Risser, A. H. (2003). *Assessment of aphasia*. Oxford: Oxford University Press.

Stark, B. C., Dutta, M., Murray, L. L., Bryant, L., Fromm, D., MacWhinney, B., Ramage, A. E., Roberts, A., den Ouden, D. B., Brock, K., McKinney-Bock, K., Paek, E. J., Harmon, T. G., Yoon, S. O., Themistocleous, C., Yoo, H., Aveni, K., Gutierrez, S., & Sharma, S. (2021). Standardizing assessment of spoken discourse in aphasia: A working group with deliverables. *American Journal of Speech-Language Pathology*, 30(1S), 491–502.

Van Dijk, T. A. (1980). *Macrostructures*. Hillsdale, NJ: Lawrence Erlbaum.

West, J., Sands, E., & Ross-Swain, D. (1998). *Bedside evaluation screening test (BEST-2)*. Austin, TX: Pro-ed.

Whitworth, A., Perkins, L., & Lesser, R. (1997). *Conversation analysis profile for people with aphasia*. London: Whurr Publishers Ltd.

Wright, H. H., & Capilouto, G. J. (2009). Manipulating task instructions to change narrative discourse performance. *Aphasiology*, 23, 1295–1308.

Yazu, H., Kong, A. P. H., Yoshihata, H., & Okubo, K. (2021). Adaptation and validation of the Main Concept Analysis of spoken discourse by native Japanese adults.

Clinical Linguistics & Phonetics. ePub ahead May 14. https://doi.org/10.1080/02699206.2021.1915385

Yeh, C. & Kong, A. P. H. (2014, October 5–7). *Development of the Taiwanese Mandarin Main Concept Analysis (TM-MCA): Normative and preliminary aphasic data* [Poster presentation]. Fifty-second annual meeting of Academy of Aphasia, Miami, FL, USA. doi: 10.3389/conf.fpsyg.2014.64.00003

Yorkston, K. M., & Beukelman, D. R. (1980). An analysis of connected speech samples of aphasic and normal speakers. *Journal of Speech and Hearing Disorders, 45,* 27–36.

Youse, K., & Coelho, C. (2006, May 29–June 2). *Treatment of conversational discourse following closed-head injury* [Paper presentation]. Thirty-sixth annual Clinical Aphasiology Conference, Ghent, Belgium.

Youse, K. M., Gathof, M., Fields, D. D. Lobianco, T. F., Bush, H. M. & Noffsinger, J. T. (2011). Conversational discourse analysis procedures: A comparison of two paradigms, *Aphasiology, 25*(1), 106–118.

Appendix 3.1

Main Concept Analysis — Scoring Form

Patient name: _____
Date of birth/Age: _____
Gender: M / F
Onset of aphasia: _____
Etiology: _____

Speech therapist: _____
Date of MCA testing: _____
Date of WAB testing: _____
WAB AQ: _____
Aphasia type: _____

Remarks:

Complete language sample:

Time = [   ] min [   ] sec = [   ] minute

	AC	AI	IN	AB

1   Target main concept: _____
| | | | | |

2   Target main concept: _____
| | | | | |

3   Target main concept: _____
| | | | | |

4   Target main concept: _____
| | | | | |

5   Target main concept: _____
| | | | | |

6   Target main concept: _____
| | | | | |

7   Target main concept: _____
| | | | | |

8   Target main concept: _____
| | | | | |

		AC	AI	IN	AB
9	Target main concept: _____				
10	Target main concept: _____				
11	Target main concept: _____				
12	Target main concept: _____				
13	Target main concept: _____				
14	Target main concept: _____				
15	Target main concept: _____				

	AC	AI	IN	AB
Index 1, 2, 3, 4 –				
Index 5 – Main concept score (MC) = (3×**AC** + 2×**AI** + 1×**IN**)				
Index 6 – AC per minute =				

Chapter 4

Research-Oriented Frameworks for Narrative Analysis

Chapter Objectives

The reader will be able to:

1. explain the significance of research-oriented analytic systems for disordered discourse
2. compare and contrast the general principles of various measurements on lexical diversity of discourse samples
3. describe the procedures of eliciting discourse samples, extracting propositional speech, segmenting extracted samples into utterances, and evaluating performances on the lexical content and sentence structure of a narrative sample, as described in the Quantitative Production Analysis (QPA)
4. describe the procedures of quantifying sentential characteristics in a discourse
5. describe the components of discourse grammar and how they are quantified
6. describe the procedures of estimating the degree of discourse cohesion and coherence of an oral discourse
7. describe the principles and procedures of natural language processing (NLP).

Introduction

Systematic analyses and sophisticated quantification of disordered language samples, together with careful comparison with the performance of healthy controls, allow researchers to capture the essential clinical characteristics of speakers with acquired language impairments at the discourse level. Not only can the results inform scientists of important information for the testing and proposal of language models or processing theories of narrative production, but also provide users with suitable guidelines to facilitate clinical applications on the evaluation of discourse deficits, such as those commonly

DOI: 10.4324/9781003254775-4

exhibited by speakers with aphasia. A few approaches of research-oriented narrative analyses will be discussed in this chapter. These systems were mainly developed in a research context to enable an examiner to objectively and systematically quantify oral narratives, and to better understand the linguistic characteristics beyond the sentential level among individuals with impaired spoken output.

Recent emergence of new tools for discourse measurement from the field of computational linguistics has facilitated the research of narratives by speakers with neurogenic language disorders. As most of these research-oriented systems generally involve complex data collection and analytic procedures, as well as extensive amount of time for data transcription and analyses by linguistically trained researchers, they are less likely to be widely used for the purpose of daily clinical evaluations. However, with a good understanding of these methodologies and theories behind the computation principles, one can easily appreciate their value for adoption in everyday clinical assessment and planning of remediation directions. Use of a sub-group of these evidence-based measures can also enhance daily clinical practice involving discourse analyses. Three major classic frameworks of discourse performance with a focus on various levels of language production, i.e., from the use of lexical items within a discourse, to the range of using different utterance types as well as the corresponding sentential and grammatical characteristics of output, and finally to the overall coherence of a text, are discussed here. This is followed by a summary of a recent report on natural language processing (NLP) and its application to discourse analysis.

Measurement of Lexical Diversity

The high prevalence of word-finding difficulties among speakers with aphasia and related neurogenic communication disorders has motivated the investigation of measurement of lexical diversity in oral discourse. Fergadiotis and Wright (2011) defined lexical diversity as "the range of vocabulary deployed in a text by a speaker that reflects his/her capacity to access and retrieve target words from a relatively intact knowledge base (i.e., lexicon) for the construction of higher linguistic units" (p. 1415). Various measures of lexical diversity, such as Type-Token Ratio (TTR), **Number of Different Words (NDW)**, or **voc-D**, have been applied to individuals with aphasia. A majority of these measures have been used to determine the impact of acquired language impairment on the overall lexical richness of narrative production. For example, Lind et al. (2009) found a lower degree of lexical variation of both nouns and verbs among speakers with aphasia, as compared to control speakers. Wright et al. (2003) were also able to demonstrate the discrepancy of lexical diversity between speakers with fluent and non-fluent aphasia. Furthermore, the change in lexical diversity has been used as a factor to indicate treatment efficacy of semantic feature analysis (SFA) (see

Chapter 7 for more details on this treatment paradigm) and its generalization to discourse production (Rider et al., 2008).

Researchers in computational linguistics who are interested in lexical diversity have, however, claimed that identifying a robust measure in this aspect has been challenging in the field (e.g., Malvern et al., 2004) and have proposed additional computation methods of lexical diversity, some of which have been applied in the field of speech–and–language pathology. In this section, a number of measures for quantification of lexical diversity in disordered discourse will be introduced.

Honoré's R statistic

Honoré's R statistic (Honoré, 1979) has been used to indicate lexical richness of a language output by highlighting the proportion of vocabulary that are used only once with reference to the total number of vocabularies in the text. It is calculated using the formula:

$$100 \times \frac{\text{Log} N}{1 - \dfrac{V1}{V}}$$

where N is the total number of words, V is the number of different words in the sample, and $V1$ is the number of words spoken only once in V. Lexical performance of 100 speakers with aphasia and their controls was analyzed using this measure (Holmes & Singh, 1996). The results showed that Honoré's R could successfully distinguish between the lexical performance of the normal and pathological groups. However, its application to other studies involving language impaired participants may be limited by the fact that it yields stable results only when a language sample contains 1300 words or more. Given that the text length collected from a picture description, story-telling, or conversation task (or even a combination of these tasks) is unlikely to reach the minimum word production requirement, Honoré's R may not be a suitable clinical measure.

Type-Token Ratio (TTR) and Number of Different Words (NDW)

Type-Token Ratio (TTR) is the ratio of unique lexical items in a transcript (i.e., the Number of Different Words, or NDW) to the total number of words. It is computed by dividing the NDW by the total word numbers of a language sample. Both the TTR and NDW are the most widely used and extensively reported measures to indicate the diversity of discoursal vocabulary in healthy adults as well as speakers with aphasia, although the

TTR has gained relatively more attention for its value for research and clinical applications. A description of how these two measures are calculated is described in Box 4.1.

Box 4.1 An Example of Type-Token Ration (TTR) and Number of Different Words (NDW) Calculation

The following is a transcript of a speaker with fluent aphasia in the sequential description task using the "Refused Umbrella" picture in the Aphasia Bank testing protocol (MacWhinney et al., 2011).

> this looks like um... is that a boy... um and this looks like his mom...
>
> and she's saying to her son... you better take the umbrella because it's going to rain... and of course he doesn't want her to... you know he doesn't want it... aww it's fine outside and you know it's ok... and she lets him get away with it (mumble)... [long pause]
>
> and then of course it's now raining and he's going... I wish I had it now... I'm wet... now what am I gonna do here I am in the buddles... mud... mud... what's that word... I can't answer that... whatever they're called... mud... mud holes... anyway so of course now he's drenched... now he has to go back home... to get the umbrella... mom is not happy about him because now he's wet...

After removing the mumble and fillers "um" and "aww" in the transcript, a simple count of the remaining words above yields a total of words 145. Note that contractions are counted as two words, i.e., the contraction "I'm" will be treated as two words, "I" and "am." The total number of words in a transcript is often referred to as the number of tokens. However, several of these tokens are repeated. The following table displays all the tokens in the above transcript, together with their frequency of occurrence:

Rank	Word	Frequency	Rank	Word	Frequency	Rank	Word	Frequency
1	is	11	24	like	2	47	had	1
2	and	7	25	looks	2	48	happy	1
3	it	7	26	mom	2	49	has	1
4	I	6	27	she	2	50	here	1
5	now	6	28	this	2	51	his	1

Rank	Word	Frequency	Rank	Word	Frequency	Rank	Word	Frequency
6	her	5	29	umbrella	2	52	holes	1
7	to	5	30	want	2	53	home	1
8	mud	4	31	wet	2	54	in	1
9	am	3	32	what	2	55	lets	1
10	course	3	33	a	1	56	ok	1
11	does	3	34	about	1	57	outside	1
12	he	3	35	answer	1	58	rain	1
13	not	3	36	are	1	59	raining	1
14	of	3	37	back	1	60	saying	1
15	that	3	38	better	1	61	so	1
16	the	3	39	boy	1	62	son	1
17	you	3	40	buddles	1	63	take	1
18	anyway	2	41	called	1	64	then	1
19	because	2	42	cannot	1	65	they	1
20	get	2	43	drenched	1	66	whatever	1
21	going	2	44	fine	1	67	wish	1
22	him	2	45	go	1	68	with	1
23	know	2	46	gonna	1	69	word	1

Of the total of 145 tokens in this transcript, there are 69 different words, i.e., 69 "types." The Number of Different Words (NDW) is therefore 69. The relationship between the number of types and the number of tokens is known as the Type–Token Ratio (TTR), calculated using the equation:

$$\frac{NDW}{Number\ of\ tokens} \times 100$$

$$= \frac{69}{145} \times 100 = 0.476$$

One limitation of the TTR and NDW is that they are highly sensitive to the length of speech samples (Owen & Leonard, 2002; Singh & Bookless, 1997) because as a language sample increases in length, it is less probable for a speaker to produce new words. In other words, if the length of a transcript is not standardized across speakers, the measure itself can be flawed given the fact that it varies as a function of the transcript length. As a result, shorter samples would appear to be richer. In addition, TTR calculated based on small samples is not sensitive to the repetition of words and therefore masks the performance of speakers (Richards & Malvern, 1997). To illustrate, in a sample of ten tokens, a speaker who produces five types with two tokens in each type will obtain a TTR value of 0.5 (i.e., 5÷10); on the other hand, if another speaker, who also produces ten tokens with five types, has one type repeated six times and the other four used only once will also obtain the same TTR value of 0.5. According to Richards and Malvern (1997), this masking effect can be avoided when there are at least 100 tokens in the language sample.

A number of studies have reported the use of a standardized sample size to measure the lexical diversity in speakers with aphasia. For example, Wright et al. (2003) used a fixed number of words in the middle portion of the entire speech samples of 23 English speakers with aphasia to compare the performances of fluent and non-fluent speakers. They obtained two sets of truncated samples, one set with 100 words and another set with 200 words, to examine if either one would result in a different lexical diversity between groups. It was found that as long as the number of words in the speech samples were fixed, the vocabulary diversity in the fluent aphasia group, as shown in both the TTR and NDW values, was significantly greater than that in their non-fluent counterparts. Owen and Leonard (2002) suggested that the employment of TTR was a simpler and more clinically feasible method to measure the degree of lexical variability. Nevertheless, one potential problem of the truncated analysis was that the selected sample might not be the most representative of the speakers' production because only a portion of the speech sample was considered.

Kong and Law (2009) have also used the method of using a pre-set sample to calculate TTR of 60 speakers with aphasia and 60 controls, with another sampling procedure. In particular, the sample size of each speaker in this study was fixed at 160 words for describing four sets of single colored picture stimuli. The speech sample elicited from each picture was trimmed to 40 words and these words were counted toward the final text. A method that considered the entire speech sample was used and each picture contributed equally towards the final TTR value. To do so, each of the four transcripts from a speaker was divided into 40 chunks, with the size of each unit calculated by dividing the total number of words by 40, and the first word from each chunk was selected. For example, in an 80-word transcript, every second word is discarded and in a 120-word transcript, every second and third word is deleted. In the case where the word number is not a multiple of 40, chunks of words are pooled such that the combined chunk would approach a whole number. Then the same number of words as the number of chunks combined would be selected. Following this "even distribution" sampling principle, the words selected should be equally spread out. For example, in a 130-word transcript, each word chunk is supposed to contain 3.25 words. The method of selecting words would involve combining four chunks together and picking up the first, fourth, seventh, and tenth words. Box 4.2 shows more examples of the sampling guidelines presented in Kong and Law (2009).

Box 4.2 Sampling Guidelines for TTR Suggested by Kong and Law (2009)

Number of words in the transcript	Way to trim the sample to 40 words
41	Delete the 21st word.
42	Delete the 21st and last word.
54	Divide the sample into two 27-word chunks. Delete the 3rd, 7th, 11th, 15th, 19th, 23rd, and last word in each chunk.
59	Delete every 3rd word in the sample.
60	Divide the sample into twenty 3-word chunks. Delete the last word in each chunk.
67	Delete the 34th word. Then divide the sample into two 33-word chunks. In each chunk, delete the 3rd and 5th word in every five words.
74	Delete the 37th and last word. Then divide the sample into eight 9-word chunks. Delete the 2nd, 4th, 6th, and 8th word in each chunk.
83	Delete the 42nd word. Then divide the sample into two 41-word chunks. Include every 2nd word in each chunk.
84	Divide the sample into four 21-word chunks. Include every 2nd word in each chunk.
85	Divide the sample into five 17-word chunks. Include every 2nd word in each chunk.
93	Delete the 47th word. Then divide the sample into four 23-word chunks. Include the 1st, 3rd, 6th, 8th, 11th, 13th, 16th, 18th, 21st, and last word in each chunk.
100	Divide the sample into twenty 5-word chunks. Include the 1st and 4th word in each chunk.
106	Divide the sample into two 53-word chunks. Include the 1st, 3rd, 6th, 9th, 12th, 15th, 18th, 21st, 24th, 26th, 28th, 30th, 33rd, 36th, 39th, 42nd, 45th, 48th, 51st, and last word in each chunk.
109	Delete the 55th word. Then divide the sample into four 27-word chunks. Include the 1st, 4th, 7th, 10th, 13th, 15th, 18th, 21st, 24th, and last word in each chunk.
119	Delete the 60th word. Then divide the sample into two 59-word chunks. In each chunk, include the 1st word in every three words.
126	Divide the sample into two 63-word chunks. Include the 1st, 4th, 7th, 10th, 13th, 16th, 19th, 23rd, 27th, 31st, 33rd, 37th, 41st, 45th, 48th, 51st, 54th, 57th, 60th, and last word in each chunk.
134	Divide the sample into two 67-word chunks. In each chunk, include the 1st and 4th word in every seven words.
142	Divide the sample into two 71-word chunks. In each chunk, include the 3rd and 7th word in every seven words.
150	Divide the sample into ten 15-word chunks. Only include the 1st, 5th, 9th, and 13th word in each chunk.
154	Divide the sample into two 77-word chunks. In each chunk, include the 1st word in every four words. Also include the last word in each chunk.
160	Divide the sample into forty 4-word chunks. Delete the 2nd, 3rd, and last word in each chunk.

Note: See Kong (2006) for a full list of sampling methods involving other transcript lengths.

The biggest challenge of computing the TTR using a standardized sample size is that different studies have used different lengths as their "standard." Currently there is not a common consensus in terms of the "best" or "golden" predetermined number of tokens for TTR calculation. Although Brookshire and Nicholas (1994) and Prins and Bastiaanse (2004) have proposed the use of a standard of 300 tokens for calculating the TTR in the population with aphasia, obtaining this amount of oral production for the purposes of both clinical evaluation and data collection in research projects is not always possible (Gordon, 2008), especially for speakers who are non-fluent or with a more severe degree of aphasia.

With the intention to overcome the inherent problem of TTR being sensitive to sample size, Holmes (1994), Malvern and Richards (2002), and Jarvis (2002) have reviewed the use of some algebraic transformations of the TTR, such as $\dfrac{logType}{logToken}$ or $\dfrac{(logToken)^2}{logToken - logType}$ (Herdan, 1960). Other reports attempting to reduce the impact of sample size included transformations such as Root TTR ($\dfrac{Type}{\sqrt{Token}}$) by Guiraud (1960) and corrected TTR ($\dfrac{Type}{\sqrt{2 \times Token}}$) by Carroll (1964). Readers who are interested in these transformed TTR indices may refer to the original articles for more details on their computation assumptions and research implications.

voc-D

To address the effect of sample length on the TTR and NDW, the measure voc-D was developed by transforming the TTR as an alternative index (Malvern & Richards, 1997). Comparison of lexical diversity of different texts was based on a curve-drawing approach. Differences in lexical diversity could be reflected in the different shapes of the curves plotted by computer software, such as the CLAN language analysis programme (MacWhinney, 2000). Conceptually, the voc-D performs a series of random samplings of type (i.e., lexical items) for each transcript to plot a curve for its empirical TTR and another curve reflecting the sample's number of tokens. The TTR is estimated based on 35 randomly selected tokens in the transcript without replacement. After repeating this process 100 times, the mean of the TTR is obtained and plotted. Subsequently, the same algorithm is repeated for subsamples of 36 to 50 tokens. By doing so, the average TTR for each subsample of increasing token size is plotted to form the empirical curve. By default, a sample must contain a minimum of 50 tokens for it to be estimated on the voc-D. Otherwise, the empirical TTR curve involved in the computation process cannot be established. For a sample with a lower degree of lexical diversity, a poorer voc-D value should result in a steeper theoretical curve that fits the empirical curve of the sample. The whole process of curve plotting is repeated three times, and the final voc-D value is the average of the three runs. With reference to these procedures, the voc-D can reflect how fast a TTR decreases in a sample. Specifically, a transcript with more type repetition should lead to a faster TTR decrease as a function of the token size. One should note that generating curves for voc-D has been reported to be a time-consuming procedure as it requires examiners to have some knowledge of algebra and statistics in order to manipulate the variables within the computer programs (Jarvis, 2002). For this reason, the voc-D is more common for use in research.

On the other hand, a few research papers in the literature of communication sciences and disorders have reported the potential clinical values of applying the voc-D. In particular, the advantage of the voc-D is that the measure was not sensitive to sample size and, therefore, discarding of speech samples was not needed. In other words, the voc-D considered the entire sample. According to the study by Wright et al. (2003), it was found that the use of voc-D values could successfully differentiate the lexical diversity of language samples of spontaneous discourse (conversation and picture description) from a group of nine speakers with fluent aphasia from another group of nine non-fluent speakers. Silverman and Ratner (2002) also applied the voc-D to evaluate the expressive lexical skills of young children who stutter. Their findings indicated that voc-D values correlated well with standardized measures of expressive vocabulary, while TTR values did not. The voc-D was also able to reflect a significantly poorer expressive lexical skill in the participant group of young children who stutter. Suggestions of promoting the application of the voc-D to general clinical settings for use by clinicians or speech-and-language pathologists were given. The primary argument was that its computation could be achieved through the use of the CLAN language analysis (see more detail in Chapter 5), which is a fairly common software in the field of speech-and-language pathology and linguistics. Moreover, the voc-D was claimed to offer some flexibility in data coding and manipulation, on top of a wide range of automatic analyses that are of interest to both researchers and clinical practitioners.

HD-D

Another measure of lexical diversity called the HD-D was proposed by McCarthy and Jarvis (2007). A feature of this measure is that it does not require a minimum of 50 tokens, as in the case of the voc-D, for estimation of lexical richness. The HD here stands for "hypergeometric distribution," which is an approach to calculate probabilities that involves sampling without replacement. The estimation of lexical diversity using the HD-D is, therefore, based on probabilities of word occurrence in a language sample. The underlying assumption is that if a particular type (i.e., lexical item) in the transcript is repeated many times (such as the pathological or stereotyped repetition of a particular single word in an aphasic discourse), there is a higher probability of drawing a sample that will contain at least one token of that type. To obtain a HD-D of a language sample, the probability of the first lexical type in the transcript encountering any of its tokens in a random sample is first estimated. The estimations of probabilities for all remaining lexical types are then added together. The final sum becomes the HD-D value for the transcript (McCarthy & Jarvis, 2010).

Measure of Textual Lexical Diversity (MTLD)

McCarthy (2005) proposed the **Measure of Textual Lexical Diversity (MTLD)** to reflect the degree of lexical richness in an oral discourse. This measure does not involve the need to discard any data in a transcript because the MTLD employs a sequential analysis of the entire language sample to estimate its degree of lexical diversity. An MTLD value is generated based on calculating the recurrent TTR of increasingly longer segments of a transcript. As mentioned earlier, the numeric value of TTR tends to decrease as the length of the transcript increases. When the TTR value of a particular segment is lower than a predetermined magnitude, a factor count will increase by 1, and the calculation of TTR is reset. This algorithm will resume the TTR calculation from the item where the factor count is added and will stop until the last token of the sample has been added, where the TTR at this point has been estimated. The total number of tokens in the transcript is then divided by the number of factor counts in the calculation process. This is followed by repeating the same algorithm with the text of the language sample reversed, so that a backward MTLD score is obtained. The final MTLD value is computed by averaging the forward and the reversed MTLD scores.

Moving Average Type Token Ratio (MATTR)

Subsequent to the McCarthy (2005) report, Covington (2007) and Covington and McFall (2010) have introduced the **Moving Average Type Token Ratio (MATTR)**. This measure estimates the lexical diversity of a language sample based on computing successive non-overlapping segments of the text using a smoothly moving window. This is done by first choosing a window length (say 100 words) and then computing the TTR for a word segment of the 1st to 100th word. The TTR computation is repeated for the next word segment of the 2nd to 101st words, and then segment of the 3rd to 103rd words, and so on for the entire sample. The final MATTR score can be obtained by averaging all the estimated TTRs. According to Covington and McFall (2010), the MATTR is not affected by accidental interactions between segment boundaries and text unit boundaries.

Which Measure on Lexical Diversity is Better?

A study by Fergadiotis et al. (2013) has evaluated the effectiveness of four of the above measures, including the voc-D, HD-D, MTLD, and MATTR, in assessing the lexical diversity among 101 people with aphasia. This was motivated by the lack of validity evidence on applying these methodologies to aphasic discourse. Results drawn from a confirmatory factor analysis revealed that the MTLD and MATTR were valid measures to reflect lexical diversity in this disordered population. In particular, they provided the strongest evidence to yield unbiased scores to reflect the degree of lexical diversity. Furthermore, it was suggested that the voc-D and HD-D provided equivalent estimation, based on their close-to-perfect relationship. Therefore, any one of the four measures can be used to reliably capture lexical diversity in aphasia, provided that the language samples contain a minimum of 50 tokens.

Quantitative Production Analysis (QPA)

One of the most comprehensive and detailed quantitative systems for analyzing aphasic production in English is the Quantitative Production Analysis (QPA), which was outlined in Saffran et al. (1989). Procedures for eliciting appropriate language samples from individuals with aphasia, extracting propositional speech from the samples and segmenting the extracted samples into utterances, as well as a system for evaluating performances on the corresponding lexical content and sentence structure were described. The development of the QPA was motivated by the lack of systematic analytic methods to clearly distinguish between speakers with agrammatic and **paragrammatic** production where the structural quality of the production could be closely examined without consideration of the differences in fluency between the two aphasia groups. Given that the blurred distinction of syntactic breakdown of aphasic sentence production has made prediction of deficit patterns following brain deficits a difficult job for clinicians (Caramazza & Berndt, 1978), the QPA was reported to be able to objectively quantify the characteristics of syntax in terms of its appropriateness and complexity.

According to Saffran et al. (1989), for a system to be considered as objective and quantitative for measuring aphasic sentence production, there are at least six requirements:

1. There is a clear, objective, and detailed procedure about elicitation of speech samples and their analytic methods, so that the same method can be replicated across studies (and/or clinical settings).
2. There is a valid way to identify propositional speech and to segment the output into units, so that the "noisy background" of the discourse

performance, such as false-starts, perseverations, or stereotyped utterances, can be removed from the final analysis.

3.   The content of the analysis should be focused on the structural elements that have been found to be disruptive or to be at risk of being disruptive in aphasia.

4.   There is a set of objective and quantifiable measures, such as in the form of numerical descriptions of relevant components, of the analyses in (3) above.

5.   The measures in (4) can be utilized for comparing between-group performances of examinees, analyzing group differences, and for reflecting changes within an examinee across time.

6.   The nature of the errors or disruption in sentences should be analyzed based on the actual structural elements present in an examinee's output. Although a list of targets related to the stimuli for speech elicitation (which in turn can assume common errors as manifested as structural deficits in an output) is often available, minimal assumptions should be made on an examinee's intended target utterance (and hence the nature of the errors committed).

Procedures about the elicitation and transcription of language samples, extraction of narrative words, segmentation of utterances, and computation of QPA indices are given below. More detailed illustration of this method is given in Saffran et al. (1989).

STEP 1: ELICITATION OF LANGUAGE SAMPLES

A well-known story (e.g., the Cinderella story), fairytale, television show, or plot of a TV drama or movie can be used to elicit a language sample. The target for analysis is a corpus of at least 150 words that represents the narrative core of an examinee's attempts to tell the story. The examinee is encouraged to use his or her own words when producing the output. It is crucial to include a relatively extensive sample because non-propositional speech will be removed from analysis (see Step 2 below). Note that the sample, at the same time, should also include recognizable targets for subsequent analysis. In case the examinee forgets or do not know a particular story, a story book with printed words deleted or covered can be used as a reminder of the story details. An examiner may talk about the picture illustrating the story with the examinee, but use of direct verbal structures that the examinee may imitate should be avoided. In most cases, collection of the sample, i.e., recording of the production, should only be started when all visual or written stimuli (such as the story book) are removed. Only minimal verbal prompts or cues should be used. In addition, specific questions that an examinee can answer in a single word or close-ended questions must be avoided.

STEP 2: TRANSCRIPTION OF ELICITED LANGUAGE SAMPLE

Standard orthography of English is used to transcribe an examinee's production, except for phonemic paraphasias and neologisms, but no punctuation should be used. English gloss should be given to all interpretable or recognizable phonemic paraphasias. Obvious pauses of one second or longer can be marked in the transcription. From time to time, an examiner may provide comments or ask questions to facilitate the production. These should also appear in the transcript but marked clearly in a new line as the examiner's speech, instead of mixing it with the examinee's output. If possible, prosodic contours can also be marked in the transcript to provide additional information for determining utterance boundaries. The total number of complete words is counted for the whole transcript, including recognizable paraphasias (but not false starts or partial production of words). Contractions should be treated as two words. Finally, the total duration of the language sample should be counted in minutes. Pauses between utterances are included in the total time but the time taken by the examiner's comments or questions should be subtracted.

STEP 3: EXTRACTION OF NARRATIVE WORDS

The aim of this step is to extract a total of 150 words or more that contain the propositional output an examinee produced (see illustration in Box 4.3). This can be done by deleting or excluding the following from the orthographically transcribed language sample:

1. neologisms
2. direct responses to a specific question by the examiner
3. comments made by the examinee on the narration or the task
4. starters or habitual statements and utterances
5. conjunctions that function to join utterances that are scored as separate sentences
6. direct discourse markers
7. repetitions (e.g., struggling) of single words, fragments of a sentence, or whole sentences that are finally produced
8. interruptions, such as a clause or fragment of a sentence
9. amendments of single words, fragments of a sentence, or whole sentences
10. elaborations of a sentence.

STEP 4: SEGMENTATION OF NARRATIVE WORDS TO UTTERANCES

Words that appear to form a coherent unit are bracketed in the transcript as one utterance (see illustration in Box 4.4). The segmentation process often involves the consideration of the following factors: (1) syntactic indicators,

Box 4.3 An Example of Narrative Word Extraction

An example of extracting narrative words in a transcript of the Cookie Theft picture description is given below. Notice that pauses of one second or longer are indicated in the transcript. Punctuation is absent and the examiner's verbal prompt is given on a new line.

> oh my god ... well .... *(2 seconds)* I mean to say for this picture... this is a regular picture... okay... *(1 second)* there is a jar ... of ... *(2 seconds)* cookies ...and ... a boy is stealing from the the coo... cookie jar.... the cookie jar .... the cookie jar... *(5 seconds)*
>
> *Examiner: please go on*
>
> what happens next is ... *(1 second)* ah ... is ... *(1 second)* ah.... *(1 second)* the girl... *(1 second)* the boy ... *(1 second)* falls down ... *(4 second)* oh ... how can I call it

- "oh my god ... well ...." can be excluded, based on the consideration that this is a comment made by the speaker on the narrative or the task
- "okay" is excluded, considering that it is a starter
- the utterance of "a boy is stealing from the the coo...cookie jar.... the cookie jar .... the cookie jar..." contains false start "coo..." for cookie and multiple direct repetitions of "cookie jar" which should be deleted
- the conjunction "and" between the utterance of "there is a jar of cookies" and another utterance "a boy is stealing from the cookie jar" is deleted
- "the girl" can also be excluded from "the girl... the boy ... falls down," given that it is an amendment to the target "the boy"

Notice that some degree of subjective judgment is always involved in this extraction process, because there may be disagreement across raters. This is especially the case if a language sample being analyzed was not collected by the rater himself or herself. The use of a video recording of the examinee's performance will be helpful in this situation. An examiner should be consistent in following the standard QPA extraction procedures when conducting analysis across speakers and/or narrative tasks. The following displays the final narrative sample that contains propositional words of the output:

> I mean to say for this picture... this is a regular picture... there is a jar of cookies...a boy is stealing from the cookie jar... what happens next is.... the boy falls down ... how can I call it

---

Box 4.4 An Example of Segmenting Words Into Utterances

The extracted words from Box 4.3 are segmented into six utterances for subsequent analysis using the QPA indices in Step 5.

(I mean to say for this picture)... (this is a regular picture)... (there is a jar of cookies)...(a boy is stealing from the cookie jar) ... (what happens next is.... the boy falls down) ... (how can I call it)

---

in which a well-formed sentence is counted as one utterance; (2) prosodic indicators, in which a falling intonation usually indicates the end of an utterance; (3) pauses, which are often present before the start of a new utterance; and (4) semantic criteria. Notice that the last two criteria may not be as reliable in disordered speech, especially in the cases with abundant pauses in the middle of an utterance or with many incidents of lexical misuse. Therefore, when in doubt, boundaries should be created to generate shorter, instead of longer, utterances. The total number of utterances is then tallied.

STEP 5: COMPUTATION OF QPA INDICES

Each utterance is categorized into one of the following three types: (a) "sentences" with structural types of "Noun + Main Verb," "Noun + **Copula** + Adjective," or "Noun + Copula + Prepositional Phrase;" (b) "topic/comment structures" with proposition-bearing structures that do not meet the criteria for (a); and (c) "others".

With reference to the basic counts and index computation shown in Table 4.1, the language sample is quantified by 17 variables reflecting the rate of speech production, the use of grammatical morphemes, the distribution of lexical items of different form classes, sentence structure, sentence complexity, and the elaboration of narratives. Particular remarks in treating specific groups of lexical or structural items include the following:

- Open-class words (basic count − D) include nouns, verbs, adjectives, and adverbs, except for degree and quantificational adverbs without −ly (e.g., very, quite, all, or most). "Be," "do," and "have" are classified as open class only when they function as a main verb. Numerals are counted as open class in the QPA, unless they function as pronoun (e.g., "There is *one* on the ground").
- Verb particles (basic count − E) are classified as closed class (e.g., "Stand *up*"). "Going to" or "have to" is classified as closed class when used as an auxiliary.

Table 4.1 Count measures and lexical and structural indices of the Quantitative Production Analysis (QPA)

Basic counts	QPA (1989) index computation	QPA (2000) index computation
(A) Total number of words		
(B) Number of narrative words		(xviii) Proportion of narrative words to total words uttered: B ÷ A
(C) Total narrative time in minutes	(i) Speech rate: B ÷ C	
Lexical content		
(D) Number of open-class words		
(E) Number of **closed-class words**: B − D	(ii) Proportion of closed-class words: E ÷ B	
(F) Number of nouns		
(G) Number of nouns requiring determiners (NrDs)		
(H) Number of NrDs with determiners	(iii) Determiner index: H ÷ G	
(I) Number of pronouns	(iv) Noun to pronoun ratio: F ÷ I	(xix) Pronoun to noun ratio: I ÷ (F+I)
(J) Number of verbs	(v) Noun to verb ratio: F ÷ J	(xx) Noun to verb ratio: J ÷ (F+J)
(K) Number of inflectable verbs		
(L) Number of inflectable verbs inflected	(vi) Inflection index: L ÷ K	
Auxiliary analysis		
(M) Number of matrix verbs		
(N) Total auxiliary (AUX) score	(vii) Auxiliary complexity index: (N ÷ M) − 1	
Structure analysis		
(O) Number of sentences		
(P) Number of words in sentences	(viii) Proportion of words in sentences: P ÷ B	
(Q) Number of words in topic/comment structures	(ix) Proportion of words in sentences and topic/comment structures: (P+Q) ÷ B	
	(x) Mean length of sentences: P ÷ O	
(R) Number of well-formed embedded sentences	(xi) Proportion of well-formed sentences: R ÷ O	
(S) Number of subject noun phrases (SNP)		

Table 4.1 Cont.

Basic counts	QPA (1989) index computation	QPA (2000) index computation
(T) Number of words in SNP	(xii) Mean length of SNP: T ÷ S (xiii) SNP elaboration index: (T ÷ S) − 1	
(U) Number of verb phrases (VP)		
(V) Number of words in VP	(xiv) Mean length of VP: V ÷ U (xv) VP elaboration index: (V ÷ U) − 1 (xvi) Embedded sentence elaboration index: (xiii+xv)	
(W) Number of embeddings	(xvii) Embedding index: W ÷ O	
		(xxi) Median length of utterance

Source: Saffran et al. (1989) and Rochon et al. (2000).

- Proper nouns generally do not require determiners (basic count − H). In ambiguous cases, do not consider a determiner obligatory.
- Only personal pronouns (e.g., "he," "she," "them," "my," "itself," or "themselves') are counted towards pronouns (basic count − I). Regular pronouns that serve a syntactic function (e.g., "that," "who," "which") are excluded here, but those replacing a noun (e.g., "I want to eat *that*") should be counted.
- Verbs (basic count − J) include main, infinitive, and gerundive verbs.
- A **matrix verb** (basic count − M) is counted when it is used as a main verb in a matrix sentence.
- The auxiliary (AUX) score (basic count − N) indicates the morphological complexity of matrix verbs. It is computed with reference to whether a matrix verb is inflected (e.g., "he leaves"), the presence of elements additional to a main verb (e.g., tense markers), or the use of **modal auxiliaries** or **auxiliary verbs** (e.g., "can," "shall," "will").
- Structural measures (basic counts − P to W) are scored only on utterances designated as "sentences," i.e., "topic/comment structures" and "others" do not involve computation of structural measures.
- In determining the degree of well-formedness in sentences (basic counts − R), any sentences with syntactic violations or missing obligatory arguments are classified as ill-formed.

Based on the performance of five agrammatic aphasic, five non-fluent, non-agrammatic aphasic, and five control speakers in a story-telling task of the Cinderella story, Saffran et al. (1989) was able to successfully apply the QPA to quantify their output. Specifically, this system was found to be able to distinguish agrammatic production from normal speech as well as from non-agrammatic aphasic speech, as reflected by indices such as speech rate and proportion of words in sentences. In addition, the performance on variables reflecting sentence complexity among individuals with non-agrammatic aphasia was found to be significantly inferior to that of their normal counterparts. More importantly, the system was also able to highlight the dissociation of morphological omission and structural simplification in one of their agrammatic participants, M.E., whose performance on verb inflections (bound grammatical morphemes) was close to normal. The distribution of the scores of morphological indices demonstrated a continuum across the two aphasic groups. This preliminary report, which indicated the validity of the tool, also included information on its inter-rater, transcription, and cross-sample reliabilities. Given its capability to capture the essential characteristics of morphological and structural disruptions of aphasic output, the QPA has become the basis for a number of other studies of English aphasic sentence production (e.g., Bird & Franklin, 1996; Byng, 1988; Byng & Black, 1989; Byng et al., 1994; Edwards, 1995; Hesketh & Bishop, 1996; Martin, et al., 1989; Schwartz et al., 1994).

Rochon et al. (2000) believed that the small sample size and the restricted data set used in the Saffran et al. (1989) study was a potential limitation. They, therefore, used the data of eight participants from the Saffran et al. (1989) study together with a new set of samples from 20 agrammatic aphasic, 9 non-fluent, non-agrammatic aphasic, and 12 normal speakers to perform a cluster analysis to investigate whether different speaker groups showed distinctive patterns of performance on the QPA variables. They also modified the calculation of two measures from the original method of calculation, the "Pronoun to noun ratio" and "Noun to verb ratio" (basic counts – I and J, respectively), and added two new indices, the "Proportion of narrative words to total words uttered" and the "Median length of utterance," to measure the efficiency and elaboration of production, respectively. The results revealed that the three groups of speakers performed significantly differently, with the measures on sentence elaboration and speech rate being the most discriminating indices between the agrammatic and control participants. Moreover, it was found that quantitative differences with respect to the morphological and structural QPA measures existed within the group of non-fluent Broca's speakers, thus providing some empirical evidence about the heterogeneity of impairment in this aphasic syndrome. The continuity in morphological and structural performance across the aphasic and control groups also extended Saffran et al.'s (1989) previous findings. The inter-rater and test-retest reliability on utterance assignment and index scoring of this revised

QPA continues to demonstrate high agreement for both the disorder and control data.

Sentential and Discourse Grammar

Another approach for analyzing aphasic narrative discourse is to quantify sentential and discourse grammars within a narrative as highlighted in Ulatowska et al. (1981), Ulatowska et al. (1983), and Olness (2006). In particular, sentential grammars can be evaluated on the number of words and morphemes as well as the complexity and types of clauses, using the following measures:

1. Length of T-units: Expressed in terms of the mean number of words and/or morphemes (see Chapter 3 for details on definition and computation of T-units).
2. Amount of embedding: Expressed in number of clauses per T-unit.
3. Ratio of coordinate to subordinate conjunctions.
4. Percentage of dependent clauses (i.e., ratio of dependent to total clauses).
5. Percentage of nonfinite clauses (i.e., ration of nonfinite to total clauses).

Discourse grammars are measured in terms of the length and occurrence of narrative superstructures as follows:

1. Length of discourse as measured by the number of T-units.
2. Occurrence of elements of superstructures and how well the clauses of the narratives are ordered in an appropriate temporal sequence:

	SUPERSTRUCTURE	EXAMPLES
a.	Abstract:	What is the story about?
	↓	
b.	Setting involving time and location, background, and identification of participants:	When? Where? What? Who?
	↓	
c.	Complicating action involving events:	What are the episodes of the story? What happened next? What is the sequence of events?
	↓	
d.	Evaluation:	So what?
	↓	
e.	Result or resolution:	What happened at the end?
	↓	
f.	Coda:	What is the moral of the story?

3. Length of elements of the narrative superstructures in (2), as measured by the number of T-units.
4. Propositional analysis of the story and its summary.
5. Amount of evaluation as measured by the number of clauses containing evaluation on the narrative task.
6. Amount of adverbial modification as measured by the number of adverbial phrases.

There are also two sets of subjective three-point rating scales, one set on the clarity and the other on the content of the discourse, to estimate the degree of discourse cohesion and coherence, respectively. Most research involves the use of naïve listeners to provide ratings on each of the two scales. More specifically, in response to the question "How comprehensible is the language of the story?" the clarity of language rating was rated on the scale:

1 (not at all clear) ------ 2 (not completely clear) ------ 3 (completely clear)

As for content rating, the questions varied slightly with reference to the nature of the narrative task as below:

1. Do you know what is happening in the story?

    1 (no) ------ 2 (for the most part) ------ 3 (yes)

2. Does the sequence of events make sense?

    1 (no) ------ 2 (for the most part) ------ 3 (yes)

3. Is the story unambiguous as to what each of the participant did?

    1 (no) ------ 2 (for the most part) ------ 3 (yes)

4. Is the story accurate with reference to the stimulus materials?

    1 (no) ------ 2 (for the most part) ------ 3 (yes)

5. Is the story complete in the sense that it does not omit any necessary information?

    1 (no) ------ 2 (for the most part) ------ 3 (yes)

6. Do you as a listener know what the examinee is talking about?

    1 (no) ------ 2 (for the most part/with difficulty) ------ 3 (yes)

7. Could you follow the procedures of this story?

    1 (no) ------ 2 (with difficulty) ------ 3 (yes)

In the Ulatowska et al. (1981) and (1983) studies, 10 mildly impaired and 15 moderately impaired speakers with aphasia (classified based on a clinical severity rating adapted directly from the Boston Diagnostic Aphasia Examination: rating scale of "0 = severe impairment" to "5 = minimum impairment") were recruited, respectively. The same numbers of unimpaired speakers were used as controls. Based on the language samples of narrative discourses elicited from a task of story-telling and another of story-retelling, a recall task of personal events, and a sequential picture description task, it was found that the structure of the discourse samples from the speakers with aphasia was largely comparable to that of the controls. In particular, narrative superstructures were largely present, except for the absence of summaries and morals. However, aphasic discourses had a tendency to contain fewer episodes with sentences being shorter in length and less elaborated. The contents within the samples were also less complete than those produced by the controls. These two studies provided useful information regarding the difference between the narrative structures of aphasic and normal discourse and procedurals. Nevertheless, the results would have been more informative if the speakers with aphasia were further classified into fluent and non-fluent groups or even into different aphasia types. The latter would provide more specific information on the disruption patterns of sentential grammars among various aphasia syndromes.

Natural Language Processing (NLP)

Natural language processing (NLP) refers to the branch of computer science specialized in **artificial intelligence (AI)** that makes use of computers to understand text and spoken words in much the same way humans are capable of. In other words, NLP involves the simulation of human intelligence in machines that are programmed to process language like human beings and mimic their actions to understand (i.e., to make sense of) spoken output. It combines the rule-based modeling of human language in computational linguistics with other models of statistics, machine learning, and deep learning to achieve the final understanding. To allow a machine to ingest and interpret human language, several NLP tasks are typically involved:

1. Speech-to-text conversion (or speech recognition): This is the process of converting spoken data (i.e., voice) into written transcripts (i.e., text data), and is required for any applications that follow voice commands or answer spoken questions. The accuracy and efficiency of speech recognition depends on many factors, including, but not limited to, voice quality of the data, signal-to-noise ratio of original sound data, speakers' speech characteristics such as intonation or accents, and the grammatical accuracy of the spoken data (see Chapter 6 for more details on a computerized approach to analyzing speech prosody).

2. Annotation of part-of-speech (or morphological tagging): This is the process of determining and assigning one or more part-of-speech to each recognized word, based on how it is used within the linguistic context (and neighbor constituents) in the text (see Excerpts 3a and 3b in Chapter 5 for examples of different morphological annotations, such as nouns, verbs, or grammatical items of pronouns or prepositions). According to Kong and Law (2019), one major challenge of annotating disordered discourse, such as an aphasic output, is the potential disagreement of parsing part-of-speech in the non-fluent or grammatically ill-formed sentences by speakers with aphasia.

3. Named entity recognition (NER): This is the process of identifying words or phrases as useful entities. For example, NER identifies "Orlando, Florida" as a location but "Orlando Magic" as a basketball team and "Orlando Bloom" as an actor's name.

4. Word sense disambiguation: This is the process of selecting the correct part-of-speech for tagged items in (2) with multiple annotations (and therefore multiple meanings or grammatical types). An automated semantic analysis will help determine the word that makes the most sense in the given context. Note that disambiguators are language specific. In order to "train" a disambiguator to ensure accurate disambiguation, a hand-annotated training set for discourse samples (with 1000 to 5000 utterances) in a particular language is suggested.

5. Co-reference resolution: This is the process of identifying if and when two words refer to the same entity. For example, a particular pronoun within the text data is identified and then determined to be referring to a certain person or object.

6. Sentiment analysis: This is the process of extracting subjective qualities of the text data, such as the attitudes or emotions of a speaker, as well as whether a speaker is showing suspicion, confusion, or using sarcasm.

Yeung et al. (2021) have recently reported a feasibility study that examined how well the technology of NLP could be applied to objective evaluation of the speech-language characteristics in ten speakers with mild cognitive impairments, another ten individuals with Alzheimer's disease, and ten healthy controls. In particular, speech recordings from these participants describing the Cookie Theft picture were extracted from the DementiaBank project (https://dementia.talkbank.org/), transcribed, and manually annotated on speaker differentiation and utterance segmentation by trained raters using customized transcription software. These transcripts were then handled using NLP with automatic feature extraction, performed using a combination of standard language processing libraries (e.g., spaCy, an open-source software library for advanced NLP, written in the programming languages Python and Cython) and customized code. Examples of the extracted variables included the following:

- *Lexical* aspect of the transcripts, such as average word length, number of words, ratio of subordinate to coordinate words, average word frequency, use of demonstrative words, average **arousal** score of nouns.
- *Semantic* aspect of the transcripts, such as proportion of subject words used, semantic similarity of description to picture content, average valence score of all words, proportion of subjects in picture described.
- *Syntactic* aspect of the transcripts, such as syntactic complexity, use of past tense verbs, use of noun phrases with determiners and nouns, use of conjunctive verb phrases, use of singular present verb phrases with prepositional phrases, number of coordinate phrases per clause, or use of coordinate phrases.

The same set of speech recordings was also rated by expert clinicians on the characteristics of word-finding difficulty, incoherence, perseveration, and speech errors. Yeung et al. found that NLP could detect objective speech-language changes in both the speakers with mild cognitive impairments and Alzheimer's disease. More importantly, these negative changes shown by the NLP variables directly correlated to clinicians' ratings. It was concluded that further research and validation through larger datasets and more clinician raters were warranted; this would lead to the development of disorder-specific digital speech and language markers that can inform the presence, types, and severity of discourse deficits. Future evidence supporting this novel approach of discourse assessment may also promote its clinical application.

Conclusions

In this chapter, a number of research-oriented approaches of discourse analyses were presented with discussion of their theoretical frameworks, computational procedures, and potential implications for clinical use. Many of these analytic methods have become the basis for developing other evaluation methods that are more clinically applicable. A good appreciation of these discourse quantification methodologies will provide readers with important fundamental knowledge on conducting objective analyses of narrative samples.

References

Bird, H., & Franklin, S. (1996). Cinderella revisited: A comparison of fluent and non-fluent aphasic speech. *Journal of Neurolinguistics, 9*(3), 187–206.

Brookshire, R. H., & Nicholas, L. E. (1994). Speech sample size and test-retest stability of connected speech measures for adults with aphasia. *Journal of Speech and Hearing Research, 37*(2), 399–407.

Byng, S. (1988). Sentence processing deficits: Theory and therapy. *Cognitive Neuropsychology, 5,* 629–676.

Byng, S., & Black, M. (1989). Some aspects of sentence production in aphasia. *Aphasiology*, *3*, 241–263.

Byng, S., Nickles, L., & Black, M. (1994). Replicating therapy for mapping deficits in agrammatism: Remapping the deficit? *Aphasiology*, *8*, 315–341.

Caramazza, A. & Berndt, R. S. (1978). Semantic and syntactic processes in aphasia: A review of the literature. *Psychological Bulletin*, *85*(4), 898–918.

Carroll, J. B. (1964). *Language and thought*. Englewood Cliffs, NJ: Prentice-Hall.

Covington, M. A. (2007). MATTR user manual (CASPR research report 2007–05). Atheus, GA.

Covington, M. A., & McFall, J. D. (2010). Cutting the Gordian knot: The moving-average type–token ratio (MATTR). *Journal of Quantitative Linguistics*, *17*, 94–100.

Edwards, S. (1995). Profiling fluent aphasic spontaneous speech: A comparison of two methodologies. *European Journal of Disorders of Communication*, *30*, 333–345.

Fergadiotis, G., & Wright, H. H. (2011). Lexical diversity for adults with and without aphasia across discourse elicitation tasks. *Aphasiology*, *25*(11), 1414–1430.

Fergadiotis, G., Wright, H. H., & West, T. M. (2013). Measuring lexical diversity in narrative discourse of people with aphasia. *American Journal of Speech and Language Pathology*, *22*(2), 397–408.

Gordon, J. K. (2008). Measuring the lexical semantics of picture description in aphasia. *Aphasiology*, *22*(7–8), 839–852.

Guiraud, P. (1960). *Problèmes et méthodes de la statistique linguistique*. Dordrecht: D. Reidel.

Herdan, G. (1960). *Type-token mathematics: A textbook of mathematical linguistics*. The Hague: Mouton.

Hesketh, A., & Bishop, D. V. M. (1996). Agrammatism and adaptation theory. *Aphasiology*, *10*, 49–80.

Holmes, D.I. (1994). Authorship attribution. *Computers and the Humanities*, *28*, 87–106.

Holmes, D. I., & Singh, S. (1996). A stylometric analysis of conversational speech of aphasic patients. Literary and Linguistic Computing, 11(3), 133–140.

Honoré, T. (1979). Some simple measures of richness of vocabulary. *Association of Literary and Linguistic Computing Bulletin*, *7*, 172–177.

Jarvis, S. (2002). Short texts, best-fitting curves and new measures of lexical diversity. *Language Testing*, *19*(1), 57–84.

Kong, A. P. H. (2006). A Cantonese linguistic communication measure for evaluating aphasic narrative production [Unpublished doctoral dissertation]. The University of Hong Kong, Hong Kong SAR.

Kong, A. P. H., & Law, S. P. (2009). Cantonese Linguistic Communication Measure (CLCM): A clinical tool for assessing aphasic narrative production. In S.P. Law, B. Weekes, & A. Wong (Eds.), *Disorders of Speech and Language in Chinese* (pp. 255–272). Clevedon, UK: Multilingual Matters.

Kong, A. P. H. & Law, S. P. (2019). Cantonese AphasiaBank: An annotated database of spoken discourse and co-verbal gestures by healthy and language-impaired native Cantonese speakers. *Behavior Research Methods*, *51*(3), 1131–1144.

Lind, M., Kristoffersen, K. E., Moen, I., & Simonsen, H. G. (2009). Semi-spontaneous oral text production: Measurements in clinical practice. *Clinical Linguistics & Phonetics*, *23*(12), 872–886.

MacWhinney, B. (2000). *The CHILDES project: Tools for analyzing talk.* Hillsdale, NJ: Erlbaum.

MacWhinney, B., Fromm, D., Forbes, M., & Holland, A. (2011). AphasiaBank: Methods for studying discourse. *Aphasiology, 25*(11), 1286–1307.

Malvern, D. D., & Richards, B. J. (1997). A new measure of lexical diversity. In A. Ryan & A. Wray (Eds.), *Evolving models of language* (pp. 58–71). Clevedon, UK: Multilingual Matters.

Malvern, D., & Richards, B. (2002). Investigating accommodation in language proficiency interviews using a new measure of lexical diversity. *Language Testing, 19*(1), 85–104.

Malvern, D. D., Richards, B. J., Chipere, N., & Dura´n, P. (2004). *Lexical diversity and language development: Quantification and assessment.* Basingstoke, UK: Palgrave Macmillan.

Martin, R. C., Wetzel, F., Blossom-Stach, C., & Feher, E. (1989). Syntactic loss versus processing deficit: An assessment of two theories of agrammatism and syntactic comprehension deficits. *Cognition, 32*, 157–191.

McCarthy, P. M. (2005). *An assessment of the range and usefulness of lexical diversity measures and the potential of the measure of textual, lexical diversity* [Doctoral dissertation]. Available from Proquest Dissertations and Theses (UMI No. 3199485).

McCarthy, P. M., & Jarvis, S. (2007). Voc-D: A theoretical and empirical evaluation. *Language Testing, 24*(4), 459–488.

McCarthy, P. M., & Jarvis, S. (2010). MTLD, voc-D, and HD-D: A validation study of sophisticated approaches to lexical diversity assessment. *Behavior Research Methods, 42*(2), 381–392. doi:10.3758/BRM.42.2.381

Olness, G. S. (2006). Genre, verb, and coherence in picture-elicited discourse of adults with aphasia. *Aphasiology, 20*, 175–187.

Owen, A. J., & Leonard, L. B. (2002). Lexical diversity in the spontaneous speech of children with specific language impairment: Application of D. *Journal of Speech, Language, and Hearing Research, 45*, 927–937.

Prins, R., & Bastiaanse, R. (2004). Analyzing the spontaneous speech of aphasic speakers. *Aphasiology, 18*(12), 1075–1091.

Rider, J. D., Wright, H. H., Marshall, R. C., & Page, J. L. (2008). Using semantic feature analysis to improve contextual discourse in adults with aphasia. *American Journal of Speech-Language Pathology, 17*(2), 161–172.

Rochon, E., Saffran, E. M., Berndt, R. S., & Schwartz, M. F. (2000). Quantitative analysis of aphasic sentence production: Further development and new data. *Brain and Language, 72*, 193–218.

Saffran, E. M., Berndt, R. S., & Schwartz, M. F. (1989). The quantitative analysis of agrammatic production: Procedure and data. *Brain and Language, 37*, 440–479.

Schwartz, M. F., Saffran, E. M., Fink, R. B., Myers, J. L., & Martin, N. (1994). Mapping theory: A treatment program for agrammatism. *Aphasiology, 8*, 19–54.

Silverman, S., & Ratner, N. B. (2002). Measuring lexical diversity in children who stutter: Application of vocd. *Journal of Fluency Disorders, 27*, 289–304.

Singh, S. & Bookless, T. (1997). Analyzing spontaneous speech in dysphasic adults. *The International Journal of Applied Linguistics, 7*(2), 165–182.

Ulatowska, H. K., Freedman-Stern, R., Doyel, A. W., Macaluso-Haynes, S., & North, A. J. (1983). Production of narrative discourse in aphasia. *Brain and Language, 19*, 317–334.

Ulatowska, H. K., North, A. J., & Macaluso-Haynes, S. (1981). Production of narrative and procedural discourse in aphasia. *Brain and Language, 13*, 345–371.

Wright, H. H., Silverman, S. W., & Newhoff, M. (2003). Measures of lexical diversity in aphasia. *Aphasiology, 17*(5), 443–452.

Yeung, A., Iaboni, A., Rochon, E., Lavoie, M., Santiago, C., Yancheva, M., Novikova, J., Xu, M., Robin, J., Kaufman, L. D., & Mostafa, F. (2021). Correlating natural language processing and automated speech analysis with clinician assessment to quantify speech-language changes in mild cognitive impairment and Alzheimer's dementia. *Alzheimer's Research & Therapy, 13*(1), 109.

Chapter 5

Multi-Linear Transcription and Analysis of Oral Discourse

Chapter Objectives

The reader will be able to:

1. describe the components in a multi-linear transcription and explain their significance for discourse analysis
2. describe the procedures and specific considerations in preparing a transcript
3. discuss the considerations needed in preparing an orthographic transcription in English versus in any other non-English languages
4. compare and contrast the different layouts of transcripts in relation to their use for discourse analysis
5. provide examples of typical or conventional transcription symbols for unimpaired as well as disordered language samples
6. discuss the considerations needed in preparing a transcription with segmental and supra-segmental information of a discourse
7. discuss the considerations in annotating non-verbal behaviors in a transcription
8. explain and justify the clinical use of multi-linear transcriptions
9. explain the research values of multi-linear transcriptions
10. discuss the use of computational tools for transcription of spoken discourse.

Introduction

Discourse is a form of communication with the unique feature of being dynamic and occurs naturally during a speaker's use of language. A comprehensive and systematic record of a communication between a speaker and a listener can ensure effective studying of the verbal as well as non-verbal interactions involved.

A carefully prepared transcription containing information about how a person is using spoken language to communicate will facilitate clinical

DOI: 10.4324/9781003254775-5

observation and subsequent linguistic analyses of language deficits. Depending on how the spoken language is recorded, an orthographic transcript usually accompanies a video or audio recording. Since human communication is a complex process and often includes more than one modality of communicative language output, recent studies have emphasized the need to capture and document as many details in the interaction as possible. This is especially the case if one attempts to identify the breakdown among individuals with acquired language disorders, who may often rely on non-linguistic forms of communication to compensate for their verbal limitations.

In this chapter, we first discuss some conventional methods used for transcribing language samples, with illustrations of how multi-linear transcriptions can be done. Why multi-linear transcription is important for conducting research in discourse production, as well as clinically relevant for understanding discourse deficits, will be addressed. We then discuss the components of different levels of annotations for conducting a multi-linear transcription of disordered language samples. To conclude, we explore the use of some existing web-accessible archiving software for preparing multi-linear transcriptions and evaluate their potential challenges for clinical usage.

Principles of Multi-Linear Transcription

According to Müller et al. (2006), to transcribe something refers to the process of "transferring or translating speech, spoken language, and non-verbal aspects of human interaction from audio or video recordings to a written (or graphic) medium" (p. 3). This process of transcribing not only can reflect both the linguistic and paralinguistic aspects within verbal communications, but also the use of gestures, body postures, gaze, touch, and/or facial expressions in the non-verbal aspects of communication. The end product is usually called a transcript, which can be considered as a representation of a transcriber's perspective on a speaker's use of verbal language and non-verbal communication, together with the transcriber's interpretation of the corresponding data.

Considerations for Preparing a Transcription

In Chapter 2, we presented different strategies to obtain language samples from speakers with neurogenic communication disorders. Factors that are often considered, such as choice of the right medium of record(s), selection of recording equipment and their positioning during the time when sample is collected, and appropriate length of a representative sample, have been discussed in the context of collecting various types of oral discourse. Once an examiner is ready to prepare a transcription, it is crucial to determine the purpose of using this transcription and the level of detail needed for its subsequent analyses. Knowing how much detail is to be included in the final transcript will also help an examiner to select the most appropriate layout to display the content of an oral discourse.

To illustrate, if an examiner is evaluating the narrative performance of a speaker with aphasia, it is common to identify the typical language characteristics and aphasic symptoms that can assist the clinical classification of the aphasia syndrome (e.g., fluent versus non-fluent) as well as the determination of severity level (e.g., mild, moderate, or severe). When transcribing the examinee's production, one should, therefore, consider as much detail as possible, including all the intelligible words and sentences spoken, errors, unintelligible speech and non-speech content, pausing or fillers, false starts, hesitation or struggling during incidents of word finding or sentence construction, as well as self-corrections. Irrespective of whether an examiner is working from the video or audio recordings of an unscripted and open-ended interaction (such as a conversation) or another narrative task (such as a describing a single picture or telling a story), the transcription process would likely involve the segmentation and numbering of the spoken text into information units or utterances. Any temporal and sequential relationships of the language content, which can inform us how different parts of the production are related in time, will be highlighted. In addition, prosodic aspects of the speech output (such as changes in intonation or loudness as well as emphasis on certain syllables, words, or phrases) and other non-verbal activities in the interaction (such as the use of gestures or eye gazes) can be simultaneously represented in the transcript.

Ideally, a multi-linear transcription should include as much detail as possible, so that it contains sufficient information to highlight the salient features of a narration. This will subsequently ensure that the examiner conducts any specific analyses without the need to go back into the original audio or video recordings. In other words, discourse analysis can be readily done by referring to only a well-prepared transcript. However, as transcribing a video or audio file can be an extremely time-consuming process, one must also set a limit on the level of detail required. A transcript should only contain content as it is produced by a speaker, not as it might have been intended by or as it "should have been said" by the speaker. The easiest and most useful way to determine the amount of detail needed is to revisit the purpose of a discourse analysis. One should also note that a transcript with unnecessary information can be distracting to those who attempt to understand the language functioning, skills, or deficits simply by reading the transcript but have no immediate contact with the examinee.

Selecting an Appropriate Transcript Layout

Various layouts have been used and reported in the literature to display the multi-faceted features of an oral discourse. A standard layout for transcripts in English uses the left-to-right and top-to-bottom convention. All participants (i.e., examiner, examinee, and, if relevant, other speakers such as family members or other communication partners) are identified. The time point where there is a speaker transition indicates a speaker's turn at talking and each turn is numbered sequentially in a transcript. An example is given in Excerpt 1 below.

Excerpt (1)

```
01  W:  Ready?
02  P:  uhh. Yes!
03  W:  Okay.
04  W:  Can you tell me about this series of three pictures?
04  P:  uh. (2s) Tree, uh, lake.
05  W:  Okay. What about [this one?]
06  P:               [Lakes    ] ummm. (1s) Pools.
07  W:  Okay.
08  P:  I don't know why that is (2s) [ummm.]
09  W:                              [And?   ]
10  P:  hold on. Water. Water.
11  P:  And they were, was at twelve o'clock
```

The sample in Excerpt 1 is part of a conversation dialog between the examiner (W) and a person with aphasia (P) during a clinical session when they discuss the content of three photos taken by P (see Whiteside et al., 2010). Each line of the transcript is numbered in order to facilitate the referencing to specific points within the interaction. While any pauses with duration in seconds are indicated by parentheses (see lines 04, 06, and 08), overlapping speech between the two participants (i.e., simultaneous talk by the two interlocutors) is indicated by square brackets (see lines 05+06 and lines 08+09), with visual alignment of the overlapped portion. The intonation of both speakers is represented by conventional punctuation marks. The same extract can be displayed using another layout as in Excerpt 2, in which the examiner and speaker with aphasia are allotted in separate columns of the transcript. Note that the overlapped talk is aligned on the same parallel line (see lines 07 and 11) in the two speaker columns.

Excerpt (2)

Line	W:	P:
01	Ready?	
02		uhh. Yes!
03	Okay.	
04	Can you tell me about this series of three pictures?	

05		uh. (2s) Tree, uh, lake.
06	Okay. What about	
07	this one?	Lakes
08		ummm. (1s) Pools.
09	Okay.	
10		I don't know why that is
11	And?	ummm.
12		hold on. Water. Water.
13		And they were, was at twelve o'clock

Another layout of transcription and coding of disordered discourse is presented by MacWhinney et al. (2011). Transcription follows the Codes for the Human Analysis of Talk (CHAT) format (MacWhinney, 2000), which was designed to operate closely with the Computerized Language ANalysis (CLAN) program (MacWhinney, 2000). Excerpts 3a and 3b show examples of production from two different participants with aphasia, who were asked to describe their stroke, and Excerpt 3c shows another example of an extract from a description task using a set of sequential pictures depicting a child refusing an umbrella and getting caught in the rain. (These samples were selected from Kong et al., 2014 and Reres et al., 2014). There are two types of speaker line, the *INV tier and *PAR tier for record of output from the investigator (i.e., examiner) and participant (i.e., person with aphasia), respectively. Utterances are segmented following the analysis of Saffran et al. (1989) and Berndt et al. (2000), with reference to the syntactic and semantic criteria as well as intonation and pauses of the language output (see Quantitative Production Analysis in Chapter 4). Unlike Excerpts 1 and 2, these transcripts contain coding of the use of co-verbal and non-verbal behaviors, as indicated by the &= symbols in CHAT. Examples include (1) &=head:yes for head nodding (see line 02 in both Excerpts 3a and 3b), (2) &=head:no for head shaking (see line 04 in Excerpt 3b), (3) &=fingers:five for showing five fingers (see line 12 in Excerpt 3b), and (4) &=ges:downpour for indicating pouring rain (see line 18 in Excerpt 3c). Additional CHAT symbols are also used in the *PAR tier to represent other specific linguistic events that happened during the discourse task. For example:

- [/] for repetition (e.g., line 14 in Excerpt 3b)
- [//] for revision (e.g., line 02 in Excerpt 3c)
- & for simple events, such as &um and &mm (e.g., line 06 in Excerpt 3a)
- & for sound fragments or fillers, such as &s (e.g., line 09 in Excerpt 3a)
- +"/ and +" in combination for using a direct quotation, commonly found in a story-telling task (e.g., lines 03 and 06 in Excerpt 3c)
- [+ gram] for incomplete utterances due to agrammatic aphasic speech (e.g., line 04 in Excerpt 3a)

- [+ jar] for utterance level error coding of jargons (e.g., line 04 in Excerpt 3c)
- +.. for incomplete or interrupted utterances (e.g., line 05 in Excerpt 3b)
- www for untranscribed materials (e.g., line 07 in Excerpt 3a)

Also notice that a %mor line can be found below each speaker line. This line indicates the morphological annotation for the part-of-speech for each item on the speaker line. Some common part-of-speech codes include n for nouns (e.g., n | stroke), n:prop for proper nouns (e.g., n:prop | Maddie), v for verbs (e.g., v | hear), aux for auxiliaries (e.g., aux | have), det:num for numbers (e.g., det:num | nine), co for communicators (e.g., co | yes), det for determiners (e.g., det | a), coord for conjunctions (e.g., coord | and), prep for prepositions (e.g., prep | about), and pro for pronouns (e.g., pro | you). Suffixes are also attached to the word (e.g., -PAST for regular past as in v | have&PAST on line 11 in Excerpt 3b, or -PL for plural as in n | year-PL on line 05 in Excerpt 3a). A %exp tier can also be seen in Excerpt 3a (see line 07), which is used in conjunction with the www CHAT symbol to indicate material that a transcriber does not know how to transcribe, does not want to transcribe, or when a speaker says something that has no relevance to the interactions taking place that can be ignored. With the %exp tier, a transcriber can include some remarks in the transcript on what was happening during the time the discourse sample is collected. Additional annotations (and therefore tiers) can also be added to the transcriptions, such as error or syntax coding, depending on the level of detail one would like to include in the transcript. As illustrated, the detailed coding can further elaborate a transcript by highlighting the relevant linguistic and non-linguistic behaviors one would like to focus on for analysis.

Excerpt (3a)

01	★INV:	and do you remember your stroke?
	%mor:	coord | and mod | do pro | you v | remember pro:poss:det | your n | stroke?
02	★PAR:	&=head:yes yes.
	%mor:	co | yes.
03	★INV:	can you tell me what happened?
	%mor:	mod | can pro | you v | tell pro:obj | me pro:wh | what v | happen-PAST?
04	★PAR:	a long time ago . [+ gram]
	%mor:	det | a adj | long n | time adv | ago.
05	★PAR:	years and years. [+ gram]
	%mor:	n | year-PL coord | and n | year-PL.
06	★PAR:	five &um &um &um +..
	%mor:	det:num | five +..

07   *INV: www.
     %exp: the participant opens her notebook, to objections from
              both the offscreen supervisor and the investigator, who asks
              the participant not to write .
08   *PAR: okay .
     %mor: co|okay .
09   *INV: because we're [//] what we're looking for is <we want to>
              [/] &s we want to hear your language .
     %mor: Conj|because pro:wh|what pro:sub|we~aux|be&PRES
              part|look-PRESP prep|for |be&3S pro:sub|we v|want
              inf|to v|hear pro:poss:det|your n|language.

Excerpt (3b)

01   *INV: &um <do you> [//] did you have a stroke?
     %mor: mod|do&PAST pro|you v|have det|a n|stroke?
02   *PAR: &=head:yes yes.
     %mor: co|yes.
03   *INV: do you remember about it?
     %mor: mod|do pro|you v|remember prep|about pro|it?
04   *PAR: &um &=head:no no.
     %mor: co|no.
05   *PAR: &um my +..
     %mor: pro:poss:det|my +..
06   *PAR: let's see.
     %mor: v|let~pro:obj|us v|see.
07   *PAR: <do you want me to> [/] do you want me to +..?
     %mor: mod|do pro|you v|want pro:obj|me inf|to +..?
08   *PAR: okay.
     %mor: co|okay.
09   *INV: yeah go ahead and talk about it.
     %mor: co|yeah v|go adv|ahead coord|and n|talk prep|about
              pro|it.
10   *PAR: okay &um &=raises:hand well &=ges:high Florida. [+
              gram]
     %mor: co|okay co|well n:prop|Florida.
11   *PAR: &m and then &=points:over we had Bevard which was
              nine months.
     %mor: coord|and adv:tem|then pro:sub|we v|have&PAST
              n:prop|Bevard rel|which cop|be&PAST&13S
              det:num|nine n|month-PL.
12   *PAR: &=points:behind Ashville &=fingers:five five days stroke
              &=points:right_side. [+ gram]
     %mor: n:prop|Ashville det:num|five n|day-PL n|stroke.

13	*INV:	&mm.
14	*PAR:	and <I didn't> [/] &um I didn't +..
	%mor:	coord | and pro:sub | I mod | do&PAST~neg | not +..
15	*PAR:	well and that was +..
	%mor:	co | well coord | and pro:dem | that cop | be&PAST&13S +..
16	*PAR:	had my +..
	%mor:	v | have&PAST pro:poss:det | my +..
17	*PAR:	Jason is my &=points:self &um &huths husband.
	%mor:	n:prop | Jason cop | be&3S pro:poss:det | my n | husband.
18	*PAR:	and my &=fingers:two two girls Maddie and Story. [+ gram]
	%mor:	coord | and pro:poss:det | my det:num | two n | girl-PL n:prop | Maddie coord | and n:prop | Story.
19	*PAR:	and <they were> [/] <they were going away> [//] &= ges:airplane they're going a plane. [+ gram]
	%mor:	coord | and pro:sub | they~aux | be&PRES part | go-PRESP det | a n | plane.

Excerpt (3c)

01	*INV:	take a look at all of them and when you're ready tell me the story you see happening here with a beginning, a middle, and an end.
	%mor:	v | take det | a n | look prep | at qn | all prep | of pro:obj | them coord | and conj | when pro | you~cop | be&PRES adj | ready v | tell pro:obj | me det | the n | story pro | you v | see part | happen-PRESP adv | here prep | with det | a n | beginning cm | cm det | a n | middle cm | cm coord | and det | a n | end.
02	*PAR:	well he's [//] <a little> [//] another little boy is saying +..
	%mor:	co | well qn | another adj | little n | boy aux | be&3S part | say-PRESP +..
03	*PAR:	he's +"/.
	%mor:	pro:sub | he~cop | be&3S +"/.
04	*PAR:	+" &=head:no &=dismisses no no no I don't need it (.) to ʌst@u [: x@n] [* n:uk] the rain. [+ jar]
	%mor:	co | no co | no co | no pro:sub | I mod | do~neg | not v | need pro | it prep | to neo | x det | the n | rain.
05	*PAR:	or to the +..
	%mor:	coord | or prep | to det | the +..
06	*PAR:	and the mother is +"/.
	%mor:	coord | and det | the n | mother cop | be&3S +"/.
07	*PAR:	+" &=ges:umbrella please please.
	%mor:	co | please co | please.

08   *PAR: ask [//] &um has she brɛrə@u [: umbrella] [* n:k-ret]
                        [//] &b &u ʌbrɛlə@u [: umbrella] [* p:n-ret] [//]
                        umbrella. [+ gram]
       %mor: v|have&3S pro:sub|she n|umbrella.
09   *PAR: and the [//] they said.
       %mor: coord|and pro:sub|they v|say&PAST.
10   *PAR: and so the [//] they set out again +"/.
       %mor: coord|and co|so pro:sub|they v|set&ZERO adv|out
                        adv|again +"/.
11   *PAR: +" &=dismisses no we got it.
       %mor: co|no pro:sub|we v|get&PAST pro|it.
12   *PAR: +" no problem.
       %mor: qn|no n|problem.
13   *PAR: they have +..
       %mor: pro:sub|they v|have +..
14   *PAR: you_know <the sun is there> [//] the sun is out.
       %mor: co|you_know det|the n|sun cop|be&3S adv|out.
15   *PAR: and they've +..
       %mor: coord|and pro:sub|they~aux|have +..
16   *PAR: but &=points:picture_3 the little girl [//] no [//] guy [/]
                        guy (.) &um is +..
       %mor: conj|but det|the adj|little n|guy cop|be&3S +..
17   *PAR: &=ges:checking_for_rain his little (.) drip drip drop. [+
                        gram]
       %mor: pro:poss:det|his adj|little n|drip n|drip n|drop.
18   PAR: and then it was raining &=ges:downpour at [//] a &bu
                        &um bunch.
       %mor: coord|and adv:tem|then pro|it aux|be&PAST&13S
                        part|rain-PRESP det|a n|bunch.
19   *PAR: <when he's> [//] I mean he [//] he's [/] he's sopping.
       %mor: pro:sub|I v|mean pro:sub|he~aux|be&3S
                        part|sop-PRESP.

While the conventions for transcribing English language samples are quite well established, researchers working with speakers of other languages face unique challenges. (A more in-depth discussion about the consideration of discourse assessment and treatment for multilingual speakers or a culturally diverse population is given in Chapter 8.) To illustrate, an extract of describing the Cookie Theft picture by a bilingual English-Shanghainese speaker with logopenic variant primary progressive aphasia (see Hilger et al., 2014 and Ramsberger et al., 2014) is shown in Excerpt 4. Shanghainese, or the Hu dialect, is one of the dialects in the Chinese language family widely spoken in the city of Shanghai and the surrounding region. Each speaker line (*CLN for the clinician and *APH for the speaker with primary progressive aphasia) contains up to six layers. The use of multiple layers can facilitate the labelling of the following information:

1. main layer or speaker layer – orthographic transcription in simplified Chinese characters, each of the lexical items in the line was separated using a space, representing the original production spoken in Shanghainese
2. phon line – phonetic transcription for of each lexical item in the main line using Roman transliteration system adapted for Shanghainese
3. tran line – word-by-word English translation of the original lexical items in the main line
4. gloss-E – a brief notation written in English for the meaning of the utterance in the main line
5. gloss-C – a brief notation written in traditional Chinese characters with the same meaning corresponding to the gloss-E line
6. comm – comments or remarks by the transcriber during the transcription process (see line 05)

Note that square brackets are used for marking a transcriber's description of events or interpretation of the speaker's intention

Excerpt (4)

01	★CLN:	现在		是	上海		闲话.	
	phon	y'an z'ai	s'i	s'ang		hai ai wo		
	tran	Now	is	shanghai	leisure word			
	gloss-E	Now [it's time for] Shanghainese.						
	gloss-C	现在是(時候)說上海話了。						
02	★APH:	哎	我	講.				
	phon	Ai	ngwo	gang				
	tran	Aih	I	speak.				
	gloss-E	Um, I'll speak [Shanghainese].						
	gloss-C	哪我說了						
03	★CLN:	喏 先问问看张图片高头有啥事体.						
	phon	Nao xian meng zang d'u pian gao d'ou you sa s'i ti						
	tran	(starting filler to accompany pointing) first ask ask see this piece picture on have what matter						
	gloss-E	Now, first let me ask you what is happening in this picture.						
	gloss-C	現在，我先問問你，看看這張圖片裡面發生什麼事情?						
04	★APH:	呃	咽	女人	么.			
	phon	e	g'e	nü ningme				
	tran	(filler) this	woman (filler)					
	gloss-E	Er— for this woman mm—						
	gloss-C	這個女人						

05 ★APH: 叻啦 汏 盤 盤 哎 呃 汏
碗 碗 .

phon le la d'a b'uan b'uan ai e d'a
wuan wuan

tran Being wash dish dish (filler pause hesitating) wash
bowl bowl

gloss-E She is washing dishes dishes uh— er— wash bowls bowls
gloss-C 她在洗碗，碗，哎，在洗碗，碗
comm Number marking is not always obligatory in Chinese
and there is no marking in this Chinese text. There is
no information as to whether the best English rendition
would be singular or plural.

06 ★APH: 呃 水 么 .
phon e s'i' me
tran (filler) water (filler)
gloss-E er— water, mm—
gloss-C 呃，水

07 ★APH: 的个 自来水 滴 落 到 的个 地
浪 呃 .

phon d'i' ge z'i lai s'i' di' luo dao d'i' ge
d'i lang e

tran this self-coming-water drip down onto this floor
above (filler pause hesitating)

gloss-E The water is dripping onto the floor – uh—
gloss-C 這個自來水滴落到這個地上了。

08 ★APH: 伊 呢 叻浪 做 梦 呃 .
phon yi ne le lang zu mong e
tran She (filler) being make dreams (filler)
gloss-E She mm — is daydreaming uh—
gloss-C 她呢在作白日夢

Research Values and Clinical Use of Multi-Linear Transcriptions

An important feature of preparing a transcript is that one will need to make ongoing decisions at every step of the transcribing process (Müller et al., 2006). Apart from deciding the most appropriate task for eliciting a language sample and the best recording method to capture the performance, translating the spoken data to a written format requires careful interpretation of the speaker's action along the way. These interpretations can be more tricky and complicated if the speaker demonstrates multiple deficits that involve the verbal and non-verbal aspects of communication.

For decades, use of transcripts has been a common approach to investigate the language abilities and characteristics among typical healthy speakers encompassing a wide range of age as well as among individuals with deficits across various developmental and acquired language disorders (e.g., Marini et al., 2011; Wright & Capilouto, 2012). Clinically, we can use transcripts to visually present specific language features and symptoms that clinicians would like to address. With a sufficient amount and enough depth of information, a transcript can serve as the basis of further analysis. A multi-linear transcription should, in theory, contain more clinically relevant and important content, and thus becomes more powerful when it comes to assessment of discourse-specific deficits.

A good transcript should be accurate, meaning that it truly reflects a speaker's performance. It can become an important record of one's discourse activity at a given time, such as the time of an initial assessment or a particular point of a discourse treatment. An accurate transcript should contain the appropriate amount of detail required for subsequent analyses and the translated data should closely correspond to the original spoken data. A reader can therefore understand how a speaker has performed based on a transcript that is carefully prepared, without the need to meet an examinee face-to-face. A reliable transcript should also contain the least amount of ambiguity.

A good transcriber should be consistent in applying the same convention of transcribing spoken data across different speakers or different disorder groups. This is related to the intra-rater reliability of preparing a transcript. As expected, a transcriber's experience and previous training may affect the accuracy as well as consistency of the transcription process. However, when more than one transcriber is involved in the transcription process, we should aim for a good reliability across transcribers (or inter-rater reliability), so that the individual difference is minimal across those who contribute to a single transcript (or a set of transcripts in the case of establishing a database or an archive of language). The degree of inter-transcriber reliability is often evaluated using the percentage of agreement (or disagreement) using a subset of the whole dataset, such as 5% to 10% of the total amount of data (see Chapter 2 for more details on the computation method).

Methodologies for preparing a transcript have evolved over the past two decades. With the advance of technology and integration of research evidence, it is believed that more sophisticated frameworks of transcription that are also user-friendly and clinically feasible will continue to evolve. Nevertheless, one should keep in mind that transcribing is a complex process involving multiple levels of interpretation of communication behaviors on the part of the transcribers. Selection of the level of detail to be included in a transcript, which in turn will affect the use of layout for display, should be determined by the research or clinical agenda of those who will use the transcripts.

Levels of Annotations

At times, a researcher or a clinician may be more interested in one or more specific aspects of communication depending on the context of investigation.

These scenarios may typically be clinical observation or studies of language deficits, sampling of language impairments, or evaluation of discourse disorders. The purpose of this section is to provide readers with some basic guidelines for establishing a multi-linear representation of spoken discourse. The number of layers within a multi-linear transcript can be expanded as desired. Examples will also be given to illustrate selective transcription process.

Orthographic Records

Orthographic representation of connected speech is often considered to be the core of most linguistic analyses. In principle, all utterances produced by a speaker should be included in the transcript using the exact wording spoken. With the use of transcribed verbatim, a transcript should reflect the exact words recorded. Punctuation marks may still be used in most transcripts, but application of the regular rules of punctuation that govern conventional written text may not be as straightforward. This is especially the case for oral discourse, which is more colloquial and often contains spontaneous and acceptable behaviors of retracing, reformulations, or grammatically ill-formed sentences. Non-speech behaviors, such as hesitation noises, fillers, pauses, or silence, should not be excluded nor be replaced. Transcribers should also refrain from alternating or substituting any portion of the original speech. We may expect the use of non-standard features of speech and language in the disordered population; they can be captured by employing specific symbols in the transcript, such as parentheses for non-conventional lexical items. Finally, each speaker's turn should be chronologically numbered to facilitate any qualitative description of the language performance (Guendouzi & Müller, 2006).

If the transcript contains non-English languages, such as in the case of Excerpt 4 or when studying multi-lingual speakers with languages that are not written with Roman alphabets, the transcriber will need to decide the best way to represent these languages orthographically. Hepburn and Bolden (2013) suggested three options as follows:

1. Use the writing system of the target language (for languages that have a standard written form).
2. Use a standard phonetic system, such as the International Phonetic Alphabet (IPA) symbols. (Note that the most recent revision by the International Phonetic Association was carried out in 2015 and the latest version of the IPA symbols published can be found at: www.internationalphoneticassociation.org/content/ipa-chart). Downloadable IPA charts with different fonts (dated 2020 with updated copyright symbols), resolutions, formats, and sections of the whole chart can also be found

at: www.internationalphoneticassociation.org/IPAcharts/IPA_chart_
orig/IPA_charts_E.html.
3.   Use a Roman transliteration system adapted for the languages being
investigated.

A potential problem with option 1 is that users who have no prior knowledge about the non-English languages being investigated will not be able to
read and understand the transcript. As for option 2, its major strength is that
the use of IPA symbols is universally understood, but the IPA symbols may
not necessarily be universal among dictionaries for some languages. Input
of IPA symbols and their encoding in computers can also be a challenge
for some computer software. The last option has its advantages of being
relatively more accessible to native English speakers. When presenting non-
English data to an English-speaking reader, use of a multi-linear transcription is in order and therefore encouraged (e.g. Sidnell, 2009). For languages
that follow the English word order relatively closely, the transcript can be as
simple as a two-line transcription, one containing the orthographic representation of the original sample and another with glosses in idiomatic English.

In most cases, however, a common practice is to provide a three-line transcription (as in the examples of two conversations in Japanese and Korean in
Excerpts 5 and 6, respectively). The first line contains the orthographic transcription of the talk in the original language (see Excerpts 5a and 6a) or in
the orthography adopted for English (see Excerpts 5b and 6b). For example,
the top lines in Excerpt 6b display Korean romanized according to the Yale
system (Lee, 2006), representing actual sounds rather than standard orthography. The second line (gloss-morp) is a morpheme-by-morpheme English
gloss of the original items in the first line, which may include a combination of
word translations and grammatical information. Alternatively, an abbreviated
form of the grammatical words can be used. The third line (gloss-E) contains
information in the form of an idiomatic English gloss that can capture the
local and interactional meaning of the original script. The advantage of using a
three-layered transcript is that it allows a reader to better understand how each
utterance of the script unfolds at the word level. Such information is particularly useful when one examines languages that violate the conventional word
order in English, as in the case of Japanese and Korean we illustrate here.

Excerpt (5a)

01   A: 何   を   します   か?
     gloss-morp   what   (particle)   do   (question particle)
     gloss-E   Should we do something?
02   B: 動物園   に   行き   たい
     gloss-morp   zoo   (particle)   go   want
     gloss-E   (I) want to visit a zoo

03 B:　　　　　　私　は　　　　　動物　が　　　　　大　　好き
です

| gloss-morp | I (particle) animal (particle) very like (particle) |
| gloss-E | I love animals a lot. |

04 B:　　　　　　かわいい　です　　　から

| gloss-morp | cute (particle) because |
| gloss-E | Because (they are) cute |

Excerpt (5b)

01 A:　　　　　nani　o　　shimasu　ka?
gloss-morp　what　PRT　do　　　Q-PRT
gloss-E　　Should we do something?

02 B:　　　　　dobutsuen　ni　　iki　tai.
gloss-morp　zoo　　　　　PRT　go　want
gloss-E　　(I) want to visit a zoo

03 B:　　　　　watashi　wa　　dobutsu　ga　　dai　suki　desu.
gloss-morp　I　　　　PRT　animal　PRT　very　like　PRT
gloss-E　　I love animals a lot.

04 B:　　　　　kawai　desu　kara.
gloss-morp　cute　PRT　because
gloss-E　　Because (they are) cute

Excerpt (6a)

01 A:　　　　　안녕하세요.　이름　은　　　　무엇　입니
까?

| gloss-morp | hello name (particle) what is (question particle)? |
| gloss-E | Hello. What is your name? |

02 B:　　　　　저　는　　　켈리　입니다.
gloss-morp　I (particle) Kelly is
gloss-E　　My name is Kelly

03 B:　　　　　홍콩　　　에서　학생　　입니다.
gloss-morp　Hong-Kong　from　student　is
gloss-E　　(I am) a student from Hong Kong

Excerpt (6b)

01 A:　　　　　annyeonghaseyo　ileum　eun　mueos　ibni kka?
gloss-morp　hello　　　　　　name　PRT　what　is　Q-PRT?
gloss-E　　Hello. What is your name?

02	B:	jeo	neun	Kelly	ibnida.	
	gloss–morp	I	PRT	Kelly	is	
	gloss–E	My name is Kelly				
03	B:	Hong-Kong	eseo	hagsaeng	Ibnida.	
	gloss–morp	Hong-Kong	from	student	is	
	gloss–E	(I am) a student from Hong Kong				

A more condensed approach to represent multiple forms of information in one single layer is shown in Excerpt 7, which is an extract of a story-telling task of "The Hare and the Tortoise" by a Cantonese Chinese speaker with aphasia. Each item on the %mor line corresponds to the relevant item on the speaker line and contains information about morphological part-of-speech, phonetic transcription, and gloss in English. For example, in the ★mor item "v | teng1=listen" (line 01), the part-of-speech of verb and phonetic romanization "teng1"of the corresponding lexicon are indicated on the left and right side, respectively, of the " | "delimiter. Its morphemic gloss in English (to listen) is also given following the " = " sign. The gloss line further provides the overall meaning of each utterance of the transcript.

Excerpt (7)

01 ★CLN: 你 有 冇 聽 過 龜兔賽跑 嘅 故事 呀?
    %mor: pro | nei5=you v | jau5=have neg | mou2=not_have v | teng1=
    listen asp | gwo3=experience n:prop | gwai1tou3coi3paau2=
    the_tortoise_and_the_hare ptl | ge3=ptl n | gu3si6=story
    sfp | aa3=sfp?
    gloss: Have you heard of the story of "The Hare and the Tortoise"?
02 ★APH: 係.
    %mor: adv | hai6=yes.
    gloss: Yes
03 ★CLN: 噉 你 而家 <可> [/-] 可 唔 可以 試 吓 講 番 一 次 嗰 個
    故仔 俾 我 聽 呀?
    %mor: fil | gam2 pro | nei5=you adv | ji4gaa1=now aux | ho2=
    can neg | m4=not aux | ho2ji5=can v | si3=try asp | haa5=
    casual v | gong2=say ptl | faan1=ptl num | jat1=one cl | ci3=
    cl det | go2=that cl | go3=cl n | gu2zai2=story v | bei2=give
    pro | ngo5=I v | teng1=listen sfp | aa3=sfp?
    gloss: Can you try to tell me the story again?
04 ★APH: eh (.1) <一> [/-] 有 個 eh eh 白兔 同埋 eh eh 龜 嘅 <同>
    [/-] 同埋 佢 嗰 eh <喺>
    [/-] 喺 <樹> [/-] 樹林 eh 裡面 個 eh 好多 好多 eh <嗰
    啲> [/] 嗰 啲 eh (.1) <嗰 嗰> [/-] 嗰 啲 eh (.1) eh 動物
    eh 話 eh (.1) eh <搵> [/-] 搵 佢地 eh 兩 個 eh比賽.

%mor: fil|eh v|jau5=have cl|go3=cl fil|eh fil|eh n|baak6tou3=
          rabbit conj|tung4maai4=and fil|eh fil|eh n|gwai1=
          turtle ptl|ge3=ptl conj|tung4maai4=and pro|keoi5=it
          det|go2=that fil|eh prep|hai2=at n|syu6lam4=glade fil|eh
          loc|leoi5min6=inside cl|go3=cl fil|eh quant|hou2do1=
          much quant|hou2do1=much fil|eh det|go2=that cl|di1=
          some fil|eh det|go2=that cl|di1=some fil|eh fil|eh
          n|dung6mat6=animal fil|eh v|waa6=say fil|eh fil|eh
          v|wan2=find pro|keoi5dei6=they fil|eh num|loeng5=two
          cl|go3=cl fil|eh v|bei2coi3=to_compete_with.

gloss: there is a rabbit and a tortoise. And there are a lot of animals
          in the wood. The animals asked them to have a race.

05 *APH: <噉> [/-] eh 噉 <咽 個> [/] 咽 個 eh 白兔 同埋 eh eh
           (1.) eh 龜 eh eh <地> [?]
           <開頭> [/] 開頭 呢 咽 個 白兔 eh eh 好 快 eh 可以 eh
           <個> [/-] 噉呢 佢 就 eh <去> [/-] 去 到 eh 咁上下 呢 佢
           就 eh 特登 <喺> [/-] 喺 咽度 eh 等 佢.

%mor: fil|eh fil|gam2 det|go2=that cl|go3=cl fil|eh
          n|baak6tou3=rabbit conj|tung4maai4=and fil|eh
          fil|eh fil|eh n|gwai1=turtle fil|eh fil|eh n|dei6=floor
          adv|hoi1tau4=in_the_beginning fil|ne1 det|go2=that
          cl|go3=cl n|baak6tou3=rabbit fil|eh fil|eh adv|hou2=very
          adj|faai2=quick fil|eh aux|ho2ji5=can fil|eh fil|gam2ne1
          pro|keoi5=it fil|zau6 fil|eh v|heoi3=go v|dou3=arrive
          fil|eh adv|gam3soeng6haa2=nearlyfil|ne1 pro|keoi5=it
          fil|zau6 fil|eh adv|dak6dang1=deliberately prep|hai2=at
          pro|go2dou6=there fil|eh v|dang2=wait pro|keoi5=it.

gloss: The rabbit and the tortoise. The rabbit was faster at first, but
          after a while... But (the tortoise) stopped to wait for him
          (the rabbit).

Segmental and Supra-Segmental Records

To record the segmental features in a transcript, one should pay attention to the phonetic details of the speech being annotated. In general, a phonetic segment should include a portion of speech with relatively constant phonetic features, i.e., phonological units of a language sample that are usually short in duration, such as vowels or consonants. Phonetic segments are combined to form a syllable. Simply using ordinary orthography to represent the range of pronunciation patterns that we encounter in the clinical population is insufficient. Most researchers will agree that orthographic convention of English is inadequate to display the phonetic distortion caused by speech impairments or deficits. Therefore, a transcriber should employ phonetic transcriptions to record the impaired pronunciation patterns identified in a language sample. In other words, transcribing the segmental level of speech provides users of the resultant transcript with important information about the phonology of an examinee. A standard methodology adopted by speech-and-language therapists is using the IPA symbols to conduct a phonetic transcription, with special attention to the following five principles (Ball, 2006). While consonants are considered with reference to the place and manner of articulation, vowels are considered using parameters of the tongue height and position and lip shape.

1. A single sound is represented by using one IPA symbol.
2. Any one sound can only be transcribed by one IPA symbol.
3. All single sounds in a language sample are denoted by single IPA symbols.
4. All sound combinations in a language sample are denoted by combined IPA symbols.
5. The full set of IPA symbols should cover contrastive sounds of all the world's languages.

Notice that a set of extended IPA (extIPA) symbols for disordered speech (Ball et al., 2018), recently updated in 2015, is available at www.internationalphoneticassociation.org/sites/default/files/extIPA_2016.pdf. Examples of using the extIPA symbols can be found in Excerpt 3c, i.e., in the case of phonemic paraphasia on line 08 ("umbrella" /ʌmˈbrɛlə/ → [brɛɾə] or [ʌbrɛlə]) or in the case of a jargon on line 04 /ʌst/. Hence, an accurate phonetic transcription, with the use of IPA and extIPA symbols lined up with the relevant parts of the orthographic transcription, can be clinically important because it facilitates the subsequent analysis of the language samples in terms of the patterns of the disordered speech demonstrated by a speaker. More sensitive and effective remediation of the speech problems can then be addressed.

Supra-segmental features of speech largely refer to the combined phenomena of intonation pattern of speech, speed of speaking, and loudness of output. Ideally, separating the supra-segmental from the segmental layer to form a multi-linear transcript can best represent the interaction among various level of speech production (Rahilly, 2006). In particular, speech intonation can be further annotated relative to its tone (or pitch patterns used), prominence (or the markedness of syllables of in terms of pitch, length, and loudness), and segmentation (or the division of speech into relevant units) of the speech signal. For example, the IPA convention for characterizing level and contour tones and word accent can be applied as one of the multi-layered representations:

- Level
  - extra high
  - high
  - mid
  - low
  - extra low
  - downstep
  - upstep
- Contour
  - rising
  - falling
  - high rising
  - low rising
  - rising-falling
  - global rise
  - global fall

Together with other additional information, such as the stress and length of syllable segments, a transcript will reflect aspects of speech characteristics other than individual articulation of speech sounds, which will have significant clinical implications on indicating how well a speaker can make relevant linguistic and communicative distinctions. Note that many of these supra-segmental features are inherently tied to the segmental level of speech production, but some of them can be independent from the segmental content and convey information on their own.

The phonological patterns of speech intonation can be illustrated using the "tadpole" notation method described by Tench (1996). Excerpts 8a to 8c indicate three intonation patterns with different emphases of the phrase "Ken wants the apple". The first line contains information about the timing of speech, and the third line displays the orthographic transcriptions of the output. The second line indicates the pitch shape of the utterance, with the dot representing the location of the segment of prominent syllable. Tench (1996) defined this dot as the nucleus of the utterance. The pitch range of the utterance is represented by the highest and lowest point of the line. In Excerpt 8a, the prominence is located in the initial syllable of the utterance, emphasizing Ken, instead of someone else, wants the apple. The intonation in Excerpt 8b represents a neutral statement as the location of prominence is at the end of the utterance. In Excerpt 8c, the prominence occurs at the segment when the action word "wants" is spoken. With the question contour at the end of the utterance, the prominence in this position can imply the indirect meaning of questioning if Ken really wants the apple.

Excerpt (8a)

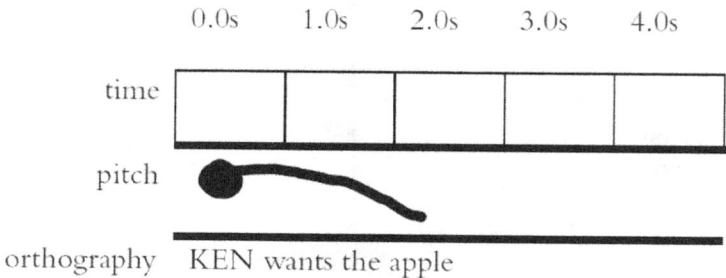

| 0.0s | 1.0s | 2.0s | 3.0s | 4.0s |

time

pitch

orthography   KEN wants the apple

Excerpt (8b)

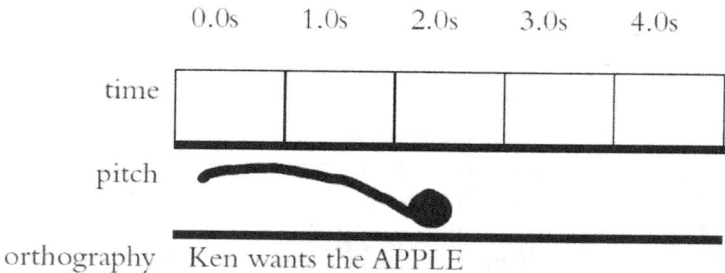

| 0.0s | 1.0s | 2.0s | 3.0s | 4.0s |

time

pitch

orthography   Ken wants the APPLE

Excerpt (8c)

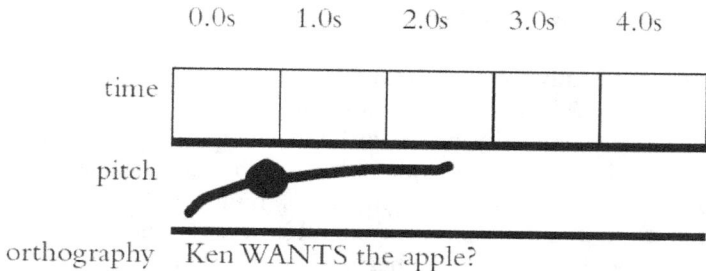

| 0.0s | 1.0s | 2.0s | 3.0s | 4.0s |

time

pitch

orthography   Ken WANTS the apple?

In English, the prosody of segmental unit final or utterance final is an important pragmatic indicator. Therefore, annotation of final intonation contours can be important for a speech transcript. This is more apparent in analyses such as Conversation Analysis (CA; see also Chapter 3) because the final prosody carries clinically relevant information on how well a turn is completed or accomplished (Hepburn & Bolden, 2013). Conventional punctuation marks can be used to represent the utterance final intonation (e.g., Drew, 2013; Raymond, 2009). For example, in Excerpt 9, an extract of telling the Cinderella story by a speaker with aphasia (PAR), utterance final intonation is marked as follows:

- . – a period to indicate a falling intonation contour (lines 03, 08, and 20)
- _ – an underscore to indicate a level intonation at the end of a turn (lines 01 and 04)
- ? – a question mark to indicate a rising intonation (line 21)
- , – a comma to indicate a slightly rising intonation, but not necessarily to mark the continuation of speaking (the middle of lines 07 and 08)
- ¿ or ?, – an inverted question mark or a question mark followed by a comma to indicate a pitch rise at the level between a comma and a question mark (lines 05 and 06)

Excerpt (9)

01	PAR:	the son of the king_
02		(1s)
03	PAR:	he is dancing her the young girl.
04	PAR:	and really. uh. she likes, he likes her really_
05	INV:	anything else?
06	PAR:	and all of a sudden twelve o'clock¿
07	PAR:	she's leav, she's gotta get home¿
08	PAR:	she's gotta be, um. it. She's gonna go back to what it was.
:		
:		
20	PAR:	so he's out in the hou, in the, in the, in the town checking everybody.
21	PAR:	did it foot, fit on the woman on the, on the shoe?

Tempo is related to the overall speed of the utterance, which can be affected by the length of pausing and the number of syllables per unit of time within a speech sample. Loudness, on the other hand, is related to the speech intensity. To indicate some form of stress or emphasis by increased volume (or pitch, or both), use of underlining, such as "What?", or upper-case letters, such as "Okay. STOP!", can be considered. Terminology used in notating music is also borrowed from the extIPA system and adopted for transcribing both speech tempo and loudness, as follows:

- Tempo
  - (.) for short pause
  - (..) medium pause
  - (...) long pause
  - allegro for fast speech
  - lento for slow speech

- Loudness
    - f, or forte, for loud speech
    - ff, or fortissimo, for louder speech
    - p, or piano, for quiet speech
    - pp, or pianissimo, for quieter speech
    - diminuendo for a gradual decrease in speech loudness
    - crescendo for a gradual increase in speech loudness

In terms of marking the voice quality using the IPA and/or extIPA diacritic symbols in a transcript, some researchers have argued that this information can inform readers about the speaker's mood or physical state (e.g., Crystal, 1997) but can be optional in language analyses. This is due to its lack of direct connection with the semantics or content of speech. Although voice quality is considered as a paralinguistic feature of spoken language, additional guidelines for grading voice quality are given in Ball et al. (1999) on their description of the Voice Quality Symbols (VoQs). Excerpt 10 is an example of representing various segmental and supra-segmental features of connected speech proposed by Rahilly (2006).

Excerpt (10)

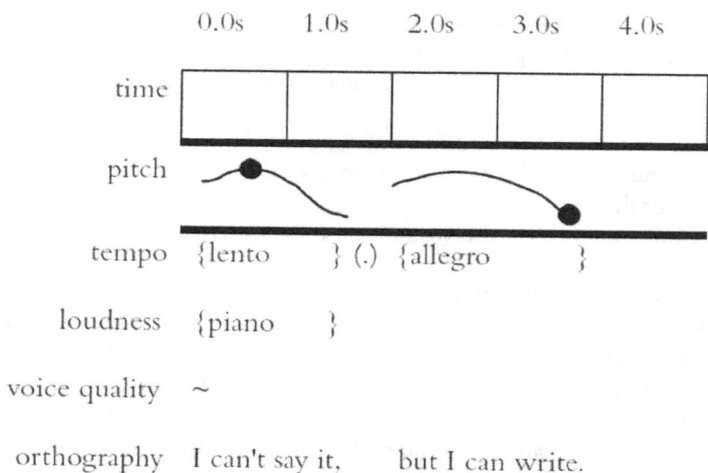

It is worth mentioning that approximately 4% of the world's languages are tonal languages, including Chinese, Thai, and Vietnamese (Maddieson, 2013). A unique feature of tonal languages is that pitch variations, which are expressed in tones, are phonemic in nature that change word meanings. In other words, tonal changes involve the use of pitch patterns to distinguish individual words or the grammatical forms of words. This is in contrast to its pragmatic function as they are in English mentioned above.

Consistent with the earlier discussion about tone in English, a syllable of a tonal language may have its own tonal pattern, which may be a relatively flat pitch at a particular level or may involve a contour tone where the pitch rises or falls over the duration of the syllable. For example, in Mandarin Chinese (or Putonghua), the syllable "ma" has four different meanings depending on tone (Tone 1 – high level: 媽 "mother," Tone 2 – mid rising: 麻 "numb," Tone 3 – mid falling then rising:馬 "horse," and Tone 4 – High falling: 罵 "to scold"). In Cantonese Chinese, there are six different meanings for syllable "si" (Tone 1 – high level: 師 "master," Tone 2 – mid rising: 史 "history," Tone 3 – mid level: 試 "examination," Tone 4 – low falling: 時 "time," Tone 5 – low rising: 市 "market," and Tone 6 – low level: 是 "yes"). When combined with the coda –k, the syllable "sik" has an additional three meanings with three different entering tones of tones 7 to 9: 色 "color," 惜 "worried," and 食 "to eat"). While tone 1 of Mandarin and tones 1, 3, and 6 of Cantonese are level tones, the others are contour tones. Because earlier transcription systems were developed for English, which is a non-tonal language, there is no one standard way to represent tones in a transcript. Lexical tones may be represented using a number system. See example of Cantonese in Excerpt 7 to represent tones using numbers within the phonetic romanization of individual lexicons.

Records of Non-Verbal Behaviors

Recognizing that communication is a complex process that often involves the use of non-verbal behaviors, one would agree that characterizing a speaker's language on just the verbal aspects can be inadequate and, in some cases, misleading. To illustrate, the compensatory role that gestures play in communication among speakers with aphasia has been reported (e.g., Lanyon & Rose, 2009; Rose & Douglas, 2001). Individuals with different types and degrees of aphasia may also exhibit various patterns and frequencies of using co-verbal gestures accompanying spoken discourse (Kong et al., 2017; Kong et al., 2019). Speakers with acquired language disorders also have a tendency to use eye gaze within a clinical (assessment or treatment) session to seek for assistance from individuals other than the clinician or to act as a compensatory strategy for re-establishing a communicative turn (Oelschlaeger & Damico, 1998). As a result of the impaired language ability caused by aphasia, employment of gestures to replace lexical items within a spoken sentence or to assist the flow of oral communication is clinically very common. In some cases, use of non-verbal social actions can facilitate the initiation or maintenance of communicative interactions. A proper documentation, interpretation, and analysis of the use of non-verbal communication strategies can undoubtedly enhance our understanding of a speaker's social and communicative effectiveness during the use of oral discourse. In addition, how well the speaker can accomplish and coordinate social actions during a face-to-face conversation, when systematically represented on a transcript, can facilitate the examination of the interaction between the use of verbal and non-verbal language among different interlocutors, including both the healthy and language-impaired populations.

A number of parameters on annotating speech-accompanying non-verbal behaviors, including eye gaze, facial expressions, gestures, and body postures, have been proposed. Given that these behaviors commonly overlap with each other and/or with spoken language, various methods have been reported to offer suggestions or guidelines for transcribing them. Goodwin (1980, 1981) has suggested some systematic procedures and a coding scheme to capture the mutual orientation among different interlocutors of a verbal interaction, including a speaker, a recipient, and a listener. For example, in a situation of clinical evaluation, a speaker can be the language-impaired person, a recipient is the clinician who is conducting a narrative task, and a listener can be the family member or spouse of the speaker.

An example of representing the behaviors of eye gaze in oral discourse is given in Excerpt 11a, which is an extract of a conversation between a clinician (*INV) and a speaker with aphasia (*PAR) discussing the PAR's perception of his language abilities. Note that a line is placed below the main utterance line of orthographic transcription to indicate a recipient's gaze toward the speaker. The absence of such a line indicates that the recipient has directed the gaze elsewhere. A letter X is used to connect to the speaker line using a bracket sign to mark the precise point at which the recipient's gaze reaches the speaker. Therefore, as indicated in line 02, the person with aphasia shifted the gaze that was originally towards the clinician before he laughed.

Excerpt (11a)

```
01   *INV:   I'm gonna be asking you to do some talking.
             [x-------------------------------------------
02   *PAR:   oh yeah definitely &=laughs.
             [x---------------- [ x--------
```

An adapted version of the above transcription method was reported by Damico and Simmons-Mackie (2006) where they suggested the use of four useful symbols to transcribe gaze and gestures:

1. x------x to indicate the maintenance of a gaze
2. ,,, to indicate a shift of a gaze from one direction to another
3. adding interlocutor information on the line in (1) to indicate the specific gaze direction
4. (( )) to indicate the use of gestures noted

Simply referring to Excerpt 11a alone, one may not readily notice that the conversation between the clinician and speaker with aphasia was recorded in the presence of the caregiver (C). Such information can be found in line 02 of Excerpt 11b, which is an extension of the same extract in Excerpt 11a. Specifically, each orthography line now contains two x---x lines, with the one above indicating the gaze of the speaker towards the recipient and vice versa for the one below. An asterisk is used in this section to indicate more clearly who the speaker is on each line. Line 02 shows that when the speaker with aphasia laughed, he actually shifted the gaze towards the caregiver. A gesture was used on line 04 when the speaker with aphasia was expressing his perception of using language to communicate. Moreover, line 08 displays how both the speaker with aphasia and clinician shifted the gaze to the caregiver, but at different time with reference to the speech content. The manner in which interlocutors are oriented to the turn during a conversation can be better specified with this approach.

EXCERPT (11B)

```
              x---------PAR-------------------------x
01  *INV:  I'm gonna be asking you to do some talking.
    PAR:   x---------INV-----------------------x
              x---------INV----,,,-------x
02  *PAR:  oh yeah definitely &=laughs.
    INV:   x---------PAR---,,,---C--x
                 x-----------PAR---------------x
03  *INV:  how do you think your speech is these days?
    PAR:   x---------INV-------------------------x
           x---INV---((ges:so_so))---x
04  *PAR:  mm (1s) like okay I guess.
    INV:   x--------PAR-----------x
           x-PAR--x
05  *INV:  okay?
    PAR    x-INV--x
           x-INV--x
06  *PAR:  yeah.
    INV    x-PAR--x
           x-----PAR---------x
07  *INV:  can you say any more?
    PAR    x-----INV---------x
           x--------INV---,,,----C---------------------x
08  *PAR:  I guess um (2s) like whenever I'm talking it's okay.
    INV:   x--------PAR--------------,,,---C--------------x
```

Transcriber's Comments or Queries

Those who have experience transcribing disordered speech will understand how difficult it can be when working with samples containing a high proportion of unintelligible or dysfluent speech. A similar degree of difficulty applies to audio or video files with high level of interference from room or background noise or with recorder malfunction.

If a transcriber is uncertain about what he or she hears or has queries about a particular sample unit, the "best guess" can still be included in the transcript, but the use of a specific coding to indicate uncertainty that involves the transcriber's "best guess" or a remark or comment from the transcriber must be included (see lines 02 and 03 in Excerpt 12). In addition, a transcriber's description of events that are present in the sample but unrelated to the discourse task can be included in a "comment" or "remark" line, rather than representing them in the main lines of a transcript (see the comm tier in lines 04 and 05 of Excerpt 12). Hepburn and Bolden (2013) have suggested the use of single and double parentheses to represent the above in a transcript as follows: single parentheses to be used in main tiers to indicate a transcriber's "best guess" and double parentheses to be used in the comm tiers to elaborate what was happening during the discourse task.

EXCERPT (12)

```
01   *INV:   can you tell me what you remember about that day?
02   *PAR:   uh e uh and uh /hɑspəlɪd/ (hospital) /hɑbəlɪd/ (hospital).
03   *PAR:   and uh the you know wa walkin(g) (waking) up.
04   *PAR:   and uh work              I can't hear.
     comm                  ((phone rings))
05   *PAR:   here                         uh y you know.
     comm              ((PAR points to own legs))
```

Use of Web-Accessible Archiving Software

The process of performing transcription and conducting manual analyses of discourse samples is extremely time-consuming and often unreliable. A number of computational tools, some freely downloadable from individual developers' websites and some requiring a license fee, have been designed to increase the reliability of transcriptions and automate the process of data analysis. With the use of computerized procedures, the final transcripts obtained using these products can greatly enhance data consistency and facilitate the sharing of transcript data. In this section, a number of software programs are introduced. Readers who are interested in learning more about these tools or in using these products should refer to the corresponding developers.

CHILDES (Child Language Data Exchange System)

The Child Language Data Exchange System (CHILDES) was first established by Brian MacWhinney for researching child language acquisition. A number of empirical studies of child language production and the majority of theoretical papers on language development that make reference to production data are now based on the use and analysis of data from this CHILDES database. The system provides users access to the Computerized Language Analysis (CLAN) program that can perform automated computation of linguistic analyses of transcripts in the CHAT (Codes for the Human Analysis of Talk) transcription format. More information about CHILDES can be found at https://childes.talkbank.org/. Since 2007, the CHILDES has been applied to transcription and analysis of discourse samples from individuals with aphasia (see MacWhinney et al., 2011). For example, MacWhinney et al. (2010) illustrated the use of CLAN to perform automated analysis of the lexical frequency and error production in a Cinderella story-retelling task. Performance on lexical diversity of a group of 25 speakers with aphasia was compared with 25 healthy adults, and the top ten nouns and verbs across both groups were computed. It was found that the aphasic group had a greater use of light verbs and a marked reduction in lexical diversity. The AphasiaBank website at https://aphasia.talkbank.org/ is the primary source for all AphasiaBank related materials, including transcripts, videos, computer programs, manuals, and transcript training. In addition, comparable databases on dementia (https://dementia.talkbank.org/), traumatic brain injury (https://tbi.talkbank.org/), right hemisphere damage (https://rhd.talkbank.org/), and conversations between adults (CABank) (https://ca.talkbank.org/) are also available.

Aiming to help make the discourse analysis process more efficient and reliable among clinical researchers and practitioners, Fromm, Forbes et al. (2020) have recently discussed and illustrated the use of the CLAN program to perform automated analyses of discourse. Advanced tools to automatically compute measures from the Quantitative Production Analysis (QPA; see details in Chapter 4) can readily reflect aspects of language production (or deficits), in both the context of clinical research and assessment/treatment evaluation. Easy comparison of linguistic discourse performance is also made possible of any given individual with aphasia to that of a large reference database of speakers with and without aphasia. The authors also highlighted the additional discourse measurement tools offered on the TalkBank System (https://talkbank.org/), including Main Concept Analysis (MCA; see Chapter 3), core lexicon checklists, and correct information unit computation techniques.

Another related study was published by Fromm, MacWhinney, and Thompson (2020) who compared the Northwestern Narrative Language

Analysis (NNLA) of spontaneous speech samples, based on the original hand-coding method, with a newly proposed automated processing using CLAN. In particular, 18 manually coded NNLA transcripts (eight from people with aphasia and ten from controls) were converted into CHAT files for compatibility with CLAN commands. Computation of 50 new CLAN-NNLA measures (translated from the original NNLA manual) was carried out to automatically obtain lexical, morphological, utterance-level, sentence-level, and verb argument structure measures. The results revealed that 46 out of the 50 automated CLAN-NNLA measures (i.e., except for six measures focusing on verb argument) did not differ significantly from those generated by the original manual coding. Hence, this quantification of grammatical deficits in aphasia was claimed to be a fast, replicable, and accessible option for researchers and clinicians, without the need for extensive linguistic knowledge and training.

Systematic Analysis of Language Transcripts (SALT)

Systematic Analysis of Language Transcripts (SALT) is a computer software that manages the process of eliciting, transcribing, and analyzing spoken language samples. Used mainly in the field of child language development and disorders, clinicians can collect representative language samples and compare clients' transcripts with age or grade-matched typical speakers. The software allows users to generate measures that reflect the syntax, semantics, discourse, rate, fluency, and errors of a discourse. A number of studies have used the SALT in the adult population with acquired language disorders, such as Holland (1982) and Szaflarski et al. (2008). More information about the SALT can be found at www.saltsoftware.com/.

Python and the Natural Language Toolkit (NLTK)

The Natural Language Toolkit (NLTK) is one of the Python programs (www.python.org/) that allows users to work with human language data (Bird et al., 2009). It provides interfaces to extract information from an unstructured text and to analyze linguistic structure in a text (including word classification, tokenization, stemming, tagging, parsing, and semantic analysis/reasoning). It contains corpora and lexical resources (e.g., WordNet) and open source text processing tools and libraries for different tasks of natural language processing (NLP) (see Chapter 4 for details). More information about NLTK can be found at www.nltk.org/.

Praat

Praat is a computer program developed by Paul Boersma and David Weenink that offers a wide range of standard and non-standard procedures for transcribing, analyzing, and manipulating samples of speech signals.

Specifically, it has been widely used for transcription at the segmental (e.g., speech segmentation) and supra-segmental levels of discourse samples. Subsequent processing of speech samples can be conducted using spectral analysis (i.e., spectrograms), pitch analysis, formant analysis, intensity analysis, and so on. More information about Praat can be found at www.fon.hum.uva.nl/praat/.

EUDICO Linguistic Annotator (ELAN)

The EUDICO Linguistic Annotator (ELAN), developed by the Max Planck Institute for Psycholinguistics, is a computerized annotation software that allows the creation, visualization, editing, and searching of annotations for audio and video data. It has been widely used for the annotation, quantification, analysis, and documentation of oral language as well as gesture employment in healthy and disordered populations. The ELAN supports the display of speech and/or video signals that synchronize with linguistic annotations.

In the past decade, the ELAN has mainly been used to code conversational gestures among normal speakers. The tool is found to be objective and effective in displaying co-verbal gestures and in performing analyses of communicative gestures during speech tasks. A number of studies have also reported the use of the ELAN to study gestural behaviors (see review by Newman et al., 2011), including gesture kinetics and functions in typical speakers (Lausberg & Sloetjes, 2009), the overlap between and synchronization of hand gestures and mouth action by individuals using sign langauge (Bank et al., 2011), and co-verbal gestures in speakers with aphasia (e.g., Kong et al., 2015). More information about the ELAN can be found at https://archive.mpi.nl/tla/elan.

Conclusions

This chapter has provided guidelines for preparing multi-linear transcriptions of disordered language samples. The procedures on performing transcriptions specific to various levels of oral discourse that will facilitate the subsequent analytic process of discourse impairment were also illustrated. We have discussed the use of multi-layered annotations to unify information on the linguistic and paralinguistic aspects within verbal communications as well as non-verbal skills co-occurring in a spoken narrative. The content should equip researchers and clinicians with sufficient fundamental knowledge to deal with the complex nature of discourse production.

References

Ball, M. J. (2006). Transcribing at the segmental level. In N. Müller (Ed.), *Multilayered transcription* (pp. 41–67). San Diego, CA: Plural Publishing.

Ball, M. J., Esling, J., & Dickson, C. (1999) Transcription of voice. In R. D. Kent & M. J. Ball (Eds.), *Voice quality measurement* (pp. 49–58). San Diego, CA: Singular Publishing Group.

Ball, M. J., Howard, S. J., & Miller, K. (2018). Revisions to the extIPA chart. *Journal of the International Phonetic Association, 48*, 155–164. https://doi.org/10.1017/S0025100317000147

Bank, R., Crasborn, O., & van Hout, R. (2011). Variation in mouth actions with manual signs in Sign Language of the Netherlands (NGT). *Sign Language & Linguistics, 14*(2), 248–270.

Berndt, R., Wayland, S., Rochon, E., Saffran, E., & Schwartz, M. (2000). *Quantitative production analysis: A training manual for the analysis of aphasic sentence production.* Hove, UK: Psychology Press.

Bird, S., Klein, E., & Loper, E. (2009). *Natural language processing with Python: Analyzing text with the natural language toolkit.* Sebastopol, CA: O'Reilly Media, Inc.

Crystal, D. (1997). *A dictionary of phonetics and linguistics.* Oxford: Whurr Publishers.

Damico, J. C., & Simmons-Mackie, N. (2006). Transcribing gaze and gesture. In N. Müller (Ed.), *Multilayered transcription* (pp. 93–111). San Diego, CA: Plural Publishing.

Drew, P. (2013). Turn design. In J. Sidnell, & T. Stivers (Eds.), *The handbook of conversation analysis* (pp. 131–149). Oxford: Wiley-Blackwell.

Fromm, D., Forbes, M., Holland, A., & MacWhinney, B. (2020). Using AphasiaBank for discourse assessment. *Seminars in Speech and Language, 41*(1), 10–19.

Fromm, D., MacWhinney, B., & Thompson, C. K. (2020). Automation of the Northwestern Narrative Language Analysis System. *Journal of Speech, Language, and Hearing Research, 63*(6), 1835–1844.

Goodwin, C. (1980). Restarts, pauses, and the achievement of mutual gaze at turn-beginning. *Sociological Inquiry, 50*(3–4), 272–302.

Goodwin, C. (1981). *Conversational organization: Interaction between speakers and hearers.* New York: Academic Press.

Guendouzi, J. A., & Müller, N., (2006). Orthographic transcription. In N. Müller (Ed.), *Multilayered transcription* (pp. 19–39). San Diego, CA: Plural Publishing.

Hepburn, A. & Bolden, G. (2013). The conversation analytic approach to transcription. In J. Sidnell, & T. Stivers (Eds.), *The handbook of conversation analysis* (pp. 57–76). Oxford: Wiley-Blackwell.

Hilger, A., Ramsberger, G., Gilley, P., Menn, L., & Kong, A. P. H. (2014). Analysing speech problems in a longitudinal case study of logopenic variant PPA. *Aphasiology, 28*(7), 840–861.

Holland, A. (1982). Remarks on observing aphasic people. In Clinical Aphasiology Conference (Ed.), *Clinical aphasiology conference* (pp. 1–3). Minneapolis: BRK Publishers.

Kong, A. P. H., Law, S.-P., & Chak, G. W.-C. (2017). A comparison of co-verbal gesture use in oral discourse among speakers with fluent and non-fluent aphasia. *Journal of Speech, Language, and Hearing Research, 60*, 2031–2046.

Kong, A. P. H., Law, S. P., & Cheung, C. K.-Y. (2019). Use of co-verbal gestures during word-finding difficulty among Cantonese speakers with fluent aphasia and unimpaired controls. *Aphasiology, 33*(2), 216–233.

Kong, A. P. H., Law, S.-P., Kwan, C. C .Y., Lai, C., & Lam, V. (2015). A coding system with independent annotations of gesture forms and functions during verbal communication: Development of a Database of Speech and GEsture (DoSaGE). *Journal of Nonverbal Behavior, 39*(1), 93–111.

Kong, A. P. H., Reres, A., & Whiteside, J. (2014, November 20–22). *Analysis of macro-linguistic structures in narrative discourse of aphasia* [Poster presentation]. The 2014 American Speech-Language-Hearing Association (ASHA) Convention, Orlando, FL, USA.

Lanyon, L., & Rose M. L. (2009). Do the hands have it? The facilitation effects of arm and hand gesture on word retrieval in aphasia. *Aphasiology, 23*, 809–822.

Lausberg, H., & Sloetjes, H. (2009). Coding gestural behavior with the NEUROGES-ELAN system. *Behavior Research Methods, 41*(3), 841–849.

Lee, S. H. (2006). Second summonings in Korean telephone conversation openings. *Language in Society, 35*, 261–283.

MacWhinney, B. (2000). *The CHILDES Project: Tools for analysing talk* (3rd ed.). Mahwah, NJ: Lawrence Erlbaum Associates Inc.

MacWhinney, B., Fromm, D., Forbes, M., & Holland, A. (2011). AphasiaBank: Methods for studying discourse. *Aphasiology, 25*(11), 1286–1307.

MacWhinney, B., Fromm, D., Holland, A., Forbes, M., & Wright, H. (2010). Automated analysis of the Cinderella story. *Aphasiology, 24*(6–8), 856–868.

Maddieson, I. (2013). Tone. In M. S. Dryer, & M. Haspelmath (Eds.), *The world atlas of language structures online*. Leipzig: Max Planck Institute for Evolutionary Anthropology.

Marini, A., Andreetta, S., del Tin, S., & Carlomagno, S. (2011). A multi-level approach to the analysis of narrative language in aphasia. *Aphasiology, 25*, 1372–1392.

Müller, N., Damico, J. S., & Guendouzi, J. A. (2006). What is transcription, and why should we do it? In N. Müller (Ed.), *Multilayered transcription* (pp. 1–18). San Diego, CA: Plural Publishing.

Newman, J., Baayen, H., & Rice, S. (2011). *Corpus-based studies in language use, language learning, and language documentation*. New York, NY: Rodopi.

Oelschlaeger, M., & Damico, J. S. (1998). Joint productions as a conversational strategy in aphasia. *Clinical Linguistics and Phonetics, 12*, 459–480.

Rahilly, J. (2006). Transcribing at the suprasegmental level. In N. Müller (Ed.), *Multilayered transcription* (pp. 69–91). San Diego, CA: Plural Publishing.

Ramsberger, G., Kong, A. P. H., & Menn, L. (2014, October 5–7). *Speech deterioration in an English-Shanghainese Speaker with Logopenic Variant Primary Progressive Aphasia* [Poster presentation]. Fifty-second Annual Meeting of Academy of Aphasia, Miami, FL, USA.

Raymond, G. (2009). Grammar and social relations: Alternative forms of yes/no type initiating actions in health visitor interactions. In A. F. Freed & S. Ehrlich (Eds.), *Why do you ask?: The function of questions in institutional discourse* (pp. 69–107). Oxford: Oxford University Press.

Reres, A., Kong, A. P. H., & Whiteside, J. (2014, October 5–7). *Proposing a clinical quantification framework of macro-linguistic structures in aphasic narratives* [Poster presentation]. Fifty-second Annual Meeting of Academy of Aphasia, Miami, FL, USA.

Rose, M., & Douglas, J. (2001). The differential facilitatory effects of gesture and visualization processes on object naming in aphasia. *Aphasiology, 15*, 977–990.

Saffran, E. M., Berndt, R. S., & Schwartz, M. F. (1989). The quantitative analysis of agrammatic production: Procedure and data. *Brain and Language, 37*, 440–479.

Sidnell, J. (2009). *Conversation analysis: Comparative perspectives*. Cambridge: Cambridge University Press.

Szaflarski, J. P., Ball, A., Grether, S., Al-fwaress, F., Griffith, N. M., Neils-Strunjas, J., Newmeyer, A., & Reichhardt, R. (2008). Constraint-induced aphasia therapy stimulates language recovery in patients with chronic aphasia after ischemic stroke. *Medical Science Monitor, 14*(5), CR243–250.

Tench, P. (1996). *The intonation systems of English*. London: Cassell.

Whiteside, J., Kong, A. P. H., Helm-Estabrooks, N., Queen, J., Roe, D., & Drew, R. (2010, November 18–20). *"The Photograph as Language" workshops for people with chronic aphasia* [Conference seminar]. The 2010 American Speech-Language-Hearing Association (ASHA) Convention, Philadelphia, PA, USA.

Wright, H. H., & Capilouto, G. J. (2012). Considering a multilevel approach to understanding maintenance of global coherence in adults with aphasia. *Aphasiology, 26*(5), 656–672.

Chapter 6

Multi-Modal and Multi-Level Analysis of Oral Discourse

Chapter Objectives

The reader will be able to:

1. provide examples of non-verbal behaviors and apply different methodologies for coding gestures, facial expressions and/or bodily actions accompanying oral discourse
2. conduct an independent coding of gesture forms and functions
3. compute simple measures to reflect the relationship between oral discourse performance and co-verbal gestures
4. explain the prosodic deficits demonstrated by speakers with aphasia and related cognitive communicative disorders
5. discuss and evaluate existing methodologies for coding speech prosody
6. describe the components critical for a multi-modal and multi-level analysis of oral discourse
7. explain the strength and justify the need and clinical value of performing a multi-modal analysis of oral discourse
8. discuss the use of computational tools for annotation of non-linguistic behaviors in spoken discourse.

Introduction

People with acquired neurogenic communication disorders, especially those with a moderate to severe grade of impairment, such as global aphasia or a later stage of dementia, characteristically demonstrate pervasive language deficits that affect their oral communication (Bayles & Yomoeda, 2007; Collins, 1986; Nicholas & Helm-Estabrooks, 1994). As a result, their using of the primary language modality of oral expression and secondary language modality of writing to convey specific propositional information is often impaired (Holland, 1984). In other words, these speakers' skills and abilities to verbally express ideas or needs are compromised. Consequently, they may

DOI: 10.4324/9781003254775-6

need to rely on the employment of alternative communicative techniques to assist their conveying of meanings.

Based on earlier studies that investigated the use of symbol-based treatment to severe aphasia (e.g., Beck & Fritz, 1998; Enderby & Hamilton, 1983), it is believed that how well persons with aphasia can learn and perform iconic encoding tasks reflects their capability to use alternative mode of communication. Individuals with impaired syntactic and grammatical abilities but a relatively intact conceptual system of semantics should demonstrate some capacity for symbolization and primitive linguistic functions (Glass et al., 1975), which is crucial for independent use of a multi-modal system to communicate. Recent studies by Kong et al. (2013) and Kong, Law, Wat, and Lai (2015) also supported this notion by showing that persons with aphasia who have relatively intact non-verbal semantic skills were able to use gestures. This was especially the case for those who had lower verbal semantic skills because Kong et al. found a higher rate of using co-verbal gestures (or gestures commonly found to accompany oral production) among these speakers. Impaired prosody, or the deficits of appropriate use of pitch, loudness, tempo, stress, intonation, and rhythm in speech to convey information about the structure and meaning of an utterance, is also a clinical feature of some disorder groups, such as right hemisphere damage. These prosodic deficits can occur alone or in combination with oral expression and can lead to devastating effects on human interaction.

In this chapter, we first review some common linguistic parameters for assessing disordered oral discourse. This is followed by a discussion of the use of various speech-accompanying non-verbal behaviors, such as gestures and facial expressions, in oral discourse. A recently published framework containing independent annotation of gesture forms and functions employed during spontaneous oral discourse is then presented. Finally, speech prosody and some methods for analyzing expressive aprosodia for acquired neurogenic communication disorders will be discussed.

Linguistic Parameters of Oral Discourse

As discussed in Chapters 3 and 4, various approaches of linguistic analysis of oral discourse have been proposed for clinical and research application. A brief review of some of these systems in relation to other modalities of verbal communication is given in this section.

Spoken discourse develops in time when a speaker talks. Since speaking is a spontaneous phenomenon, utterances within a discourse are not always rephrased, which may be more prone to one or more of the following characteristics:

1. pauses or stutters
2. repetition of individual lexical items, phrases, or sentences

3. lexical, morphological, or syntactic errors
4. inappropriate cohesive ties
5. incoherent sentences (Crystal, 1992)

Acquired neurogenic communication disorders can disrupt a speaker's capacity to manage micro-linguistic components of verbal output, such as the informativeness, morphology, grammaticality, and syntax of an oral narrative. Depending on the severity of the communication disorder, macro-linguistic skills of cohesion (such as grammatical relationship between parts of a sentence essential for content interpretation) and coherence (such as the order of statements in a logical sequence) may also be impaired. In addition, when another interlocutor is involved in a conversation with the language-impaired person, problems in the lexical and communication efficiency of verbal output, as well as the pragmatics of speech, will become more apparent. Evaluation of discourse breakdown needs to adequately describe speaker characteristics and the interference demonstrated. With reference to the above-mentioned linguistic aspects, a patient's overall communicative strength and weakness can be more holistically identified.

Non-Verbal Behaviors and Affective Communication

Non-verbal behaviors for human communication include a wide range of activities, such as gestures, body postures and movements, touching behaviours, facial expressions, eye gaze, as well as vocal cues that accompany spoken words (Knapp et al., 2014). They are commonly used in daily interactions to serve different communicative purposes. Different non-verbal behaviors can also carry emotional or attitudinal information that supplements the verbal content (Jagoe & Wharton, 2021). According to Verderber et al. (2012), non-verbal communication involves bodily actions and vocal qualities that accompany verbal messages, which is characterized by its continuous and multi-channeled nature that can help a speaker convey his or her ideas and emotions. It is continuous because as long as a speaker is in presence of another communication partner (or a listener), any kind of non-verbal behavior can be perceived as a form of communication. Non-verbal communicative behaviors can be intentional or unintentional and, therefore, may be ambiguous in some social contexts as a result of different interpretation by the person perceiving these behaviors.

Human Gestures

According to McNeill (1992), gesture can be defined as the arm and hand movements that synchronize with verbal output. They are commonly used together with spoken language in human communication. Research on gesture employment has been conducted from different perspectives and approaches, each with different aims and emphases. For example, researchers in the field of linguistics, psychology, and social sciences are interested in the association between language and human thoughts. In the discipline of neuroscience and neurolinguistics, gesture research mainly focuses on exploring gestures that accompany oral production and their neural correlates. In the field of communication sciences, such as studies involving speakers with aphasia or hearing impairment, researchers examine the relationships between gestures and deficits in oral language. Scientists with a background in computer sciences and computer engineering, on the other hand, have evaluated and reported various methods and algorithms for real-time gesture and posture recognition, which can then contribute to the translation of human movements into computer information.

Various frameworks in classifying co-verbal gestures have been proposed. In general, these gestures can be largely divided into two types: Referent-related gestures and Functional gestures. Tables 6.1 and 6.2 contain detailed descriptions about the definitions, examples, and sources of these two groups of gestures, respectively. One should keep in mind that the terminology of different gestures is not entirely consistent in the literature. Overlapping of one or more types of gestures in terms of their usage during oral discourse is also not uncommon (e.g. iconic gestures versus kinetographic and panto-mimic gestures or beat gestures versus batons).

The term "gesticulation" was utilized in Kendon's formality-based classification (Kendon et al., 1981) for what we typically refer to as gestures. Specifically, various gestures forms are viewed on a continuum with reference to their formality and speech-dependency as shown in Figure 6.1. Following this sequence, gesticulations have the least degree of formality and more effort is required to accurately recognize and analyze them. In contrast, **emblems** and signs have the highest degree of formality because of their higher degree of certainty with little or no ambiguity in their gesture shape.

Great variability and individual differences exist in human's use of gestures. Co-verbal gestures, which are considered to be a complex performance uniquely found in humans, contain content bearing semantic and visual information (Quek et al., 2002). In a recent review article on individual gestural use and processing, Özer and Göksun (2020) explained how speakers differ in frequencies of using gestures, purposes of employing these gestures and their corresponding salient characteristics, degrees of benefits they gain from using and seeing gestures during comprehension, and facilitated learning with presence of gestures depending on their cognitive dispositions. The quantity and quality of gesture employment has been found to be influenced by a number of factors such as a speaker's age (e.g., Cohen & Borsoi, 1996; Feyereisen & Havard, 1999), gender (Knapp & Hall, 2010; Knapp et al., 2014), level of language proficiency (e.g., Kong et al., 2012), presence of language impairment (e.g., Kong et al., 2010; Lanyon &

Table 6.1 Types of different referent-related co-verbal gestures reported in the literature

Gesture types	Definition	Example	Sources
Iconic gestures	Gestures that are (1) directly relating to the semantic content of speech, (2) depicting a physical aspect of its referent, (3) used to show a physical and concrete item, or (4) used to model the shape of an object or the motion of an action	A simple concrete or abstract "description" using the hands to show the size of an item (e.g., a parcel)	Knapp & Hall, 2010; Lanyon & Rose, 2009; de Ruiter, 2000
Kinetographic gestures	Gestures that directly show a bodily action	Upward and downward movements of both arms to show the action of "flying"	Lemay et al., 1988
Pantomime	Gestures that describe objects and actions in a complex and sequential manner	Sketching the path or direction of an idea in the air or making a series of circular movements with the hand or arm to suggest meaning(s) additional to a specific word	de Ruiter, 2000; Lanyon & Rose, 2009
Handling (pantomime)	Gestures that pretend to use an object	Acting out how to use a knife to cut something	Van Nispen et al., 2016
Enacting (pantomime)	Gestures that simulate the performance of a non-object-directed (intransitive) action	Pretending to feel cold	
Object (pantomime)	Gestures that represent whole or part of an object	Two hands showing a palm up position and joined together to represent a "bowl"	
Shape (pantomime)	Gestures that outline or mold the shape of an object	A circular hand motion in the air to shape a circle	
Ideographic gestures	Gestures that trace or sketch out in the air the "paths" and "directions" of the thought pattern	Shaking an arm in the air between the locations of two mentally-imagined tasks, and then stopping the motion on one of the locations at the end	Efron, 1941; Lemay et al., 1988
Metaphoric gestures	Gestures that provide a certain degree of pictorial content to communicate an abstract idea	A circular hand motion in the air accompanying the statement "There is something else" to represent the concept of "something"	Ekman & Friesen, 1969; Jacobs & Garnham, 2007

(continued)

Table 6.1 Cont.

Gesture types	Definition	Example	Sources
Deictic gestures	Gestures that are employed to (1) refer to objects or actions by pointing at them or (2) indicate objects in a conversational space	Simple pointing actions (e.g., to an item in a story picture stimulus)	Hofemann, Fritsch, & Sagerer, 2004; McNeill, 1992
Emblems	(1) Gestures that are lexicalized and specific to a given language community, which can be used as substitutes for words (2) Gestures that are commonly understood signals, or (3) gestures with specific meaning that are consciously used and understood	(1) An "OK" sign for okay, (2) a "V" for "victory" or "world peace," or (3) thumbs-up for "good" or "all right"	de Ruiter, 2000; Knapp & Hall, 2010; Lanyon & Rose, 2009
Air writing and numbers	Gestures that are spontaneous and writing movements of single or strings of letters in the air or on an available surface	Writing letters (or characters) in the air; Finger tracing a word or writing letters with an empty hand on the desk or thigh	McNeill, 2000; Sekine et al., 2013
Numbers	Gestures that use fingers to directly display numbers	Four fingers up to display the number "4"	Kistner, 2017
Illustrators	Gestures that reinforce or supplement what is being said and (1) are used mostly in face-to-face interaction and (2) are tied to the content and/or flow of speech	Holding up two palms to signify "I don't know" or wagging a finger while making a point	Efron, 1941; Ekman, 1977
Beat gestures	Gestural movements with no clear handshape that accentuate speech segments, underline the rhythm of a speech, or the stress of a statement but do not represent a discernible meaning to the speech content	A simple beat or rhythmic beating of the hand, arm, or fingers. It can be a simple flick or a moving motion in an up-and-down or a back-and-forth fashion	Kistner, 2017; Kistner et al., 2019; Lanyon & Rose, 2009; McNeill, 1992, 2000
Batons	Gestures that are rhythmic, similar to a conductor's baton, and are used to beat the tempo of mental locomotion	Rhythmic flicking of a finger, hand, or arm during counting of different animals	Efron, 1941

Table 6.2 Types of different functional co-verbal gestures reported in the literature

Gesture types	Definition	Example	Sources
Emphasis gestures	Gestures that beat out time, accentuate, or emphasize a particular part of a statement	A flicking of a finger at a specific part of an utterance	Armstrong et al., 2007
Interactive gestures	Gestures that (1) regulate and organize the process of coming together, (2) regulate and organize the back-and-forth nature of speaking and listening, or (3) assist the process of verbal dialogues without conveying any topical information	(1) Hand movements that create emphasis and/or grab attention (e.g., an "air quotes," or "quotation" gesture with the use of the index and middle fingers involving both hands), (2) turn gestures (e.g., showing a palm to invite someone to join a conversation), or (3) greeting gestures	Bavelas et al., 1995; Knapp & Hall, 2010
Pragmatic gestures			Kendon, 2004
Conduit gestures			McNeill, 1985
Thinking gestures			Gullberg, 2011
Regulators	Gestures that (1) support the interaction and communication between sender and recipient and/or (2) structure the interaction and dialogue	Dropping an arm as a person completes what he/she is saying or raising an arm when a person wants to speak	Kendon, 1983; Malandro et al., 1989
Self-cueing gestures	Gestures that occur specifically as part of an effort to recall a word and/or to find an appropriate sentence structure	Finger tracing on the surface of a table during difficulty of finding a word	Kong et al., 2010
Facilitative gestures	Gestures that are produced during word-finding difficulties before a speaker finally resolves the problem		Kistner, 2017
Communicative gestures	Gestures that are produced during word-finding difficulties without the speaker resolving the problem	A hand motion in the air shaping a "square" at the time to say the word "iPad," but this act fails to help produce the final target word	
Augmentative gestures	Gestures that occur during a speech in the absence of any word-finding difficulties	Simple pointing actions (e.g., to an item on the dining table)	
Additional gestures	Gestures that convey information additional to speech	Acting out one of the major swimming strokes, e.g., breaststroke, when talking about a previous swimming lesson	
Compensatory gestures	Gestures that replace speech	A gesture of raising three fingers is used when there is no co-occurring speech (mentioning the quantity of three) and no signs of word-finding difficulties	
Essential gestures	Gestures that convey information absent in the speech and are essential for conveying a message		Van Nispen et al., 2017

Gesticulation → Language-like gestures → Pantomimes → Emblems → Sign languages

Figure 6.1 Kendon's continuum (from natural gesticulation to full-formed linguistic codes of sign languages)

Rose, 2009), cognitive abilities (Knapp & Hall, 2010; Knapp et al., 2014), or cultural and language background (e.g., Kita, 2009; Wilson, 1998).

Gestures and Age

Investigating age-related issues concerning the use of language and its associated co-verbal gestures may enable one to better understand the role that non-verbal behaviors play in forming impressions and in interpersonal communication (Montepare & Tucker, 1999). There seems to be a decreased proportion of spontaneous hand gestures related to the speech content as one ages. To illustrate, the use of representational gestures, such as iconic, metaphoric, or deictic gestures as compared to beats, was reported to occur significantly less frequently in conversations among older adults (Feyereisen & Havard, 1999). In another study by Cohen and Borsoi (1996), who examined the differences of employing gestures in an object description task in a group of young and another group of elderly adults, fewer descriptive gestures was found in the elderly participants. Although the two age levels were comparable in terms of the number of non-descriptive gestures, co-verbal gestures linking more closely to the content of the oral production, which may or may not carry a portion of the verbal message in a non-verbal form, were used less frequently by the older group. Finally, the patterns of using pantomimic gestures was reported to be different across age groups of normal adults speakers (Ska & Nespoulous, 1987). While younger speakers with an average age of 25 years tended to employ more self-oriented one-handed gestures in response to a verbal command of executing pantomimes, those with a mean age of 71 years were found to use a part of their body to serve as the constituents of relevant imaginary object(s).

Note that opposite findings of older speakers using more gestures have also been reported. For example, Kong, Law, Kwan et al. (2015) have suggested that unimpaired individuals aged 60 years or older used gestures more frequently than two other younger speaker groups: those aged 18–39 years as well as 40–59 years; and the differences were statistically significant. The stipulation was that because aging could decrease efficiency in allocating resources (Old & Naveh-Benjamin, 2008) and lengthen reaction time (Gooch et al., 2009) in memory tasks, it became natural for older speakers to gesture more spontaneously to alleviate the linguistic demand of a discourse task and free up additional cognitive capacity and effort for this activity.

Gestures and Demand of Linguistic Tasks

A number of research studies have attempted to examine the relationship between co-verbal gestures and daily conversation. The beneficial effects of gestures accompanying human conversations include reduction of a speaker's linguistic demand (Goldin-Meadow, 1999, 2003) and sparing of cognitive capacity for speech tasks (Rauscher et al., 1996). The increased use of gestures during speaking, therefore, helps reduce the cognitive load and allows the speakers to devote more cognitive resources to rehearsing target stimuli in speech (Clough & Duff, 2020). Note that there have also been arguments suggesting that the act of inhibiting gesture production could actually increase cognitive load during speaking, and thus reduce overall linguistic performance; this inhibition can pose more challenges to neurogenic populations with communication disorders because of their inherent reduction or impairment in attentional capacities and/or working memory.

Gestures can also promote the formulation of thoughts and ideas when one converses complicated ideas, such as explaining a mathematic problem (Goldin-Meadow, 2003), and free up capacity for retrieving words from memory. For example, unimpaired speakers were found to be able to remember more words in a word reciting task when gesturing was involved (Alibali & DiRusso, 1999), indicating that gestures might help lower the demand of working memory in a naming task. It was also suggested that a higher proportion of gestures is associated with retrieving lexical items of lower familiarity (Morrel-Samuels & Krauss, 1992).

In addition, given that gesture and spoken language are highly related and can originate from a single process (Cicone et al., 1979; Xu et al., 2009), co-verbal gestures can facilitate lexical retrieval during spontaneous speech production, at least at the conceptual level where mental lexicons are activated (Hadar & Butterworth, 1997; Krauss & Hadar, 1999). This argument can be supported by the findings in which typical speakers with a lower overall lexical diversity at the discourse level would tend to produce more co-verbal gestures (Crowder, 1996). When typical speakers were restricted from using arm and hand movements, there was an increase in non-juncture-filled pauses and a decrease in speech fluency of verbal expression involving spatial content (Rausher et al., 1996). All of the above can demonstrate the positive effects of using gestures specific to lexical access in unimpaired speakers.

Gestures and Speakers' Linguistic Competence

Knowing that both the routes of gesture and speech production can be originated from the same conceptualizing stage, similar to the initial stage proposed in many models of lexical and sentence production (e.g. Garrett, 1975; Levelt, 1989), the condition of aphasia allows one to elucidate the possible communicative, as well as non-communicative, functions that gestures serve during oral discourse production. It is reasonable to assume that if gestures and speech are both activated at the same time when one uses oral expression, speakers with aphasia with a diminished capacity to execute verbal production should have a higher tendency to use the gestural modality to assist communication. This was indeed the case as reported by Feyereisen (1987) who found that persons with aphasia had a tendency to employ more co-verbal gestures as a result of their lower degree of informativeness in the spoken output.

A number of studies have been conducted to compare the gestural profiles between individuals with and without aphasia and concluded that speakers with impaired oral ability secondary to the language deficits associated with aphasia employed gestures more frequently to compensate for their difficulties. For example, with reference to the quantity and types of gestures elicited from a conversational interview, Lemay et al. (1988) found that hand gestures (predominantly batons, ideographic, and deictic gestures) were employed more by speakers with Broca's aphasia but the least by neurologically unimpaired controls. Wernicke's aphasia also demonstrated significantly more kinetographic gestures than their non-aphasic counterparts. Speakers with aphasia have been reported to gesture significantly more frequently and for a significantly longer period of time than their unimpaired conversational partners (Herrmann et al., 1988). Those who suffered from more severe aphasia were also found to employ gestures more as a strategy to bypass their linguistic limitation and to convey messages more successfully, i.e., using gestures as an alternative means of communication (Hogrefe et al., 2012). Furthermore, speakers with severe aphasia tended to employ gestures in a manner different from the controls by using significantly fewer speech-focused hand movements. Instead, significantly more codified gestures, such as emblems containing direct non-verbal translations of a word or phrase that could represent a speaker's mind as a lexical item (Poggi, 2008), are used as speech substitutes by these individuals.

While the studies mentioned above have a focus on counting the occurrence of co-verbal gestures, a few other studies have attempted to compare the physical parameters of gestures used by speakers with aphasia and to determine how pragmatically appropriate these gestures were during communication tasks. For example, Cicone et al. (1979) found that speakers with relatively preserved expressive language ability produced more gestures than those with impaired expressive language. In other words, the gestural profile of speakers with aphasia (in terms of quantity) was found to closely parallel their speech output. Glosser et al. (1986) also revealed that speakers with a moderate degree of aphasia produced less meaningful gestures during face-to-face informal dyadic conversations than those with a mild degree of aphasia, irrespective of the quantity of gestures produced. However, a review of the complexity of these gestures suggested that speakers with more impaired language skills produced proportionally fewer complex gestures that were semantically modifying and/or communicative. More non-specific and unclear gestures also appeared in the moderately aphasic group. The observation that gestural complexity was significantly and negatively correlated with measures of linguistic impairment for the speakers with aphasia in Glosser et al.'s (1986) study seems to be contradictory to other reports in the literature but is clinically important. With these results, one can argue that the long-assumed compensatory role of employing gestures by individuals with aphasia is far from straightforward as one may assume, at least for the case when the semantic, physical, and/or pragmatic properties of gestures are considered.

While gestural profiles in speakers with aphasia vary as a function of their language integrity, it should be noted that this phenomenon was also reported among typical healthy speakers. In particular, individuals with low phonemic fluency skills, as reflected by a lower ability to generate a list of single words starting with a specific given initial consonant, but high spatial visualization skill were found to gesture more often (Hostetter & Alibali, 2007). The rate of producing representational gestures, however, was not necessarily affected by the skills of phonemic fluency alone, suggesting that individual differences in using gestures were associated with corresponding cognitive skills. Moreover, adult speakers whose oral narratives were lower in lexical diversity tended to produce more target-enhancing or content-carrying gestures to supplement and enrich their speech (Crowder, 1996). Those with a richer lexical diversity, on the other hand, were found to have fewer gestures, especially gestures that were redundant to the original speech content.

Speech fluency is another factor that has been found to impact co-verbal gesture employment, in which stuttering was found to reduce the amount of gesture production in oral speech (Mayberry & Jaques, 2000). Specifically, individuals who stuttered were reported to have significantly fewer words with gestures (30%) than those who did not stutter (78%). In terms of the proportion of time in a discourse task when speakers were using co-verbal gestures, it was found that the stuttering condition significantly lowered the percentage of gesturing behaviour (20% of the total discourse time for the stuttering group versus 70% for those who did not stutter). One explanation for this observed pattern of fewer gestures in stuttered speech was that the sentence structures tended to be simpler in stuttered output and more time was given to convey less content; hence lowering speakers' need to compensate for sentence formulation and speech content conveyance using gestures.

Finally, the use of meaningful gestures during novel word-learning tasks was found to facilitate subsequent retrieval of these words (Krönke et al., 2013). Recalling literal as well as abstract meanings in verbal messages could also benefit from the mapping of gestures and linguistic representations (Argyriou et al., 2017). In short, although speakers with aphasia tend to demonstrate a more limited range of co-verbal gesture types (Caute et al., 2021), using them can facilitate lexical access, mental representations of concepts, and exploration of ideas through transitional knowledge; all these characteristics benefit communication and can potentially lead to better learning and more lasting improvement in cognitive functions such as memory (Clough & Duff, 2020).

Gestures and Narrative Tasks

With a specific interest to examine how conversation topics and conversation partners influence the use of gestures, Kistner et al. (2020) studied narrative and procedural conversations in 20 people with aphasia and 21 unimpaired controls. Familiar conversation partners (such as family members or friends) were nominated by the participants, and unfamiliar conversation partners were also recruited to engaged in two different conversational tasks with each participant: one involving the narrative topics of "happy memory" and "busy weekend," and another two procedural topics of "how to wrap a parcel" and "how to make scrambled eggs." The results indicated that significantly more gestures were produced in procedural than in narrative conversations in both speaker groups (e.g., four times as many iconic gestures in procedural than in narrative conversations). There were also more semantically rich gestures in procedural conversations. Interestingly, both groups showed a tendency to use significantly more gestures when conversing with unfamiliar conversation partners; this could be contributed by both groups' higher degree of language formality and pragmatic demands when speaking with less familiar people.

Facial Expressions

Facial expressions are the arrangement of facial muscles to communication emotional reactions or states (Ekman, 1966; Fridlund, 1994; Verderber et al., 2012). According to Knapp and Hall (2010), facial expressions serve a regulatory function during spontaneous discourse for a speaker to provide feedback to an interlocutor and to manage the flow of interaction. Apart from conveying emotional states, they can communicate a speaker's interest and mediate responsiveness during interactions. Seven basic emotions, which are universal and do not vary much by culture, can be conveyed through human facial expressions: happiness, sadness, anger, fear, disgust, surprise, and contempt (Kohler et al., 2004; Knapp & Hall, 2010; Verderber et al., 2012). Note that the actual displays of emotions may vary between gender and across cultures (Verderber et al., 2012). Other emotions such as embarrassed, shame, guilt, pride, or jealousy that do not have a universally-agreed expression should not be excluded from analyses. Furthermore, humans can also convey a particular emotion through the use of eye contact or gaze. Table 6.3

Table 6.3 Specific facial features of seven basic co-verbal emotional facial expressions

Facial expressions	Specific facial features
Happiness	• raised inner eyebrows • tightened lower eyelid • muscle around the eyes tightens • raised cheeks • upper lip raises • lip corners turn upward
Sadness	• furrowed eyebrow • opened mouth with upper lip raised • lip corners stretch and turn down • chin pulls up
Anger	• lowered eyebrows • eyes wide open with tightened lower lid • lips exposing teeth and stretched lip corners
Fear	• eyes wide open • furrowed and raised eyebrows • stretched mouth
Disgust	• eyebrows pull down • nose wrinkles • upper lip pulls up • lips loose
Surprise	• entire eyebrow pulls up • eyelids pull up • mouth hangs open
Contempt	• often involves unilateral facial expression • neutral eyes • lip corner pulls up and back on one side

includes examples of specific facial features associated with these seven basic emotional facial expressions.

Kong et al. (2010) have investigated the use of facial expressions and other non-verbal behaviors among four Cantonese-speaking individuals with aphasia (two fluent and two non-fluent). Controls matched in gender, age, and education level were also included to compare the performance of using these non-verbal behaviors between the two groups. The results revealed that although the aphasic group used significantly more non-verbal behaviors than their normal counterparts, facial expressions were the least employed non-verbal behavior. How the employment of non-verbal behaviors was affected by fluency of producing discourse was also examined. It was found that the non-verbal behavior-to-token (total number of words produced) ratio for the non-fluent speakers was five times higher than that of the fluent speaking controls. The non-verbal behavior-to-utterance ratio was also the highest for the non-fluent group. These results suggest that persons with aphasia who were compromised in their fluency (often characterized by fragmented utterances, simpler sentence structures, and reduced oral discourse skills) tended to use more speech-accompanying non-verbal behaviors.

Bodily Actions and Adaptors (or Touching Behaviors)

Apart from decoding the meaning of a message, dynamic body movements can also provide additional cues to listeners to identify emotions within a verbal context (Montepare et al., 1999). The position, orientation, and manner of movement of different bodily actions may indicate a speaker's attention and dominance of a verbal interaction.

Gestures that are not used intentionally during a communication are called **adaptors**. They are sometimes referred to as touching behaviors and are often used unconsciously, especially when a person is tense or anxious and may occur in instances of speech failure (Beall, 2004; Geoff & Thompson, 2001; Knapp & Hall, 2010). In other words, we use adaptors, unintentionally in most cases, to lower the degree of discomfort or to pacify nervousness or anxiety. They are considered to be a kind of self-focused behavior that reflects a speaker's state of mind. There are two major kinds of adaptors reported in the literature:

1. Self adaptors, which can be further divided into:
    a. body-focused (or bodily) adaptors that are representations of own negative feelings or negative feelings toward others, such as adjusting clothes or eyeglasses, biting nails, pinching or scratching body or head (Knapp & Hall, 2010; Kendon, 1981)
    b. gesture-focused adaptors that share some common trajectory features of conventional gestures but do not necessarily carry any content, such as non-functional pointing and/or hand movements, or hand-waving in the air (Knapp & Hall, 2010).
2. Object-focused adaptors that include the unconscious manipulation of a particular object, such as fidgeting and toying with an object, playing with jewelry, or tapping a pencil (Ekman & Friesen, 1972).

Frameworks for Coding Gestures and Other Non-Verbal Behaviors Employed During Oral Discourse

A clear and comprehensive classification framework for gestures can help researchers identify the referential value of gestures in communication (McNeill, 1992). This is clinically relevant for speech-and-language pathologists or related practitioners to compare non-verbal performance across individuals with language impairments. Given the close and apparent relationship between gesture use and language production, various gesture coding systems have been reported in the literature of psychology. Many of these systems were developed for use in typical healthy speakers. However, variations among the systems in terms of their annotation categories have complicated the interpretation of gesture use as well as their function during production of spontaneous speech (Scharp et al., 2007). Examples of some gesture analytic systems are given below:

- Ekman and Friesen (1969) proposed a five-way classification of co-verbal gestures including:

  (1) pictorial gestures —movements that are used to reveal speech content by "drawing" a picture of the target, such as using the hands to mimic the shape or size of an object

  (2) spatial gestures – hand motions that are used to show spatial distances, such as using both palms facing each other to indicate the distance of platform gap in a train station

  (3) rhythmic gestures – hand movements that are used to stress particular phrases or movements of fingers along the flow of natural speech

  (4) kinetic gestures – movements that are used to perform an action related to the speech content, such as arm moving to imitate the action of running

  (5) pointing gestures – or the use of finger(s) to point to or point out specific objects.

  With reference to this annotation framework, a co-verbal gesture can be coded as one or more types of these five gestures. One critical limitation of this coding framework lies on the overlapping nature of gesture classification and, therefore, potential ambiguity of the gesture types in the system.

- McNeill (1992) later modified Ekman and Friesen's (1969) classification so that one gesture could only be coded once. More specifically, all hand movements representing actions or features of objects (i.e., kinetic and pictorial gestures, respectively) were referred to as "iconic gestures." All movements associated with the flow or rate of the output (i.e., rhythmic gestures) were classified as "beats." In addition to movements providing spatial information, those that conceptualized abstract ideas were coded as "metaphoric gestures." As for pointing gestures, they were grouped together with other movements that indicated location and identified as "deictic gestures." The author also included two new codes in the system, namely "emblems" and "pantomime." The former was defined as any conventionalized signs, such as a thumbs-up gesture, that are culturally specific with standard forms and significances but vary from place to place, while "pantomime" was defined as a single gesture or a sequence of gestures that allowed one to convey a narrative line within a story without the use of speech. McNeill believed that this modified coding system not only widened the definition for each type of gesture, but also provided a clearer framework to analyze gesture production during spontaneous speech.

- Another system focusing on the degree of information overlap between gestures and content in oral discourse was reported by Crowder (1996). In this system, co-verbal gestures were dichotomized into gesture-speech pairs and non-meaningful gestures. The gesture-speech pairs were further categorized into one of the following three sub-types,:
  (1) redundant gestures, of which no new information was added to speech content
  (2) enhancing gestures, which could function to expand existing speech content
  (3) content-carrying gestures, which could provide additional meaning absent in a verbal discourse.

Non-meaningful gestures, on the other hand, were those identified during pauses or filling of speech gaps. Mather (2005) considered these non-meaningful gestures as **"regulators,"** which were usually used during speech for filling gaps of speech initiation, continuation, shifting, or termination.

- Based on the rationale that non-verbal behaviors in speakers with aphasia contains rich information on the style and residual capabilities of communication, Kong et al. (2010) proposed a quantification system to capture the use of referent-related gestures, functional gestures, facial expressions, and adaptors (or bodily or gestural touching behaviors) during a **monologue** task about an important event of the speaker and a story-telling task. The linguistic properties of the discourse samples were also analyzed to evaluate their relations with these non-verbal behaviors. Specifically, the following measures were computed:
  (1) total number of non-verbal behaviors, which was used to obtain the percentage distribution of the four kinds of non-verbal behaviors
  (2) total number of words (or token)
  (3) total number of utterances
  (4) total number of errors produced
  (5) the ratio of non-verbal behaviors to token
  (6) the ratio of non-verbal behaviors to utterance
  (7) the ratio of errors to non-verbal behaviors.

An Innovative Coding Framework With Independent Annotation of Gesture Forms and Functions

Gesture production is an integral component of spoken communication and almost always accompanies the use of spoken language. Understanding changes in gesture usage in the presence of damage to the language network has the potential to both aid clinical diagnosis and to increase our understanding of the brain's language network. However, co-verbal gestures have not been systematically studied. This is largely due to the absence of a detailed classification of gesture use, with clear differentiation of coding of gesture forms and functions. For example, the rhythmic and pointing gestures in Ekman and Friesen (1969) and the beats in McNeill (1992) were coded based on their function served during the co-occurring speech segment, but the remaining ones were related to the gesture forms or patterns of gestural movement. Acknowledging that a particular form of gesture can serve one or more communicative functions, the mixed coding of gesture forms and functions within one quantification system can, therefore, be conceptually problematic and may create confusion when it comes to interpreting gesture employment. To illustrate, the word-finding process in normal speakers was reported to be facilitated by the use of iconic gestures because of the provision of an alternate route of lexicon access (Butterworth & Hadar, 1989); at the same time, iconic gestures were found to help listeners decode speech content more accurately (Beattie & Shovelton, 1999). Another good example is the reported functions of deictic gestures to lower demand on speakers' cognitive resource and facilitate speech formulation (Goldin-Meadow, 2003) as well as to help listeners decode messages by directly pointing to and/or illustrating objects in the real world (Ekman & Friesen, 1969). These examples clearly indicate that without a non-overlapping annotation framework, one cannot reliably classify how a particular form of gesture carries different (non-)communicative functions under various conditions.

Motivated by the limitations mentioned above, i.e., the research gap of mixed coding of gesture forms and functions, which can be conceptually problematic and may create confusion when it comes to interpreting gesture use, Kong, Law, Kwan, et al. (2015) have proposed a classification framework with independent annotation of co-verbal gestures employed during the tasks of story-telling and procedural discourse. The classification focused on two aspects: (1) physical properties of a gesture and (2) how it is used in an utterance. Following McNeill's (1992) definition, a unit of gesture in this framework is defined as the duration from the start of a movement until the hand(s) returns to its resting position (McNeill, 1992). If the hand(s) does not return to its resting position, gestures will be divided by either a pause in the movement or an obvious change in shape or trajectory (Jacobs & Garnham, 2007). During the flow of speech, self-adapting motions, such as touching the face or changing hand position from the lap to the table, are excluded from the analysis as they do not contain any semantic attachment (Jacobs & Garnham, 2007). Six forms of gestures modified based on the classification by Ekman and Friesen (1969), Mather (2005), and McNeill (1992) are proposed, as follows:

1. iconic gestures
2. metaphoric gestures

3.   deictic gestures
4.   emblems
5.   beats
6.   non–identifiable gestures, which are referred to any uncodable finger, hand, and/or arm movements due to its ambiguous connection or lack of a direct meaning to the speech content (a gesture that was partly visually obstructed but cannot be categorized as any of the above five forms is also coded as non–identifiable).

While the first four forms are content-carrying, the other two are not. In the dimension of functions, gestures can be classified by their primary role in communication. Acknowledging that sometimes a specific gesture can serve one or more communicative purposes, only the primary function in relation to the speech content is annotated. Eight functions of gestures adopted from several previous studies are used:

1.   Providing additional information to message conveyed: A gesture gives information in addition to the speech content (Goldin-Meadow, 2003), i.e., the content of the gesture contains additional information related to the speech. For example, when a speaker says the word "open," he/she gives a twisting motion in the air, representing the action to open a bottle. This gesture gives additional information to the speech content (about the manner of opening a container, but not other objects).
2.   Enhancing the speech content: A gesture contains the same meaning as the speech content (Beattie & Shovelton, 2000). This might facilitate a listener to decode speech content. For instance, a speaker uses his finger to show the action of turning on an air conditioner when saying "I switched on the AC when I walked into the house."
3.   Providing alternative means of communication: A gesture carries meaning that is not included in speech content (Lemay et al., 1988). Speech could be superseded by the gesture employed. For example, a speaker only points to the right when he or she responds to the question of "Which way shall we go?"
4.   Guiding and controlling the flow of speech: A gesture that reinforces the rhythm of the speech (Jacobs & Garnham, 2007). The rate of gesture movement is usually synchronized with the pace of speech. For example, a speaker flicks his or her finger when naming a series of related items.
5.   Reinforcing the intonation or prosody of speech: A gesture used by a speaker to emphasize his or her meaning or to intensify and/or accentuate a target element in a statement. For example, a speaker gives a strong flick at the target word.
6.   Assisting lexical retrieval: A gesture that is intended for use to facilitate lexical access (Krauss & Hadar, 1999). This is usually coded when

a speaker attempts to produce a target word after gesturing at times of word-finding difficulty, such as an observable time delay when trying to retrieve the target word(s), stating "I know that word, but I can't think of it," interjections, circumlocution, word or phrase repetitions, and word substitutions within a speech (Mayberry & Jaques, 2000). For example, this type of gestures may occur when a speaker demonstrates a notice-able pause or prolongation of speech sound in the middle of a sentence where he or she is stuck with finding a particular target word (that is finally retrieved) or when a speaker reformulates or substitutes a phrase or sentence during speech (German, 2001).

7. Assisting sentence re-construction: A gesture often used by a speaker to facilitate the modification of the syntactic structure of a sentence (Alibali et al., 2000). Alternatively, this gesture is produced when there is difficulty in sentence construction and refinement of sentence structure is noticed after the use of this gesture.

8. No specific function deduced: A gesture that does not show a specific function in relation to the speech content or an unclassifiable function other than the seven mentioned above.

The most important criteria in differentiating the first three gesture functions is to determine if the presence of a gesture, irrespective of its form, can provide non-verbal information that was additional to (functions 1 and 3) or the same as (function 2) the corresponding speech content. Function 5 differs from functions 2 and 4 in that the latter ones do not involve a speaker's intensifying or accentuating a target element in the oral output. If needed, coders can also use prosodic patterns that are specific and consistent to the speech content to make the distinction. Regarding functions 6 and 7, a particular annotated gesture should accompany a delay or struggle of word finding and sentence formulation, respectively, as described above.

Following the procedures of data processing suggested by Kong, Law, Kwan, et al.'s (2015) study, all linguistic production by a speaker should be videotaped and subsequently transcribed orthographically. Each language sample and its corresponding digitized video are then linked using the EUDICO Linguistic ANnotator (ELAN; Max Planck Institute for Psycholinguistics, 2002; see Chapter 5 for more details about this software). Annotations of a sentence or word in a language transcript can be time-aligned to the non-verbal features observed in the corresponding audio and/or video media. The orthographic transcripts in Kong et al. followed the format in the Child Language ANalyses computer program (CLAN; MacWhinney, 2003). Three independent tiers were generated in each ELAN document to annotate the (1) linguistic information of the transcript, (2) forms of gestures that appeared, and (3) function for each gesture used. Frequency count of each gesture form and function can be obtained using the "Annotation Statistics" option in ELAN. A screenshot of annotating

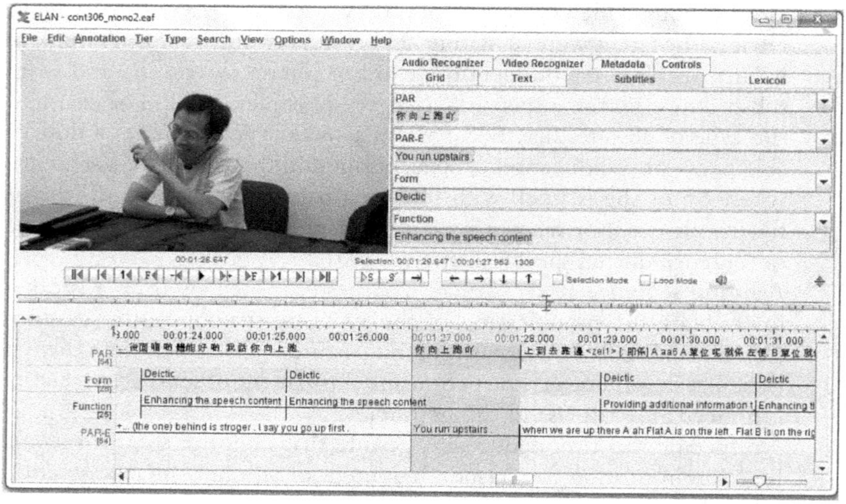

Figure 6.2 A screenshot in ELAN with annotations of a speaker's oral production and co-verbal gestures

Source: © Anthony Pak-Hin Kong, Ph.D.

a speaker's oral production and co-verbal gestures is given in Figure 6.2. Specifically, the "Video" viewer on the top left corner shows a speaker's performance in the video. The "Grid" and "Text" panels next to the video display the individual segments of a tier and their corresponding annotation values, respectively. The "Subtitles" and "Lexicon" panels on the right side display the selectable tiers as video subtitles. The "Interlinear" viewer at the bottom shows the multi-level annotations, including the speech produced by a speaker (PAR) and the associated co-verbal gesture forms (FORM) and functions (FUNCTION) used. Since the production was in Cantonese Chinese in this example, a fourth tier showing corresponding gloss in English (PAR_E) was generated and included.

Based on independent annotation of co-verbal gestures among 119 neurologically unimpaired right-handed native speakers of Cantonese (further divided into three age and two education levels), Kong, Law, Kwan, et al. (2015) reported that about one third of the normal speakers did not use any gestures at all during the spontaneous discourse tasks. The results also indicated that content-carrying gestures were mainly used for helping listeners to decode speech content, while non-content-carrying gestures primarily served the purpose of emphasizing speech content. Moreover, older speakers tended to use gestures more frequently, and speakers with a higher level of language proficiency produced fewer gestures.

The same annotation framework was applied to 48 individuals with aphasia and their controls matched in gender, age, and education level (Kong et al., 2013; Kong, Law, Wat, & Lai, 2015). It was found that the severity of aphasia and verbal-semantic impairment was associated with significantly more co-verbal gestures. Hand or arm paralysis or weaknesses (i.e., hemiplegia) were not found to affect their employment of gestures. Moreover, significantly more gestures were employed by the speakers with aphasia, although about 10% of them did not gesture. Among those who used gestures, content-carrying gestures, including iconic, metaphoric, deictic gestures, and emblems, served the function of enhancing speech content and providing information additional to the speech content. As for the non-content carrying gestures, beats were used primarily for reinforcing speech prosody or guiding speech flow, while non-identifiable gestures were used for assisting lexical retrieval or with no specific functions.

Further studies investigating the use of co-verbal gestures in native Cantonese speakers with stroke-induced aphasia have been published. For example, Kong et al. (2017) compared gesture use in three participant groups: 23 neurologically healthy speakers, 23 speakers with fluent aphasia, and 21 speakers with non-fluent aphasia. The non-fluent aphasia group was found to use communicative gestures the most while speaking. Interestingly, the rate of gesture use in speakers with fluent aphasia did not differ significantly from the control counterparts. The percentages of complete sentences and dysfluency in both aphasic groups strongly predicted the gesturing rate (i.e., the gesture-to-word ratio). In a more recent study that focused on 58 speakers with fluent aphasia and 58 controls (Kong et al., 2019), it was revealed that when word-finding difficulties occurred at the discourse level, people with fluent aphasia showed a tendency to use gestures to enhance and assist communication, although this strategy did not always improve verbal expression or resolve the anomia problem. (This seems to be contradictory to Jagoe and Wharton (2021) who believe that the association and latency between the gesture and a spoken output was indicative of the facilitating effect of gesture on lexical retrieval.) Moreover, gestures involving a rhythmic beat could improve the overall prosody (i.e., stress and intonation) of production. An example of this kind of gesture is the flicking of an arm up and down rhythmically when one lists places previously visited, as in "I have been to many cities in the US, including New York, Chicago, Los Angeles, Seattle, and Orlando!"

In addition, the methodology and/or principles of Kong, Law, Kwan, et al.'s (2015) annotation system have been applied to describe changes in gesture production under conditions of damage to the language system by other neurological disorders, such as focal brain injury (Akbiyik et al., 2018; Özer et al., 2019), as well as co-verbal gesture employment in neuro-typical younger (Fronda & Balconi, 2020) and older (Özer et al., 2019) adults, learners of a second language (Wouters, 2020), tourist guides (Cataldo et al., 2019), talk show hosts (Szabó et al., 2020), and teachers (Kartchava & Mohamed, 2020).

For speech-and-language pathologists or related clinicians who have no immediate access to the ELAN (or similar computer software) to digitally annotate co-verbal gestures, a paper and pencil-based coding method is illustrated in Example 6.1. In particular, a speaker's oral discourse is transcribed orthographically and segmented into sentences or utterances. All speech-accompanying gestures that appeared in each line are coded within the text by inserting a Δ symbol. The form and function of each gesture can then be coded independently following the guidelines in Kong, Law, Kwan, et al. (2015). Measures adapted from Kong et al. (2010) to evaluate the relationships between the gesture employment and the linguistic properties of the discourse sample can also be computed readily. A blank coding form can be found in Appendix 6.1.

Motivated by the lack of readily usable gesture assessment that can help clinicians evaluate use of gestures in people with aphasia, Caute et al. (2021) have recently proposed a **City Gesture Checklist (CGC)** that can offer a "quick and dirty" method to assess gesture through different coding categories, inform therapy targets, and measure outcomes. Specifically, the design of CGC followed the principle of independent coding of gesture forms and functions put forth by Kong, Law, Kwan, et al. (2015) and Kong et al. (2019), and aimed to help clinicians and researchers structure their observations of gesture use. This would enable a more systematic approach to (1) record observations of different types of co-gestures employed, (2) identify factors that affect gesture use, and (3) determine the effectiveness of using the observed gestures. As shown in Figure 6.3, which is part of the full CGC (freely available from https://aphasia.talkbank.org/gesture/), a clinician can observe a conversation or watch a pre-recorded video to tally in real time the number of (and further describe) each of the following gesture types: pointing (concrete), pointing (abstract), emblems/conventional gestures, iconics (shape/outlining), iconics (pretending), number, air writing, and others (e.g., gestures that do not fit into the main categories, such as gestures representing time or personalized gestures). To allow a more meaningful description and individualized summary of the observed gesture types, the next section of the CGC details questions pertaining to gesture functions and the manner they were employed (see Box 6.1).

Speech Prosody

Prosody is an important component of natural speech because it signals both linguistic and emotional information (Wells & Whiteside, 2008). Prosodic features in discourse, including pitch, tempo, loudness, tone, stress and intonation, are related to the para-verbal aspect of oral communication and are directly related to the structuring of information in discourse. According to

Example 6.1 An Example of Paper-Based Coding of Co-Verbal Gestures

Patient name: _L.A._ Date of birth/Age: _Mar 28, 1956 / 65_ Gender: _M / F_ Etiology: _Wernicke's aphasia_

Date of testing: _Oct 11, 2022_ Speech therapist: _A.K._

Complete language sample:

...From what I can tell looks like a young ... a young man ... and he's gotten a ball out there and he's thrown it in the air xxx in the air.
The next scene I see something go in there ... and I can't see the kid now but I can see like a window. So I'm just lookin (g) through, I'm tryin (g) to get in there ... catch somethin (g) ... catch a ball or somethin (g).
The third time I see somebody else is was on the outside. Now they're on the inside ... somebody's on the outside just sitting here watching tv, but looks like a ball's coming.
And the force (fourth) one is ... it looks like they saw the ball on the ball and they don't know how they didn't say they caught or anything. It's just sittin (g) here.

Sentence number	Narrative task: AphasiaBank – Protocol – Broken window. Total duration: 1 minutes 17 seconds	Number of words	Gesture form						Gesture function								Remarks for gestures
			Iconic	Metaphoric	Deictic	Emblems	Beats	Non-identifiable	Providing additional information	Enhancing speech content	Providing alternative means of communication	Guiding and controlling speech flow	Reinforcing speech intonation or prosody	Assisting lexical retrieval	Assisting sentence re-construction	No specific function	
1	from what I can tell looks like a young △ a young man	12			1					1							Points to picture 1
2	and he's gotten a ball out there and he's throw it in the air △	16	1							1							Gesture: throwing

Narrative task:
AphasiaBank
Protocol –
Broken window
Total duration: 1 minutes 17 seconds

Sentence number	Narrative task	Number of words	Iconic	Metaphoric	Deictic	Emblems	Beats	Non-identifiable	Providing additional information	Enhancing speech content	Providing alternative means of communication	Guiding and controlling speech flow	Reinforcing speech intonation or prosody	Assisting lexical retrieval	Assisting sentence re-construction	No specific function	Remarks for gestures
			Gesture form						Gesture function								
3	xxx in the air	4															
4	the next scene I see something go in there	9															
5	and I can't see the kid now but I can see like a window	14															
6	so I'm just lookin (g) through, I'm tryin (g) to get in there Δ catch somethin (g)	15			1					1							Points down
7	catch a ball or somethin (g)	5															
8	the third Δ time I see somebody else is was on the outside Δ	12			2					2							Δ1 points to picture 3 Δ2 points to picture 1
9	now they're on the inside Δ	6			1					1							Points to picture 3

									Gesture: trajectory
10	somebody's on the outside just sitting here watching tv △ but looks like a ball's coming	17	1				1		
11	and the force (fourth) one is △....	5	1			1			Points to picture 4
12	it looks like they saw the ball on the ball and they don't know how they didn't say they caught or anything	24							
13	△it's just sittin (9) here	5	1			1			Taps picture 4
14									
15									
	Total:	144	2	7	7	1	1	1	

Overall remarks: xxx = unintelligible speech / jargons; one error in sentence 11

(1) Total number of gestures: 9
(2) Total number of words (or token): 144
(3) Total number of utterances: 13
(4) Total number of errors produced: 1
(5) The ratio of gestures to token: $9 \div 144 = 0.0625$
(6) The ratio of gestures to utterance: $9 \div 13 = 0.6923$
(7) The ratio of errors to gesture: $1 \div 9 = 0.111$

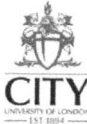

City Gesture Checklist

This checklist is for use in real time, to describe how clients with aphasia use gesture spontaneously. You could use it while watching a video or observing a conversation.

Tally the number of each gesture type you observe the client using. There is a blank space in each box for notes. Additional space for observations and further information on each coding category is given over the page.

Name/initials: Date:

Assessor: Communication partner/s:

Situation being observed/topic of conversation:

Location/setting:

Pointing-concrete	Pointing-abstract	Emblems/ conventional gestures
e.g. "you"	e.g.	e.g. "hello" / Thumbs up
Iconics - shape/outlining	**Iconics - pretending**	
e.g. "cup" / e.g. "camera"	e.g. "cold" / e.g. "scissors"	
Number	**Air writing**	**Other**

CGC developed by Anna Caute, Abi Roper, Lucy Dipper & Madeleine Pritchard [July 2017], synthesised from coding criteria used in the aphasia and gesture research literature and refined through co-design with practising UK speech and language therapists. Images used with permission from **british-sign.co.uk**

Figure 6.3 Example of the City Gesture Checklist (CGC) that summarizes gesture types and quantity

Source: © Caute, Dipper, & Roper 2021; https://aphasia.talkbank.org/gesture/CGC.pdf and https://figshare.com/s/04a60389e5ba500a88da

---

Box 6.1 Questions in the City Gesture Checklist (CGC) Pertaining to Gesture Functions and the Manner They Are Employed

Examinee's characteristics:

(1) Is there a hemiplegia or hemiparesis?
(2) Were gestures produced using both hands or arms?
(3) Were gestures produced using the dominant hand?
(4) Was there perseveration of gestures?
(5) Was there motor difficulty carrying out gestures (e.g., grouping behaviors)?

Gesture functions:

(6) Did gestures accompany speech?
(7) Did gestures replace speech?
(8) Were there other communication methods alongside gesture (e.g., drawing, writing, facial expression, etc.)?

Manner of gesture production:

(9) Was there a variety of gesture types used?
(10) Was there a missing gesture type that could extend communication?
(11) Was there an over-reliance on one type of gesture?
(12) How effective was the use of gesture?

Source: Caute et al. (2021)

Kendon (1983), prosody is one of the three components of human spoken language, in addition to verbal communication and gestures. These three components are typically used by everyday speakers simultaneously during communication to accomplish the representation of a specific meaning. Cruttenden (1986) has specified the direct links between prosodic features and non-verbal behaviours, such as a rising pitch in association with a rising head and a rising tone in association with lifting eyebrow or hands.

Framework for Analysis of Aphasic Speech

Prosody comprises a variety of supra-segmental phenomena that determine the structure of a spoken utterance, such as intonation, prominence, stress, or breaks. Three major acoustical parameters related to speech prosody, including fundamental frequency (F0), intensity, and duration, have been extensively researched in the literature.

A large body of investigations aiming to examine the prosodic characteristics of oral discourse among healthy adult speakers is available in the field of linguistics and applied linguistics. Similar studies focusing on disordered speech in aphasia, with a great majority of them looking at the prosodic dimensions of Broca's aphasia, have been conducted to establish some objective measures that could quantify the types and degrees of aphasia. For example, according to Ackermann et al. (1993), the dysprosody of English speakers with Broca's aphasia predominantly included disturbance of temporal organization of speech utterances. Secondary to the disorder in phonetic production, implementation of articulatory gestures, and/or planning of sentences, speech production in Broca's aphasia has been reported to be altered in intonation contours (Ackermann et al., 1993), restricted in the ranges of intonation (Ryalls, 1982), higher in the variation of F0 formant frequency and vowel duration (Ryalls, 1986), disturbed in production of F0 (Seddoh, 2004), impaired in the control of speech rate during vowel production (Baum, 1993), as well as disordered in temporal (durational) control of consonant and vowel production (Baum et al., 1990). A later study on speech production of native Italian speakers with Broca's aphasia revealed intrusion of long pauses within utterance, frequent F0 resetting, widened F0 range, and abnormal lengthening of syllables which distorted the overall intonation (Marotta et al., 2008). Hisham (2014) also showed that Palestinian-speaking individuals with Broca's aphasia suffered from deficits in speech planning and timing, abnormal durational patterns, impairments in the implementation of phrase-final lengthening, and exhibited a F0 range higher than unimpaired speakers.

Measurement of acoustic parameters in earlier studies, such as voice-onset-time (VOT), formant, and phoneme duration, were mainly performed by human inspection of speech waveforms and spectrograms. Some of these features were found to be contrastive between fluent and non-fluent aphasia (Baum, 1993; Wambaugh et al., 1996). In the past two decades, a small number of studies have attempted to automate assessment of aphasic speech based on machine learning techniques (e.g., Fraser et al., 2013; Le et al., 2014). Aphasic pattern classifiers were trained using both text and acoustic features extracted from manually annotated narrative recordings. These studies focused mostly on English; similar works on other languages have rarely been reported (Dahmani et al., 2008).

Aprosodia in Right Hemisphere Damage (RHD)

Apart from the disorders in the semantics, syntactic, and pragmatic aspects of language, another well-documented deficit of verbal communication associated with right hemisphere damage (RHD) is impaired prosody.

Aprosodia largely refers to the reduced ability or inability to produce or comprehend affective aspects of language (Blake, 2007).

Speakers with RHD are characterized by their flattened and monotonous speech patterns with attenuated variations in stress, duration, and fundamental frequency (Duffy, 1995). Given that language skills and motor speech abilities are fundamentally unimpaired following a pure right hemispheric brain insult, linguistic and motor speech disturbances are often not considered as the primary source of prosodic problems in RHD. According to Myers (1999), prosodic production deficits secondary to RHD can be emotional or linguistic in nature:

- Emotional prosodic production deficits have the unique features of flat, robotic, and monotone prosodic contour in spontaneous speech. The ability to use pitch variations to signal emotion tends to be reduced. Therefore, listeners may perceive these prosodic characteristics in RHD as problems in matching the appropriate prosodic contour to one's emotional status. It is, therefore, not uncommon for RHD speakers to rely on semantic information to convey emotions. One hypothesis about this impaired ability of prosody-emotion matching is that encoding of emotional behavior is affected by the brain damage among individuals with RHD (e.g., Ross, 1985), which is often accompanied by reduced emotional output in other modalities, such as facial expressions or gestures.
- Linguistic prosodic production deficits are related to the defected use of prosodic cues to signal contrastive stress. For example, speakers with RHD have been reported to be impaired in producing different sentence types (such as declaratives, interrogatives, and imperatives) with the use of appropriate pitch patterns (Weinstraub et al., 1981). At the sentence level, speakers with RHD have a tendency to use fewer and less salient cues to signal emphatic stress. The uniform pausing occurs between words, problematic inter-syllabic pausing, and reduced contrastive stress across words or syllables also leads to the signature mechanical sound characteristic in RHD.

A number of studies on remediation of aprosodia have been published (e.g., Anderson et al., 1999; Rosenbek et al., 2004; Stringer, 1996) but their treatment efficacy has been limited. This has led to some questioning of whether aprosodia is amenable to treatment (Leon et al., 2005). One challenge with behavioral treatment of aprosodia is the co-morbidity of anosognosia in many individuals with RHD.

Impaired Prosody in Traumatic Brain Injury (TBI)

Irwin (2009) summarized different prosodic impairments associated with traumatic brain injry (TBI), and concluded that almost all aspects of prosodic production are susceptible to the negative impact of TBI but detailed analysis across various specific aspects of prosody is required due to individual variations in this population. Prosodic abnormality (or dysprosody) in TBI can be caused by impaired speech subsystems (including respiration, phonation, articulation, and resonation) which subsequently lead to dysarthria. The affected word intelligibility across severity ratings in TBI has also been found to correlate with impaired prosody. Deviant speech dimensions commonly related to dysprosody are highly variable in TBI, and include rate of speech, syllable length, pitch, volume, stress, and phrase length (Theodoros et al., 1994). The type and severity level of dysarthria subsequent to TBI can affect different aspects of prosodic production; therefore, one cannot really identify a "typical" prosodic profile of speakers with TBI.

A recent systematic review by Ilie et al. (2017) has also highlighted the relationship between TBI and impaired ability to process prosody. In particular, TBI survivors were found to react statistically significantly slower than healthy individuals in identifying emotions (e.g., empathy and irony) from prosody. Apart from this longer reaction time needed to identify or label prosodic information about emotions, discrimination of emotional and non-emotional tones was also problematic. Speakers with TBI were significantly more impaired to process prosodic information that is muffled, nonsense, competing, or in conflict. It was concluded that further research is warranted to examine how factors like TBI severity, brain injury location, and time elapsed since injury would influence the extent of these confirmed prosodic processing impairments.

Impaired Affective Prosody in Alzheimer's Disease and Prosodic Characteristics in Mild Cognitive Impairments (MCI)

Testa et al. (2001) reported a study that assessed the ability of patients with Alzheimer's disease to produce and repeat affective prosody in relation to their severity of dementia and changes in emotional behaviors. To identify the patterns of deficits in affective communication, the participants were engaged in a semi-structured interview to discuss situations and activities that could trigger emotional responses (such as fear, happiness, or embarrassment). Affective-prosodic repetitions were elicited by asking the participants to repeat sentences and strings of monosyllables using renditions of various emotional intonations including "neutral," "sad," "surprised," "angry," "happy," and "disinterested." Although the patients with Alzheimer's disease maintained relatively normal performance in their spontaneous affective-prosody, significant impairments were found in their ability to repeat affective aspects of speech. Progressive decline in using affective prosody was found as the severity of dementia increased. Furthermore, patients with a higher degree of negative behavioral changes, such as depression, had a tendency to demonstrate more problematic symptoms of sensory aprosodia. This was in contrast to participants with normal affective-prosodic performance who displayed less dementia symptoms, more close-to-normal linguistic abilities, and fewer aberrant psychiatric behaviors. In summary, speakers with dementia could also be at risk for affective-prosodic deficits, which seemed to get worse in terms of their disturbances in prosodic skills and mood as they became more affected by the condition of dementia.

In a recent study by Meilán et al. (2020), speech parameters related to mild cognitive impairment (MCI) and those that may flag the presence of developing or preclinical Alzheimer's disease (i.e., an underlying neurodegenerative process) were explored. Compared with a group of 73 older people with non-degenerative MCI, the overall group performance of 13 persons with developing Alzheimer's disease demonstrated significantly longer duration of reading time and phonation time, more pauses in utterances and more syllable intervals, softer speech (i.e., lower voice intensity), more concentration of energy in low frequency sounds, and higher variability in articulatory rhythm. The authors concluded that these characteristics of more imprecise utterances, a higher degree of dysfluency, more speech pauses in syntactic boundaries of utterances, greater variability in the number of syllabic boundaries with high rhythmic variability, and lower periodicity and isochrony in speech were notable markers to more advanced dementia in the future.

Instrumental Analysis: A Computerized Approach on Analyzing Speech Prosody

The use of instrumental analysis in assessing and classifying prosodic impairments has opened a new avenue for more detailed, refined, and elaborated descriptions of these deficits associated with acquired neurogenic disorders. Together with conventional auditory-perceptual methods, this instrumental technique can provide a more thorough assessment and subsequently lead to a better understanding of these deficits. Since acoustic analyses can be conducted in computers with a relatively low cost, speech prosody of speakers with various types of disorders can also be analyzed based on factors such as disorder severity, age, or gender (Kent & Kim, 2003). Acoustic analyses of the overall speech functions in a speaker can be done by a parametric assessment of speech sub-systems as illustrated in Table 6.4. Given speech prosody is more related to duration, intensity, pitch, and fundamental frequency (F0) contour, our discussion here will focus on these aspects.

In order to perform a more detailed analysis of the prosodic characteristics of oral discourse, units of spoken words and phonemes need to be located based on their occurrences with reference to the corresponding speech signals. An alignment process linking the speech signals and their

Table 6.4 Speech sub-systems involved in parametric assessment of speech functions

Speech functions	Aspects of speech production involved in an acoustic analysis
Prosody	• analysis of intonation pattern • analysis of pitch range and duration of consonants • analysis of pitch range and duration of vowels • voice analysis
Intelligibility	• analysis of consonants • analysis of vowels • analysis of intonation • analysis of nasal resonance
Speech rate	• analysis of speech rate • analysis of **diadochokinetic (DDK) rate**
Voice quality	• analysis of nasal resonance • analysis of intonation • voice analysis, such as sustained phonation

corresponding spoken unit in a digital audio file can be done manually, by marking the time boundaries between each signal and its spoken units. However, a major drawback is that it may take a long time (i.e., many hours) to finish one short speech sample (say a few minutes) and is therefore not practically feasible. With the use of specialized programs, such as the Hidden Markov Model Toolkit (HTK) (University of Cambridge, 2003–2014) or Praat (Boersma & Weenink, 2002–2014), and suitable algorithms (e.g., EasyAlign; Goldman, 2008), a forced alignment process can be conducted automatically instead. A pre-requisite needed before conducting this alignment process is the use of existing acoustic models to ensure automatic and optimal matching between the speech signal and the corresponding spoken unit. In theory, each orthographic transcript can be aligned into phonemes, syllables, and individual orthographic words as illustrated in Figure 6.4.

Post-alignment analysis such as pitch tracking and duration measurement can then be conducted by extracting relevant information based on the aligned dataset. Using specific scripts or functions included in the Praat software, measures such as mean F0 and pitch range of each utterance, average pitch levels across the sampled utterances, duration of onset and coda of individual lexical items, etc. can be calculated. Spectrograms can also be created for each utterance to facilitate the analytic process, if needed.

Using this analytic framework, Lee et al. (2013) investigated the statistical variation of speech duration in oral discourse by 17 speakers with fluent aphasia. Specifically, the focus of the analysis was on (1) the duration of

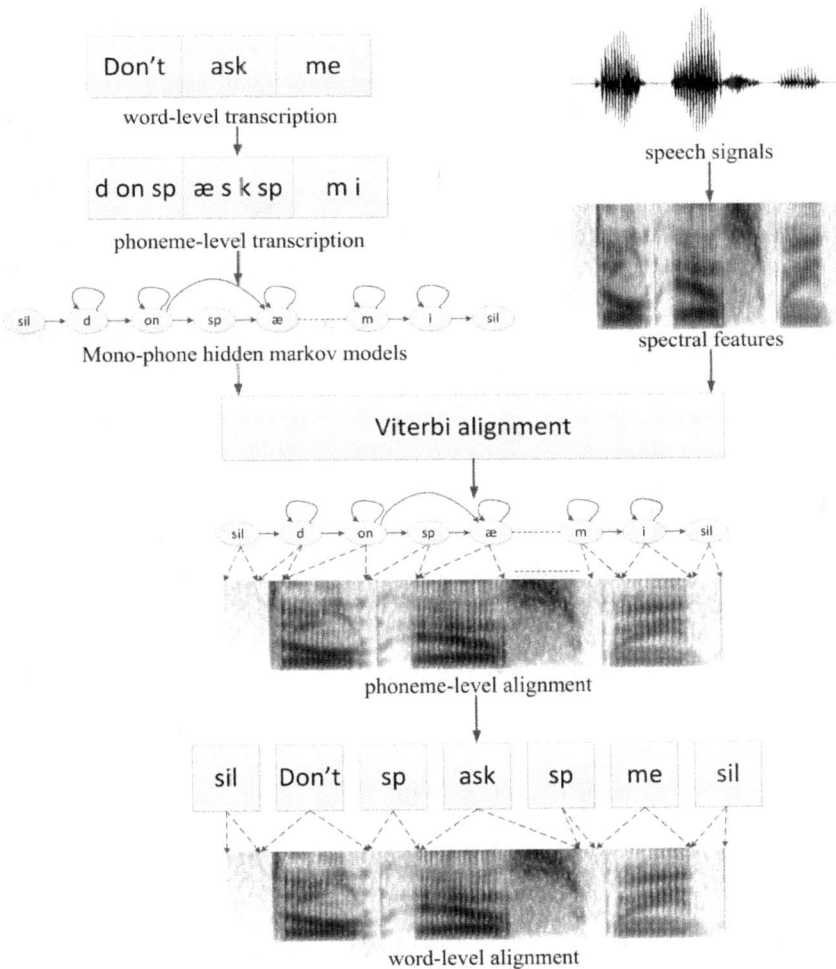

Figure 6.4 An illustration of automatic forced alignment
Source: © Anthony Pak-Hin Kong, Ph.D.

continuous speech chunks, and (2) the duration ratio of speech chunk and inter-chunk pauses. A speech chunk was defined by Lee et al. as a segment of speech samples containing propositional speech that did not contain any non-speech or unintelligible speech segments. It must be a continuous signal segment bounded by major pauses that were 0.5 seconds in length or longer. The observations on aphasic speech samples were also compared with those of unimpaired control speakers. The major observations on the characteristics of aphasic discourse duration included the following:

1. The aphasic group produced a higher number of continuous speech chunks (close to three times more) than the controls, although the normal discourse contained 50% more words than the aphasic samples. In other words, the aphasic samples were more fragmented and the overall quantity of the output tended to be lower.
2. Speech chunks in the control samples tended to be longer than the aphasic ones, with an average number of 10.5 and 5.8 words for the unimpaired and aphasic speech, respectively.
3. The average duration of a speech chunk was shorter in the aphasic group (1.73 second) compared to the controls (2.79 second).
4. The average inter-chunk pauses in aphasic speech was longer in the aphasic group (0.82 second), as compared to the normal counterparts (0.62 second).

Although speech chunks obtained using the above-mentioned definition are not necessarily related to the linguistic or prosodic structure of the utterance, the fact that (1) speakers with aphasia tended to have more silence breaks than controls and that (2) the average duration of these silence breaks was longer is consistent with the typical profile of aphasia. At the lexical level, the aphasic group produced fewer spoken characters in total, but the average duration for producing a character was significantly longer than controls. This provides further objective supports to their reduced efficiency in conveying propositions. As a result, there were more speech segments in the aphasic group, with each segment found to be shorter in duration and to contain fewer spoken characters. A follow-up investigation on the discrepancy of word durations for content and function words in fluent aphasia by the same research group was recently reported (Lee et al., 2014). On top of the overall longer word duration demonstrated by the aphasic group, which was in line with their earlier results of higher speaking rate in speech of unimpaired speakers, it was found that content words (including open-class parts-of-speech such as nouns, verbs, and adjectives) were significantly longer than function words in the aphasic speech samples. Such a difference was not statistically significant in control group.

In the past decade, there has been a fast growing interest in using natural language processing (NLP) (see Chapter 4 for details) and speech signal processing to extract speech and language features in disordered speech for clinical decision making, or – more specifically – for making a clinical diagnosis. The recent developments in the fields of computational linguistics and machine learning, as well as the advancement of technology in speech signal processing, have made it possible to apply computational methods to automate the analysis of speech and language datasets (Voleti et al., 2019).

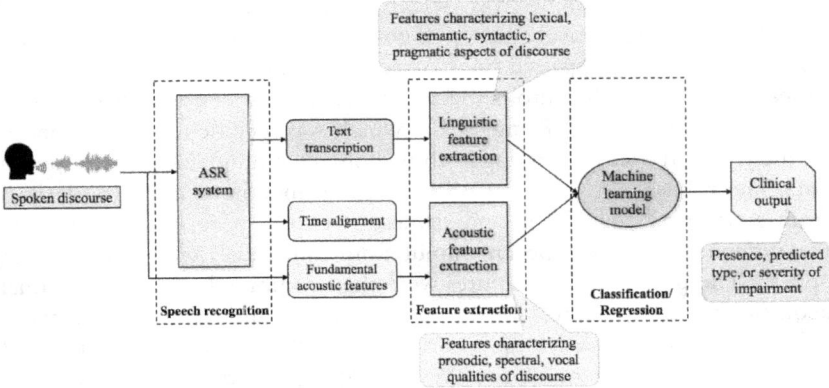

Features characterizing lexical, semantic, syntactic, or pragmatic aspects of discourse

Features characterizing prosodic, spectral, vocal qualities of discourse

Figure 6.5 An illustration of applying automatic speech recognition (ASR) and machine learning-based approaches of analysis to make a clinical diagnosis

Source: © Anthony Pak-Hin Kong, Ph.D.

Figure 6.5 provides a simplified illustration of how **automatic speech recognition (ASR)** and machine learning-based approaches of analysis is applied to make a clinical diagnosis. A language sample is first collected from a patient using one or more elicitation tasks. Instead of manual transcription, the sample is transcribed via ASR. This is followed by extracting a set of speech and language features that aim to measure different aspects of acoustic (e.g., prosodic characteristics such as loudness or fundamental frequency, spectral characteristics such as speech formant trajectories, or vocal qualities such as jitter or shimmer) and linguistic (e.g., lexical, semantic, syntactic, or pragmatic characteristics) information in the original sample. These features then become the input of a machine-learning model that aims to predict a dependent variable of interest, such as the presence of a clinical disorder (e.g., early detection of Alzheimer's dementia; Mahajan & Baths, 2021, or mild cognitive impairment; Nagumo et al., 2020) and/or the severity and type of this condition (e.g., classification of Alzheimer's dementia and prediction of related neuropsychological scores; Haulcy & Glass, 2021).

One major challenge in applying ASR to process pathological language samples is the spontaneous nature of speech, in which language impairments can be misclassified as reduced proficiency in speaking. Qin et al. (2018) demonstrated the possibility of extracting robust acoustic features of suprasegmental duration (i.e., non-speech-to-speech duration ratio, average duration of silence segments, average duration of speech segments, ratio of silence segment count to syllable count, and syllable count per second) and text features (e.g., inter-story feature of number mis-clustered story vectors, and intra-story feature of similarity with reference to unimpaired speech) from erroneous ASR output based on Chinese speakers with aphasia. A sensitivity of 89.4% and 88.6% was yielded to classify more severe and milder cases of aphasia, respectively, on top of good differentiation between speakers with aphasia and unimpaired ones. A recent investigation has described the development of a fully automated system of deep neural network (DNN) based ASR (Qin, Lee, & Kong, 2020), which was specific to aphasic speech by multi-task training involving both in-domain and out-of-domain speech data. The robust text features similar to those in Qin et al. 2018, derived from story-level embedding and siamese network, were used to quantify the difference between speech output from individuals with and without aphasia. The proposed text features were then combined with conventional acoustic features to address aspects of speech and language impairments in aphasia. Results revealed a high correlation (0.83) between predicted and official aphasia quotient of the Western Aphasia Battery, suggesting that this fully automated ASR was an efficient way of processing and analyzing aphasic speech for the purposes of diagnosis and rehabilitation. In a follow-up study, Qin, Wu et al. (2020) reported an end-to-end approach to automatic speech assessment for Cantonese speakers with aphasia. Comparisons of various neural networks (e.g., 2-layer Gated Recurrent Unit [GRU] and Convolutional Neural Network [CNN] models) to classify disordered speech were performed. It was concluded that the CNN model was able to learn duration-related features as well as acoustic features such as transitions between speech parts and silence parts or variation of formants to determine the severity of aphasia. Similar studies focusing on individuals with Alzheimer disease (e.g., Barragán Pulido et al., 2020; Lopez-de-Ipina et al., 2018) have also emerged.

With easy access to different open access or public speech and language databases, such as corpora of unimpaired speech (see, for example, Open Language Archives Community, OLA [www.language-archives.org/], Linguistic Data Consortium hosted by the University of Pennsylvania [www.ldc.upenn.edu/], or The Language Archive of Max Planck Institute for Psycholinguistics [https://archive.mpi.nl/tla/]) and disordered speech (see, for example, TalkBank [www.talkbank.org/] or Database Enterprise for Language And Speech Disorders, DELAD; Lee et al., 2021), there is an increased potential for combining extracted acoustic and text-based features from speech and language samples to help automatic assessment of communication, cognitive, and related mental (thought) disorders.

Conclusions

This chapter presented an overview of a number of multi-modal and multi-level analyses of oral discourse reported in the literature. Linguistic, extralinguistic, and prosodic information is closely tied together when one produces a spontaneous oral discourse. Performing a multi-modal analysis of oral discourse can, therefore, allow an examiner to consider multiple features of deficits demonstrated by a language-impaired person. Proper annotation of gestural and prosodic information accompanying spoken language can also provide clinicians with important insights into the management of language disorders. With more systematic and scientific investigations, it is believed that this analytic approach will gain more research attention, which will in turn allow better clinical application in the future.

Acknowledgement

Part of the research results presented in this chapter was supported by a grant from the National Institute of Health (NIH) "Toward a multi-modal and multi-level analysis of Chinese aphasic discourse" (R01DC010398) to the author.

References

Ackermann, H., Hertrich, I., & Ziegler, W. (1993). Prosodic disorders in neurologic diseases: A review of the literature. *Fortschritte der Neurologie − Psychiatrie, 61*(7), 241–253.

Akbıyık, S., Karaduman, A., Göksun, T., & Chatterjee, A. (2018). The relationship between co-speech gesture production and macrolinguistic discourse abilities in people with focal brain injury. *Neuropsychologia, 117,* 440–453.

Alibali, M. W., & DiRusso, A. A. (1999). The function of gesture in learning to count: More than keeping track. *Cognitive Development, 14*(1), 37–56.

Alibali, M. W., Kita, S., & Young, A. J. (2000). Gesture and the process of speech production: We think, therefore we gesture. *Language & Cognitive Processes, 15*(6), 593–613.

Anderson, J. M., Beversdorf, D. Q., Heilman, K. M., & Gonzalez-Rothi, L. J. (1999). Treatment of expressive aprosodia associated with right hemisphere injury. *Journal of International Neuropsychological Society, 5,* 157.

Argyriou, P., Mohr, C., & Kita, S. (2017). Hand matters: Left-hand gestures enhance metaphor explanation. *Journal of Experimental Psychology, 43,* 874–886.

Armstrong, L., Brady, M., Mackenzie, C., & Norrie, J. (2007). Transcription-less analysis of aphasic discourse: A clinician's dream or a possibility? *Aphasiology, 21*(3–4), 355–374.

Barragán Pulido, M. L., Hernández, J., Ballester, M., González, C., Mekyska, J., & Smékal, Z. (2020). Alzheimer's disease and automatic speech analysis: A review. *Expert Systems with Applications, 150,* 113213.

Baum, S. R. (1993). An acoustic analysis of rate of speech effects on vowel production in aphasia. *Brain and Language, 44*(4), 414–430.

Baum, S. R., Blumstein, S. E., Naeser, M. A., & Palumbo, C. L. (1990). Temporal dimensions of consonant and vowel production: An acoustic and CT scan analysis of aphasic speech. *Brain and Language, 39*(1), 33–56.

Bavelas, J. B., Chovil, N., Coates, L., & Roe, L. (1995). Gestures specialized for dialogue. *Personality and Social Psychology Bulletin, 21,* 394–405.

Bayles, K., & Yomoeda, C. (2007). *Cognitive-communication disorders of dementia*. San Diego, CA: Plural Publishing.

Beall, A. E. (2004). Body language speaks: Reading and responding more effectively to hidden communication. *Communication World, 21*(2), 18–20.

Beattie, G., & Shovelton, H. (1999). Mapping the range of information contained in the iconic hand gestures that accompany spontaneous speech. *Journal of Language and Social Psychology, 18*(4), 438–462.

Beattie, G., & Shovelton, H. (2000). Iconic hand gestures and the predictability of words in context in spontaneous speech. *British Journal of Psychology, 91*(4), 473.

Beck, A. R., & Fritz, H. (1998). Can individuals who have aphasia learn iconic codes? *Augmentative and Alternative Communication, 14*, 184–196.

Blake, M. L. (2007). Perspectives on treatment for communication deficits associated with right hemisphere brain damage. *American Journal of Speech-Language Pathology, 16*, 331–342.

Boersma, P., & Weenink, D. (2002–2014). Praat: doing phonetics by computer [Computer software]. www.fon.hum.uva.nl/praat/

Butterworth, B., & Hadar, U. (1989). Gesture, speech, and computational stages: A reply to McNeill. *Psychological Review, 96*(1), 168–174.

Cataldo, V., Schettino, L., Savy, R., Poggi, I., Origlia, A., Ansani, A., Sessa, I., & Chiera, A. (2019). Phonetic and functional features of pauses, and concurrent gestures in tourist guides' speech. In D. Piccardi, F. Ardolino, & S. Calamai (Eds.), *Audio archives at the crossroads of speech sciences, digital humanities and digital heritage* (Vol. 6, pp. 205–231). Milano: Officinaventuno.

Caute, A., Dipper, L., & Roper, A. (2021). The City Gesture Checklist: The development of a novel gesture assessment. *International Journal of Language & Communication Disorders, 56*(1), 20–35.

Cicone, M., Wapner, W., Foldi, N., Zurif, E., & Gardner, H. (1979). The relation between gesture and language in aphasic communication. *Brain and Language, 8*(3), 324–349.

Clough, S., & Duff, M. C. (2020). The role of gesture in communication and cognition: Implications for understanding and treating neurogenic communication disorders. *Frontiers in Human Neuroscience, 14*, 323.

Cohen, R. L., & Borsoi, D. (1996). The role of gestures in description-communication: A cross-sectional study of aging. *Journal of Nonverbal Behavior, 20*(1), 45–63.

Collins, M. (1986) *Diagnosis and treatment of global aphasia*. San Diego, CA: College Hill Press.

Crowder, E. M. (1996). Gestures at work in sense-making science talk. *The Journal of the Learning Sciences, 5*(3), 173–208.

Cruttenden, A. (1986). *Intonation*. Cambridge: Cambridge University Press.

Crystal, D. (1992). *Introducing linguistics*. Harlow: Penguin

Dahmani, H., Selouani, S., Chetouani, M., & Doghmane, N. (2008). Prosody modelling of speech aphasia: Case study of Algerian patients. In *2008 3rd International Conference on Information and Communication Technologies: From Theory to Applications (ICTTA)* (pp. 1–6). IEEE. doi: 10.1109/ICTTA.2008.4530030

de Ruiter, J. (2000). The production of gesture and speech. In D. McNeill (Ed.), *Language and gesture* (pp. 284–311). Cambridge: Cambridge University Press.

Duffy, J. R. (1995). *Motor speech disorders: Substrates, differential diagnosis, and management*. St Louis, MO: Mosby.

Efron, D. (1941). *Gesture and environment*. Morningside Heights, NY: King's Crown Press.

Ekman, P. (1966). Communication through nonverbal behavior: A source of inforamation about interpersonal relationship. In S. S. Tomkins, & C. E. Izard (Eds.), *Affect, cognition and personality* (pp. 390–442). New York, NY: Springer Publishing Company Inc.

Ekman, P. (1977). Biological and cultural constribution to body and facial movements. In J. *Blacking* (Ed.), *Anthropology of the body* (pp. 39–84). New York, NY: Academic Press.

Ekman, P. & Friesen, W.V. (1969). The repertoire of nonverbal behavior: Categories, origins, usage, and coding. *Semiotica, 1*(1), 49–98.

Ekman, P. & Friesen, W.V. (1972). Hand movements. *Journal of Communication, 22*(4), 353–374.

Enderby, P., & Hamilton, G. (1983). Communication aid and therapeutic tool: A report on the clinical trial using Splink with aphasic individuals. In C. Code & B. Muller (Eds.), *Aphasia therapy* (pp. 187–193). London: Edward Arnold.

Feyereisen, P. (1987). Gestures and speech, interactions and separations: A reply to McNeill (1985). *Psychological Review, 94*, 492–498.

Feyereisen, P., & Havard, I. (1999). Mental imagery and production of hand gestures while speaking in younger and older adults. *Journal of Nonverbal Behavior, 23*(2), 153–171.

Fraser, K. C., Rudzicz, F., & Rochon, E. (2013). Using text and acoustic features to diagnose progressive aphasia and its subtypes. In *Proceedings of Interspeech* (pp. 2177–2181).

Fridlund, A. (1994). *Human facial expression: An evolutionary view*. San Diego, CA: Academic Press.

Fronda, G., & Balconi, M. (2020). The effect of interbrain synchronization in gesture observation: A fNIRS study. *Brain and Behavior, 10*(7), e01663.

Garrett, M. F. (1975). Syntactic process in sentence production. *Psychology of Learning and Motivation, 9*, 133–177.

Geoff, R., & Thompson, R. (2001). *Understanding body language*. Hauppauge, NY: Barron's Educational Series, Inc.

German, D. J. (2001). *It's on the tip of my tongue: Word-finding strategies to remember names and words you often forget*. Chicago, IL: Word Finding Materials, Inc.

Glass, A., Gazaniga, M., & Premack, D. (1975) Artificial language training in global aphasics. *Neuropsychologia, 11*, 95–103.

Glosser, G., Wiener, M., & Kaplan, E. (1986). Communicative gestures in aphasia. *Brain and Language, 27*(2), 345–359.

Goldin-Meadow, S. (1999). The role of gesture in communication and thinking. *Trends in Cognitive Sciences, 3*(11), 419–429.

Goldin-Meadow, S. (2003). *Hearing gesture: How our hands help us think*. Cambridge, MA.: Belknap Press of Harvard University Press.

Goldman, J. P. (2008). EasyAlign: A semi-automatic phonetic alignment tool under Praat. http://latlcui.unige.ch/phonetique/easyalign.php

Gooch, C. M., Stern, Y., & Rakitin, B. C. (2009). Evidence for age-related changes to temporal attention and memory from the choice time production task. *Aging, Neuropsychology & Cognition, 16*(3), 285–310.

Gullberg, M. (2011). Thinking, speaking, and gesturing about motion in more than one language. In A. Pavlenko (Ed.), *Thinking and speaking in two languages* (pp. 143–169). Bristol: Multilingual Matters.

Hadar, U., & Butterworth, B. (1997). Iconic gestures, imagery, and word retrieval in speech. *Semiotica, 115*, 147–172.

Haulcy, R., & Glass, J. (2021). Classifying Alzheimer's disease using audio and text-based representations of speech. *Frontiers in Psychology, 11*, 624137.

Herrmann, M., Reichle, T., Lucius-Hoene, G., Wallesch, C.-W., & Johannsen-Horbach, H. (1988). Nonverbal communication as a compensative strategy for severely nonfluent aphasics? – A quantitative approach. *Brain and Language, 33*(1), 41–54.

Hisham, A. (2014). Dysprosody in aphasia: An acoustic analysis evidence from Palestinian Arabic. *Journal of Language and Linguistic Studies, 10*(1), 153–162.

Hofemann, N. N., Fritsch, J., & Sagerer, G. (2004). Recognition of deictic gestures with context. *Lecture Notes in Computer Science, 3175*, 334–341.

Hogrefe, K., Ziegler, W., Weidinger, N., & Goldenberg, G. (2012). Non-verbal communication in severe aphasia: Influence of aphasia, apraxia, or semantic processing? *Cortex, 48*, 952–962.

Holland, A. (1984). *Language disorders in adults*. San Diego, CA: College Hill Press

Hostetter, A. B., & Alibali, M. W. (2007). Raise your hand if you're spatial: Relations between verbal and spatial skills and gesture production. *Gesture, 7*, 73–95.

Ilie, G., Cusimano, M. D., & Li, W. (2017). Prosodic processing post traumatic brain injury – a systematic review. *Systematic Reviews, 6*(1), 1.

Irwin, B. (2009). Prosodic impairment associated with traumatic brain injury. *Perspectives on Neurophysiology and Neurogenic Speech and Language, 19*(3), 97–102.

Jacobs, N., & Garnham, A. (2007). The role of conversational hand gestures in a narrative task. *Journal of Memory and Language, 56*(2), 291–303.

Jagoe, C., & Wharton, T. (2021). Meaning non-verbally: The neglected corners of the bi-dimensional continuum communication in people with aphasia. *Journal of Pragmatics, 178*, 21–30.

Kartchava, E., & Mohamed, A. (2020). Investigating EAP teachers' use and perceptions of gesture in general and in corrective feedback episodes. *TESL Canada Journal, 37*(2), 51–77.

Kendon, A. (1981). *Nonverbal communication, interaction, and gesture*. The Hague: Mouton.

Kendon, A. (1983). Gesture and speech: How they interact. In J. M. Wiemann, & R. P. Harrison (Eds.), *Nonverbal interaction* (pp. 13–43). Beverly Hills: Sage Publications.

Kendon, A. (2004). *Gesture: Visible action as utterance*. New York: Cambridge University Press.

Kendon, A., Sebeok, T. A., & Umiker-Sebeok, J. (1981). *Nonverbal communication, interaction, and gesture: Selections from SEMIOTICA*. Hauge: Mouton Publishers.

Kent, R. D., & Kim, Y. J. (2003). Toward an acoustic typology of motor speech disorders. *Clinical Linguistics and Phonetics, 17*(6), 427–45.

Kistner, J. (2017). *The use of gestures in the conversations of people with aphasia*. Doctoral Dissertation City: University of London.

Kistner, J., Dipper, L. T., & Marshall, J. (2019). The use and function of gestures in word-finding difficulties in aphasia. *Aphasiology, 33*(11), 1372–1392.

Kistner, J., Marshall, J. & Dipper. L. T. (2020). The influence of conversation parameters on gesture production in aphasia. *Clinical Linguistics & Phonetics, 34*(8), 693–717.

Kita, S. (2009). Cross-cultural variation of speech-accompanying gesture: A review. *Language and Cognitive Processes, 24*(2), 145–167.

Knapp, M. L., & Hall, J. A. (2010). *Nonverbal communication in human interaction*. Boston, MA: Wadsworth/Cengage Learning.

Knapp, M. L., Hall, J. A., & Horgan, T. G. (2014). *Nonverbal communication in human interaction*. Boston, MA: Wadsworth Cengage Learning.

Kohler, C. G., Turner, T., Stolar, N. M., Bilker, W. B., Brensinger, C. M., Gur, R. E., & Gur, R. C. (2004). Differences in facial expressions of four universal emotions. *Psychiatry Research, 128*, 235–244.

Kong, A. P. H., Law, S.-P., & Chak, G. W.-C. (2017). A comparison of co-verbal gesture use in oral discourse among speakers with fluent and non-fluent aphasia. *Journal of Speech, Language, and Hearing Research, 60*, 2031–2046.

Kong, A. P. H., Law, S. P., & Cheung, C. K.-Y. (2019). Use of co-verbal gestures during word-finding difficulty among Cantonese speakers with fluent aphasia and unimpaired controls. *Aphasiology, 33*(2), 216–233.

Kong, A. P. H., Law, S.-P., Kwan, C. C.Y., Lai, C., & Lam,V. (2015). A coding system with independent annotations of gesture forms and functions during verbal communication: Development of a Database of Speech and GEsture (DoSaGE). *Journal of Nonverbal Behavior, 39*(1), 93–111.

Kong, A. P. H., Law, S. P., Kwan, C., Lai, C., Lam,V., & Lee, A. (2012, November 18–20). *A comprehensive framework to analyze co-verbal gestures during discourse production* [Poster presentation]. The 2012 American Speech–Language–Hearing Association (ASHA) Convention, Atlanta, GA, USA.

Kong, A. P. H., Law, S.P., & Lee, A. S. Y. (2010). An investigation of use of nonverbal behaviors among individuals with aphasia in Hong Kong: Preliminary data. *Procedia Social and Behavioral Sciences, 6*, 57–58.

Kong, A. P. H., Law, S., Wat, W., & Lai, C. (2013). Employment of gestures in spontaneous verbal discourse by speakers with aphasia. *Procedia Social and Behavioral Sciences, 94*, 200–201.

Kong, A. P. H., Law, S. P., Wat, W. K. C., & Lai, C. (2015). Co-verbal gestures among speakers with aphasia: Influence of aphasia severity, linguistic and semantic skills, and hemiplegia on gesture employment in oral discourse. *Journal of Communication Disorders, 56*, 88–102.

Krauss, R. M., & Hadar, U. (1999). The role of speech-related arm/hand gestures in word retrieval. In R. Campbell & L. Messing (Eds.), *Gesture, speech, and sign* (pp. 93–116). Oxford: Oxford University Press.

Krönke, K. M., Mueller, K., Friederici, A. D., & Obrig, H. (2013). Learning by doing? The effect of gestures on implicit retrieval of newly acquired words. *Cortex, 49*, 2553–2568.

Lanyon, L., & Rose, M. L. (2009). Do the hands have it? The facilitation effects of arm and hand gesture on word retrieval in aphasia. *Aphasiology, 23*(7–8), 809–822.

Le, D., Licata, K., Mercado, E., Persad, C., & Provost, E. M. (2014). Automatic analysis of speech quality for aphasia treatment. *Proceedings of Acoustics, Speech and Signal Processing (ICASSP), 2014*, 4853–4857.

Lee, A., Bessell, N., van den Heuvel, H., Saalasti, S., Klessa, K., Müller, N., & Ball, M. J. (2021). The latest development of the DELAD project for sharing corpora of speech disorders. *Clinical Linguistics & Phonetics*. Epub ahead. doi: 10.1080/02699206.2021.1913514

Lee, T., Kong, A. P. H., Chan, V. C. F., & Wang, H. (2013). Analysis of auto-aligned and auto-segmented oral discourse by speakers with aphasia: A preliminary study on the acoustic parameter of duration. *Procedia Social and Behavioral Sciences*, *94*, 71–72.

Lee, T., Kong, A. P. H., & Wang, H. (2014, October 5–7). Duration of content and function words in oral discourse by speakers with fluent aphasia: Preliminary data [Poster presentation]. Fifty-second annual meeting of Academy of Aphasia, Miami, FL, USA. doi: 10.3389/conf.fpsyg.2014.64.00039.

Lemay, A., David, R., & Thomas, A.P. (1988). The use of spontaneous gesture by aphasic patients. *Aphasiology*, *2*(2), 137–145.

Leon, S. A., Rosenbek, J. C., Crucian, G. P., Hieber, B., Holiway, B., Rodriguez, A. D., Ketterson, T. U., Ciampitti, M. Z., Freshwater, S., Heilman, K., & Gonzalez-Rothi, L. J. (2005). Active treatments for aprosodia secondary to right hemisphere stroke. *Journal of Rehabilitation Research and Development*, *41*(1), 93–102.

Levelt, W. J. M. (1989). *Speaking: From intention to articulation*. Cambridge, MA: MIT Press.

Lopez-de-Ipina, K., Martinez-de-Lizarduy, U., Calvo, P. M., Mekyska, J., Beitia, B., Barroso, N., Estanga, A., Tainta, M., & Ecay-Torres, M. (2018). Advances on automatic speech analysis for early detection of Alzheimer disease: A non-linear multitask approach. *Current Alzheimer Research*, *15*(2), 139–148.

MacWhinney, B. (2003). Child Language Analyses (CLAN) [Computer software]. https://childes.talkbank.org/

Mahajan, P., & Baths, V. (2021). Acoustic and language based deep learning approaches for Alzheimer's dementia detection from spontaneous speech. *Frontiers in Aging Neuroscience*, *13*, 623607.

Malandro, L. A., Barker, L. L., & Barker, D. A. (1989). *Nonverbal communication*. Reading, MA: Addison-Wesley.

Marotta G., Barbera, M., & Bongioanni, P. (2008). Prosody and Broca's aphasia: An acoustic analysis. *Studi Linguistici e Filologici*, *6*, 79–98.

Mather, S. M. (2005). Ethnographic research on the use of visually based regulators for teachers and interpreters. In M. Metzger & E. Fleetwood (Eds.), *Attitudes, innuendo, and regulators* (pp. 136–161). Washington, DC: Gallaudet University Press.

Max Planck Institute for Psycholinguistics. (2002). www.lat-mpi.eu/tools/elan/.

Mayberry, R. I., & Jaques, J. (2000). Gesture production during stuttered speech: Insights into the nature of gesture-speech integration. In D. McNeill (Ed.), *Language and gesture* (pp. 199–214). New York: Cambridge University Press.

McNeill, D. (1985). So you think gestures are nonverbal? *Psychological Review*, *92*(3), 271–295.

McNeill, D. (1992). *Hand and mind: What gestures reveal about thought*. Chicago, IL: The University of Chicago Press.

McNeill, D. (2000). *Language and gesture*. Cambridge: Cambridge University Press.

Meilán, J., Martínez-Sánchez, F., Martínez-Nicolás, I., Llorente, T. E., & Carro, J. (2020). Changes in the rhythm of speech difference between people with nondegenerative mild cognitive impairment and with preclinical dementia. *Behavioural Neurology*, *2020*, 4683573.

Montepare, J., Koff, E., Zaitchik, D., & Albert, M. (1999). The use of body movements and gestures as cues to emotions in younger and older adults. *Journal of Nonverbal Behavior*, *23*, 133–152.

Montepare, J. M., & Tucker, J. S. (1999). Aging and nonverbal behavior: Current perspectives and future directions. *Journal of Nonverbal Behavior*, *23*, 105–109.

Morrel-Samuels, P. & Krauss, R. (1992). Word familiarity predicts temporal asyn-chrony of hand gestures and speech. *Journal of Experimental Psychology: Learning, Memory and Cognition, 18*, 615–622.

Myers, P. S. (1999). *Right hemisphere damage: Disorders of communication and cognition.* San Diego, CA: Singular Publishing.

Nagumo, R., Zhang, Y., Ogawa, Y., Hosokawa, M., Abe, K., Ukeda, T., Sumi, S., Kurita, S., Nakakubo, S., Lee, S., Doi, T., & Shimada, H. (2020). Automatic detection of cognitive impairments through acoustic analysis of speech. *Current Alzheimer Research, 17*(1), 60–68.

Nicholas, M., & Helm-Estabrooks, N. (1994) Patterns of language preservation and loss in global aphasia. *Seminars in Speech and Language, 15*(1), 37–52.

Old, S. R., & Naveh-Benjamin, M. (2008). Differential effects of age on item and asso-ciative measures of memory: A meta-analysis. *Psychology and Aging, 23*(1), 104–118.

Özer, D., & Göksun, T. (2020). Gesture use and processing: A review on individual differences in cognitive resources. *Frontiers in Psychology, 11*, 573555.

Özer, D., Göksun, T., & Chatterjee, A. (2019). Differential roles of gestures on spa-tial language in neurotypical elderly adults and individuals with focal brain injury. *Cognitive Neuropsychology, 36*(5–6), 282–299.

Poggi, I. (2008). Iconicity in different types of gestures. *Gesture, 8*(1), 45–61.

Qin, Y., Lee, T., & Kong, A. P. H. (2018). Automatic speech assessment for aphasic patients based on syllable-level embedding and supra-segmental duration features. *Proceedings of ICASSP, 2018*, 5994–5998.

Qin, Y., Lee, T., & Kong, A. P. H. (2020). Automatic assessment of speech impairment in Cantonese-speaking people with aphasia. *IEEE Journal of Selected Topics in Signal Processing, 14*(2), 331–345.

Qin, Y., Wu, Y., Lee, T. & Kong, A. P. H. (2020). An end-to-end approach to automatic speech assessment for Cantonese-speaking people with aphasia. *Journal of Signal Processing Systems, 92*(8), 819–830.

Quek, F., McNeill, D., Bryll, R., Duncan, S., Ma, X .F., Kirbas, C., McCullough, K. E., & Ansari, R. (2002). Multimodal human discourse: Gesture and speech. *ACM Transactions on Computer-Human Interaction, 9*(3), 171–193.

Rauscher, F. H., Krauss, R. M., & Chen, Y. (1996). Gesture, speech, and lexical access: The role of lexical movements in speech production. *Psychological Science, 7*(4), 226–231.

Rosenbek, J. C., Crucian, G. P., Leon, S. A., Hieber, B., Rodriguez, A. D., Holiway, B., Ketterson, T. U., Ciampitti, M., Heilman, K., & Gonzalez-Rothi, L. J. (2004). Novel treatments for expressive aprosodia: A phase I investigation of cognitive-lin-guistic and imitative interventions. *Journal of International Neuropsychological Society, 10*, 786–793.

Ross, E. D. (1985). Modulation of affect and non-verbal communication by the right hemisphere. In M. M. Mesulam (Ed.), *Principles of behavioral neurology* (pp. 239–257). Philadelphia: F. A. Davis.

Ryalls, J. (1982). Intonation in Broca's aphasia. *Neuropsychologia, 20*, 355–360.

Ryalls, J. (1986). An acoustic study of vowel production in aphasia. *Brain and Language, 29*, 48–67.

Scharp, V. L., Tompkins, C. A., & Iverson, J. M. (2007). Gesture and aphasia: Helping hands? *Aphasiology, 21*, 717–725.

Seddoh, S. A. (2004). Prosodic disturbance in aphasia: Speech timing versus inton-ation production. *Clinical Linguistics & Phonetics, 18*(1), 17–38.

Sekine, K., Rose, M. L., Foster, A. M., Attard, M. C., & Lanyon, L. E. (2013). Gesture production patterns in aphasic discourse: In-depth description and preliminary predictions. *Aphasiology, 27*(9), 1031–1049.

Ska, B., & Nespoulous, J. (1987). Pantomimes and aging. *Journal of Clinical and Experimental Neuropsychology, 9*, 754–766.

Stringer, A. Y. (1996). Treatment of motor aprosodia with pitch biofeedback and expression modeling. *Brain Injury, 10*, 583–590.

Szabó, É., Béres, T., & Guba, C. (2020). A beszélgetőműsorokban megjelenő kézi gesztusok leírásának egy lehetséges módja [A possible way for describing hand gestures in talk shows]. *Jelentés és Nyelvhasználat, 7*(1), 51–74.

Testa, J. A., Beatty, W. W., Gleason, A. C., Orbelo, D. M., & Ross, E. D. (2001). Impaired affective prosody in AD: relationship to aphasic deficits and emotional behaviors. *Neurology, 57*, 1474–1481.

Theodoros, D. G., Murdoch, B. E., & Chenery, H. I. (1994). Perceptual speech characteristics of dysarthric speakers following severe closed head injury. *Brain Injury, 8*, 101–124.

University of Cambridge. (2003–2014). Hidden Markov Model (HTK) Toolkit [Computer software]. http://htk.eng.cam.ac.uk/

Van Nispen, K., Van De Sandt-Koenderman, M., Mol, L., & Krahmer, E. (2016). Pantomime production by people with aphasia: What are influencing factors? *Journal of Speech, Language, and Hearing Research, 59*(4), 745–758.

Van Nispen, K., Van De Sandt-Koenderman, M., Sekine, K., Krahmer, E., & Rose, M. L. (2017). Part of the message comes in gesture: How people with aphasia convey information in different gesture types as compared with information in their speech. *Aphasiology, 31*(9), 1078–1103.

Verderber, R. F., Verderber, K. S., & Sellnow, D. D. (2012). *COMM 3 (with CourseMate with Interactive Video Activities, SpeechBuilder(TM) Express Printed Access Card)*. Boston, MA: Wadsworth Cengage Learning.

Voleti, R., Liss, J. M., & Berisha, V. (2019). A review of automated speech and language features for assessment of cognitive and thought disorders. *IEEE Journal of Selected Topics in Signal Processing, 14*(2), 282–298.

Wambaugh, J. L., Doyle, P. J., Kalinyak, M. M., & West, J. E. (1996). A critical review of acoustic analyses of aphasic and/or apraxic speech. *Clinical Aphasiology, 24*, 35–63.

Weinstraub, S., Mesulam, M. M., & Kramer, L. (1981). Disturbance in prosody: A right hemisphere contribution to language. *Archives of Neurology, 38*, 742–744.

Wells, B., & Whiteside, S. (2008). Prosodic impairment. In M. J. Ball, M. R. Perkins, N. Muller, & S. Howard (Eds.), *The handbook of clinical linguistics* (pp. 549–567). Oxford: Wiley-Blackwell.

Wilson, F. R. (1998). *The hand: How its use shapes the brain, language, and human culture*. New York, NY: Pantheon Books.

Wouters, M. (2020). Gestures and speech: The role of learners' gestures in second language acquisition [Master thesis] Faculté de philosophie, arts et lettres, Université catholique de Louvain. Prom.: Gilquin, Gaëtanelle. http://hdl.handle.net/2078.1/thesis:24058

Xu, J., Gannon, P. J., Emmorey, K., Jason, F. S., & Braun, A. R. (2009). Symbolic gestures and spoken language are processed by a common neural system. *Proceedings of the National Academy of Sciences of the United States of America, 106*(49), 20664–20669.

Appendix 6.1

A Gesture Coding Form Modified From Kong et al. (2010, 2015)

Patient name: _____   Date of birth/Age: _____   Gender: M / F   Etiology: _____

Date of testing: _____   Speech therapist: _____

Sentence number	Narrative task: ___ / Total duration: ___ minutes ___ seconds	Number of words	Gesture form						Gesture function								Remarks for gestures
			Iconic	Metaphoric	Deictic	Emblems	Beats	Non-identifiable	Providing additional information	Enhancing speech content	Providing alternative means of communication	Guiding and controlling speech flow	Reinforcing speech intonation or prosody	Assisting lexical retrieval	Assisting sentence re-construction	No specific function	
1																	
2																	
3																	
4																	
5																	
6																	
7																	
8																	
9																	
10																	

Appendix 6.1 Continued

Narrative task: _____

Total duration: _____ minutes _____ seconds

Sentence number	Number of words	Gesture form						Gesture function								Remarks for gestures
		Iconic	Metaphoric	Deictic	Emblems	Beats	Non-identifiable	Providing additional information	Enhancing speech content	Providing alternative means of communication	Guiding and controlling speech flow	Reinforcing speech intonation or prosody	Assisting lexical retrieval	Assisting sentence re-construction	No specific function	
I1																
I2																
I3																
I4																
I5																
Total:																

Overall remarks:

(1) Total number of gestures:
(2) Total number of words (or token):
(3) Total number of utterances:
(4) Total number of errors produced:
(5) The ratio of gestures to token:
(6) The ratio of gestures to utterance:
(7) The ratio of errors to gesture:

Considerations for Treatment Options That Can Facilitate and Enhance Discourse Production

Chapter Objectives

The reader will be able to:

1. describe various methods to strengthen word retrieval in aphasic discourse
2. differentiate between communication-based and drill-based discourse intervention in aphasia
3. describe the significance of using multi-modal communication training in discourse treatment
4. describe the basic principles of enhancing social communication skills among speakers with brain injuries
5. describe the relationships between cognitive rehabilitation and discourse production among speakers with brain injuries
6. discuss the basic principles of discourse training among speakers with right hemisphere damage
7. discuss the basic principles of discourse training among speakers with dementia
8. explain how conversational therapy is applied to speakers with aphasia, traumatic brain injury, and dementia
9. explain how the approach of group therapy is beneficial to enhance discourse production in aphasia, traumatic brain injury, and dementia
10. discuss how communication partners can be involved in discourse treatment for aphasia, traumatic brain injury, and dementia.

Introduction

A diverse literature has addressed the need for intervention of spoken language at the discourse level for speakers with acquired neurogenic communication impairments. Many articles have been published to discuss discourse interventions involving word retrieval or conversation for aphasia (e.g., Bhogal et al., 2003; Brady et al., 2012). Some other reports have illustrated

DOI: 10.4324/9781003254775-7

behavioral and cognitive training for speakers with concurrent cognitive communicative disorders (e.g., Cicerone et al., 2011). A major conclusion for most of these review articles is that appropriate remediation for individuals with acquired communication disorders is crucial and has great benefits to the service receivers as well as their significant others or primary caregivers (see also Green, 1984).

A recent systematic review of interventions targeting discourse production in aphasia (Dipper et al., 2020) has highlighted that discourse treatments are clinically efficacious and can improve outcomes of people with aphasia. In order to provide a more comprehensive summary that organizes the information from various sources regarding discourse treatment in the adult population, this chapter will provide a description of various therapy approaches reported in the existing literature and will attempt to identify gaps on the issue of valid approaches and measures to discourse treatment. With a coherent synopsis describing various intervention practices, the content of this chapter will be a good resource for clinicians or researchers in the field.

Principles of Treatment to Facilitate Discourse in Aphasia

A great proportion of studies on discourse therapy in the literature were carried out in the population with aphasia. Therefore, a higher variety of therapeutic techniques are available for clinicians who would like to address discourse impairments associated with this condition. Most of the protocols discussed in this section are interventions that either directly and specifically address one's problematic discourse process(es) or strengthen one's linguistic ability with maintenance of residual linguistic skills.

Targeting Spoken Word Retrieval With Discourse Treatment

According to the review article by Boyle (2011), various word retrieval treatment approaches using the communication context to target structured conversations and narrative discourse have been reported to lead to positive treatment effects and/or maintenance of discourse production. In other words, positive outcomes for improved word-finding abilities can contribute to the general processes of word retrieval, as well as better and more efficient sentence construction, which then facilitates enhanced macrostructures of discourse (such as increased overall degree of informativeness) (Conroy et al., 2009). Specifically, reported treatment programs include the following:

- Phonologic and orthographic cueing (e.g., Greenwood et al., 2010; Herbert et al., 2003; Hickin et al., 2001) is usually conducted in two phases. The first phase involves intervention focusing on naming of nouns, with targets treated with phonologic and orthographic cues provided in a contingency-based hierarchy and distractors. These cues are first given with minimal information, followed by grading addition of phonemes or letters of a target until the item is named or the whole word (i.e., model) has been presented for repetition. The second phase typically includes tasks designed to systematically move from picture naming towards controlled conversational speech. Carefully structured conversations with the same targets used in phase 1 are practiced and trained in phase 2. Suitable tasks may include naming to definition, PACE activity that involves structured conversation, or production of spoken lists of treated items in goal-directed categories.

- Semantic feature analysis (SFA; e.g., Antonucci, 2009; Boyle, 2004; Peach & Reuter, 2010) is a functional therapeutic technique that has been widely used for the treatment of naming deficits at the single word level among individuals with aphasia (Davis & Stanton, 2005). With the aim of facilitating an individual with aphasia to access semantic networks and to provide self-cues during instances of anomia (Boyle & Coelho, 1995), the therapy centers at the mapping between a target concept (usually a noun) with related semantic features using a SFA diagram (see Figure 7.1; modified from Haarbauer-Krupa et al., 1985; Massaro & Tompkins, 1992), so that a 'web' of concepts related to the target written in the diagram is generated. The mapping process is initiated even if a speaker can spontaneously name the target initially. Common prompts used during a training may include "This makes me think of...", or "This can be found in...". By completing and analyzing the SFA diagram, a speaker with naming difficulties can see connections, make predictions, and master important concepts, all of which are skills crucial

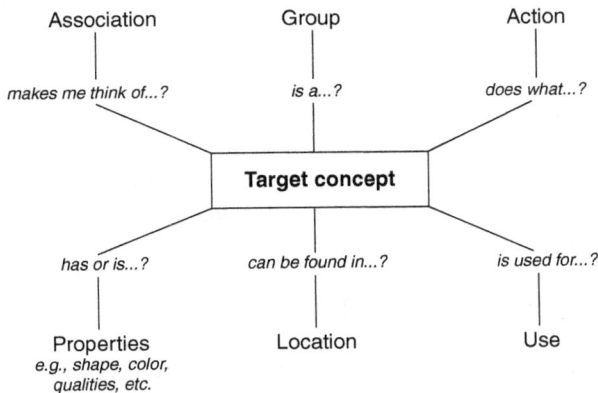

Figure 7.1 Semantic feature analysis (SFA) diagram
Source: © Anthony Pak-Hin Kong, Ph.D.

for enhancing vocabulary use and comprehension. The application of the SFA to spontaneous discourse can be done by asking a speaker to produce narratives using progressively longer picture sequences, to describe a series of events, or to produce a procedural discourse. When there is a difficulty in producing a target noun during the telling of stories, the same method of generating semantic features and similar cueing strategies mentioned above is used. The same method can be applied to other parts-of-speech, such as verbs (Peach & Reuter, 2010). Once this SFA strategy becomes internalized and is used habitually, it can help a speaker explore how sets of things are related to one another and promotes the speaker's use of key lexical items as well as important features related to a topic.

- **Phonomotor Treatment (PMT**; Kendall, Oelke, Brookshire, & Nadeau, 2015) is an intensive treatment program that focuses on phonological processing. It involves a 2-stage multi-modal training of speech sounds, first in isolation and then progressing to sound combinations and single words. Stage 1 of this treatment addresses isolated sounds and includes various perception (auditory perceptual discrimination and grapheme-to-phoneme matching) and production (oral phoneme productions, and visual feedback + verbal descriptions of motor movements) tasks through multi-modal processing of orthographic, auditory, articulatory-motor, tactile-kinesthetic, visual, and conceptual information of targets. Stage 2 proceeds with the same procedures, except that the training focuses on sound combinations, progressing to 1-, 2-, and 3-syllable phoneme sequences in both real and non-word combinations. Instead of just improvement in lexical retrieval, a recent examination (Silkes et al., 2019) reported that PMT could lead to widespread improvement throughout the language system, including the functionally critical level of discourse production in speakers with aphasia. Specifically, an immediate treatment effect post-treatment and a maintenance effect three months later were shown by a significant improvement in Correct Information Units (CIUs) per minute. Significantly better percentage of CIUs at the maintenance testing were also observed. In a follow-up investigation (Silkes et al., 2021) that aimed to compare the effects of PMT and SFA on discourse production, it was found that PMT could facilitate more long-lasting improvement of functional communication at the discourse level.

- Barrier task treatment paradigms targeting verb retrieval (e.g., Goral & Kempler, 2009; Hengst et al., 2010; Hengst et al., 2008):

  - Using modified constraint-induced aphasia therapy (CIAT) procedures, Goral and Kempler (2009) applied the treatment protocol to target verb production in the narrative task of co-constructing stories. Specifically, CIAT has been designed for people with more chronic aphasia, who may adopt a number of basic compensatory strategies to help them communicate. It involved systematic constraint of verbal as well as non-verbal communication modalities with massed practice of targeted language skills because persons with aphasia who relied on the use of compensatory strategies would diminish their previously learned communication skills and delaying their recovery. The aim of CIAT is for clinicians to identify these types of compensatory strategies (such as the use of gestures, facial expressions, pointing, writing, drawing, or making simple sound effects) demonstrated by the speakers with aphasia and constrain their use. Instead, the employment of specifically targeted communication methods (which tend to be more complex) are encouraged and trained (Balardin & Miotto, 2009; Szaflarski et al., 2008). CIAT can promote improvement of language functions through the use of the language center in the brain. Full speech may not be necessary because the final target usually depends on a speaker's severity level and spared ability. This extension of using the traditional request-response training paradigm involved the use of contingency-based cueing hierarchy similar to that in the above-mentioned phonologic and orthographic cueing approach.

- Another reported barrier task involved the construction of verbal labels for people and places in a semi-structured conversation task, with a focus on repeated engagement (Hengst et al., 2008; Hengst et al., 2010). Since the production of actual labels (or verbal items) can vary from session to session, the goal is to enhance verb production in discourse through strengthening the process of coming up with labels agreed between a clinician and a client in one single treatment session or over several sessions. The paradigm allows replication of real-life conversational repetition, but with the topic of conversation constrained for easier control on the part of the clinician. According to the authors of the above studies, these non-traditional methods to address discourse-level word retrieval deficits were viable and clinically relevant options to enhance oral discourse. Appendix 7.1 shows some suggested discourse activities.

Impairment-Based Versus Drill-Based Versus Communication-Based Treatment

Impairment-based treatments typically involve training on word or sentence production that targets specific micro-linguistic impairments, including word-finding problems, lexical errors, syntactic and paragrammatic errors, incomplete cohesive ties, limited or impaired connective forms, or reduced syntactic complexity. Intervention following this approach mainly focuses on training the specific impaired language component(s) and addresses some secondary treatment targets of incorporating strategies to compensate for the deficit(s). Improvement of micro-linguistic skills may positively affect the overall macro-linguistic structure of discourse. In addition, improved language skills at the impairment level can sometimes help its generalization to functional communication (Teasell et al., 2011). Many researchers have argued that everyday communication, such as conversation, presents a paradigm of using language that can be very different from a task-based situation. For example, Springer et al. (2000) have mentioned that daily conversation is a challenging task for speakers with aphasia because of the additional cognitive and emotional complications, on top of linguistic demand, involved in the process among these speakers. This is in contrast to the more controlled impairment-based intervention that contains primarily specific behaviors targeted in a therapy. Some patients, such as those with a more severe degree of language impairment, may benefit more from a well-structured linguistic task with targets aimed at improving a particular skill or sets of skills.

Drill-based treatments have a strong emphasis on repetition and careful selection of training items with reference to a patient's limitation, current level of language performance, and specific need(s). Howard and Hatfield (1987) called this approach the "stimulation" method because of its heavy reliance on multiple drill repetitions (or imitations) of a set of target items across different elicitation tasks in a session. This arrangement is often repeated across a number of sessions to facilitate a patient's learning through reinforcement of behaviors and strengthening of neuro-pathways that underlie target skills (Hengst et al., 2010).

Communication-based treatments, on the other hand, are often mediated using a communicative context to conduct an intervention. Use of language by a patient is often facilitated by various communication contexts to achieve the major goal of linguistic (as well as non-verbal) information transfer. Other researchers have considered this approach of training as a sociolinguistic, functional, or pragmatic method (see Kempler, 2005) and highlighted the dialogic features of this therapy technique. One important characteristic of this therapy method is its incorporation of exchange of novel information between a clinician and a patient, irrespective of the language activities or task (e.g., open-ended dialogues, one-to-one or group discussions, or structured barrier tasks).

Kempler and Goral (2011) have described two treatment protocols that targeted spoken production of well-formed sentences containing verbs:

- The first was referred to as the "drill protocol" because the principle treatment was eliciting target verbs and sentence structures through repetition, with maximum support of auditory modeling and visual stimuli. A total of 64 concrete and picturable verbs were used for the total duration of 30 treatment hours, distributed over four weeks, i.e., an average of 7.5 hours per week. The productions of targets were mediated by tasks that were highly structured to practice a list of verbs. Since the list contained a closed set of predetermined target verbs, there was no exchange of novel information between the clinician and patient. Instead, auditory models, written stimuli, and action pictures of the target verbs were practiced across a range of language activities, such as sentence repetition, sentence completion, choral reading, and picture description.

- The second protocol was the "generative protocol" that promoted verb production in sentences during less constructed communicative exchanges. This method largely adapted the pragmatically-based cooperative principle that guides conversation (Grice, 1975). The production was more spontaneous in language activities without the use of direct modeling of pre-selected targets. Depending on the nature and content of a treatment activity, any verbs deemed to be appropriate were acceptable and could be considered correct. Unlike the "drill protocol" in which the practice of pre-determined verbs was obligatory, there was no specified "correct target" for a particular action. The key was to promote functional and flexible use of language for a specific context as well as appropriate, relevant, and unambiguous use of a verb that could sufficiently distinguish that action from others.

These two protocols both determined target sentence structures for individual patients based on their linguistic competency. The ultimate goal was for the speakers to produce a verb in a well-formed sentence that was difficult, but not impossible, to produce. The target sentence structure could also be shaped throughout the course of therapy so that the clinician could potentially increase the length and complexity of sentences being treated. For example, according to Kempler and Goral (2011), the target sentence structures may progress through the following sequence with one structure targeted at a time:

1. present progressive verbs in isolation, e.g., "crying"
2. subject + intransitive verb (S–V) phrases, e.g., "The girl is crying"
3. subject + transitive verb + object (S–V–O) phrases, e.g., "The girl is reading a book"
4. subject + verb + object + prepositional phrase (S–V–O–PP) phrases, e.g., "The girl is reading a book on the bed."

A criterion of 80% performance level was suggested before a patient advanced to the next target structure, which was more complex. The accuracy was monitored by regular probing the production of verbs within the target structure every three to six treatment hours. Three levels of scaffolding in all tasks were also implemented in the following order:

1. general prompts, e.g., "Could you say that sentence with a verb?"
2. more specific prompts, e.g., "What is this person doing?"
3. models for direct repetition.

The effectiveness of these two protocols for improving narrative production in aphasia, as reflected by measures on lexical (e.g., total number of verbs or verb density) and sentential (e.g., lexical density of utterances or sentence completeness) performance as well as discourse productivity (e.g., total number of words and utterances) and narrative structures (e.g., local and global coherence and story line ratio), was evaluated. While the results based on two speakers with chronic non-fluent aphasia suggested that both methods had led to positive outcomes, the communication-based intervention was more effective in improving narrative production, primarily due to its emphasis on exchanging new information and the fact that it allowed better capitalization of one's preserved discourse knowledge.

Novel Approach to Real-Life Communication: Narrative Intervention in Aphasia (NARNIA)

Developed by Whitworth et al., (2015) to address discourse problems in aphasia, the integrated multilevel intervention of Novel Approach to Real-life communication: Narrative Intervention in Aphasia (NARNIA) has been shown to improve macrostructure use to further scaffold production of words and sentences for subsequent discourse organization. The specific steps in NARNIA include:

1. reference to a metalinguistic approach of using language, to increase a client's awareness of and attention to word-level production as well as sentence and discourse structures
2. using picture sequences, to first focus on helping the client identify the main event(s), and then to access the relevant verbs and nouns for each event (to subsequently create a complete argument structure for the corresponding main event)
3. reference to personally related real-life incidents of the client, to maximize attention to actions and corresponding nouns for future oral descriptions
4. introducing a framework for narrative discourse and the sentences required (based on story grammar) to organize a complete output with a beginning (i.e., setting of the scene), middle (i.e., events taking place), and end (i.e., coda of the story)
5. introducing frameworks for the other genres (e.g., recount, procedure, or exposition) when the client achieves a good mastery of this narrative framework

6. improving a mind-mapping approach to retrieve and then link ideas to help organize and plan of thoughts for subsequent production
7. addressing appropriate use of cohesive devices (e.g., reference and connectives) to maximize connectivity between ideas
8. promoting self-evaluation of performance across all levels of word, sentence, and discourse production after each discourse attempt.

According to the authors, the implementation of these steps should follow several principles. First, visual prompts will be used but will gradually decrease. A client's responses may be written down initially but, as the sessions progress, there should be a transition to the spoken modality of output, with feedback provided in real time. Finally, the majority of topics in the treatment sessions should be directly related to and prompted from the client's personal experiences; this will facilitate generalization of intervention.

Conversational Therapy

Conversation serves an important function to exchange information between two speakers, to maintain social relationships in humans, to negotiate a sense of self, and to manage a healthy emotional status. Many intervention programs of aphasia have the ultimate goal to increase the functional level of a patient's ability to communicate naturally through the means of everyday conversations. For example, impairment-focused therapy for aphasia has been reported to facilitate the conversational skills of persons with aphasia (Carragher et al., 2012). In a later qualitative review on conversation therapy for aphasia (Simmons-Mackie et al.,2014), the authors summarized that there are four "principle roots" that contribute to this therapy method:

1. **Life Participation Approach to Aphasia (LPAA**; Byng & Duchan 2005; LPAA Project Group, 2000; Simmons-Mackie 1998, 2000, 2008): This approach overtly aims to improve access to and participation in conversation among people with aphasia. The process of improving conversation is generally conducted in the context of social and participation models of intervention. Specifically, it is a "consumer-driven service-delivery approach that supports individuals with aphasia and others affected by it in achieving their immediate and longer term life goals" (Chapey et al., 2000; p.4). With the focus on helping individuals with aphasia to re-engage in life so that they will, in the long run, rely on minimal communication support, conversation therapy often involves the patients and their families in deciding the intervention content. This decision-making process significantly empowers the persons involved to choose and participate in the recovery process. In other words, persons with aphasia and their significant others will actively take

part in the design of conversation interventions that ultimately aim for a more rapid return to active life participation on the part of the patients.

2. Conversation analysis (CA): In Chapter 3, we discussed the use of CA, a systematic procedure to analyze conversation in human, as a mean of evaluating and assessing aphasia. It is a rigorous approach to capture the structural features and to characterize resources that speakers with aphasia use to achieve conversational goals. For example, how well a speaker can convey a meaning, negotiate ideas collaboratively, take conversational turns, and repair communicative breakdowns can be readily reflected by various measures of CA (Goodwin & Heritage, 1990). Although CA has been mainly known for its application to clinical assessment of aphasia, it can be employed to support daily talking (e.g., Beeke et al., 2007) based on the premise that a change in the conversational behavior of the speaker with aphasia will facilitate the change in the conversational behavior of the unimpaired conversational partner, and vice versa. Instead of considering intervention options to address specific language impairments or to promote compensatory strategies to overcome aphasia, a clinician will focus the interventions towards the conversational resources and troubles experienced by a speaker. More attention is paid to highlighting the conversational patterns in partnership and ensuring both the patient and unimpaired communication partner(s) are aware of their own constructive and destructive patterns, so that the need to change is acknowledged and valued in the therapeutic process. Wilkinson (1995) has also emphasized the interactive nature of CA because of the close engagement between the clinician, the person with aphasia, and the person's conversational partner in the intervention process. One common method to achieve the above is to provide both communication partners involved with options for change and an environment for them to practice and review new conversational patterns. In particular, a CA program can be divided into three stages as illustrated by Beeke et al. (2007):

I.   Stage 1: Focus on raising awareness of conversation in general, which can be done by an education and discussion of aspects of communication and repair between the parties (i.e., person with aphasia and communication partner) receiving conversation therapy and the clinician. The strength of conversation competence currently demonstrated by the language-impaired speaker and communication partner can also be addressed.

II. Stage 2: Focus on raising awareness of the parties' conversational patterns, which will often involve recording natural conversations, followed by careful reviewing of the video recordings. Discussion about the facilitatory as well as problematic conversational patterns should be done, with the aim of ensuring (1) the elimination of behaviors that have caused or may contribute to conversation breakdowns and (2) the mutual recognition of who is unhappy about the flow of a conversation and the underlying reason(s). Both partners are encouraged to discuss how they felt about the interaction and to explore options to increase and enhance more successful conversation.

III. Stage 3: Focus on strategies for change, which will involve the practice, implementation, and continuous review of effective conversation strategies. Personalized handouts may be used to identify the patterns present in their conversation and to propose helpful alternatives to be used in the training.

3. Functional and behavioral orientations (e.g., Boles, 1997, 1998; Hopper et al., 2002): This approach involves a clinician directly addressing problematic behaviors that affect the ongoing of a conversation and modifying these behaviors through appropriate training. Examples of behaviors that are commonly targeted in conversation therapy include the following:

a. Targeting persons with aphasia:
   i. increasing multi-modal or total communication
   ii. increasing initiations, turn taking, and participation in conversation
   iii. asking more questions
   iv. improving self-repair, repair during communication breakdown, introduction of new topics, and management of topics
   v. managing turns strategically.

b. Targeting communication partners:
   i. reducing unnecessary correcting or teaching behaviors
   ii. reducing asking for known information (such as "test questions" of "What is your name?"), interruptions, or restrictive discourse behaviors (such as overuse of close-ended questions)
   iii. improving repair strategies of communicative breakdown
   iv. facilitating turns by speakers with aphasia to increase their participation
   v. reducing speech rate and complexity
   vi. increasing the emphasis or repetition of key elements to facilitate the ongoing of a conversation
   vii. using appropriate and effective scaffolding techniques for revealing and acknowledging the competence of the person with aphasia
   viii. promoting multi-modal or total communication
   ix. managing turns strategically and improving topic management.

4. Counseling-oriented approaches: Given that some strategies in conversation therapy incorporate elements directly drawn from the field of counsellng, this approach is "relationship" oriented and is closely related to the therapeutic techniques mentioned in the counseling literature

(Boles & Lewis, 2003). While the primary goal of this approach is to improve conversation, conducting a therapy is based on the premise that the relationship of a communication party cannot be separated from their communicative interactions (Berstein-Ellis & Elman, 2007). Therefore, some methods in the intervention process are explicitly adapted from counseling or family therapy.

One should realize the overlapping nature of the four above-mentioned principle roots of conversation therapy. Nevertheless, similar to other reported aphasia treatment purposes, the focus of conversation therapy can vary depending on which approach a clinician follows to address the needs of a particular individual with aphasia or communication partner. For example, at different time of the therapy, the training can be generic or individualized. Depending on the specific needs of the party or the stage of intervention, the focus of the training may shift from addressing specific conversational problems to proposing solutions. From time to time, compensatory strategies may be introduced to encourage the person with aphasia and/or the conversation partner to use multi-modal (e.g., Kagan, 1998) and/or total communication, such as writing, drawing, pictographs, props, gestures, or electronic devices (Rautakoski, 2011), to assist oral conversation.

The use of computerized rehabilitation programs for conversation training have been reported by Cherney et al. (2008) and Manheim et al. (2009). The authors of these two studies reported therapeutic procedures that involved the use of computerized script training, including (1) the development of individualized scripts that were pre-recorded on the AphasiaScripts™ computer software, (2) extensive home practice for nine weeks with a daily training of 30 minutes, as well as (3) weekly follow-up meetings with clinicians to monitor practice and assess progress. The practice was divided into three stages: (1) patient observed the routine with verbal and visual input; (2) repetition of sentences in the conversation; and (3) conversation practice with a virtual therapist. Results based on speakers with chronic aphasia suggested that this training could improve their content, grammar, and conversational routines.

Beeke et al. (2018) described **Better Conversations with Aphasia (BCA)**, an intensive and tailored conversation therapy that is freely available at https://extend.ucl.ac.uk/. The BCA aims to develop, train, and promote the best conversation strategies between a person with aphasia and his or her key conversation partner with the support of a therapist. Best et al. (2016) have examined and reported how deploying video feedback in BCA was able to raise conversation partners' awareness of maladaptive conversation behaviors. Specifically, an eight-week program (of 1.5 hours per week) was conducted to actively engage eight persons with agrammatic, non-fluent aphasia and conversation partners in discussions and problem solving conversations. Video feedback, alongside written materials, was provided to focus on conversation strategies used in their dialogues. A significant decrease in barrier behaviors was found at the end of the eighth session of intervention.

Multi-Modal Communication Training

A few studies have described the simultaneous training of pre-selected stimuli in both the verbal and non-verbal modalities to strengthen links within the semantic network for word retrieval and to improve switching across both modalities to facilitate daily communication. These investigations shared the assumption that both verbal and non-verbal responses of a concept are specific extensions of the semantic representations. Furthermore, flexible movement among the verbal and non-verbal representations achieved by intensive learning and practice among speakers with language impairment can hypothetically facilitate their overall communication. Details of the general principles of some of these training protocols are as follows:

- Multi-modal Communication Training (MCT) (Purdy & Cocchiola, 2006): Purdy and Van Dyke (2011) reported the use of Multi-modal Communication Training (MCT) that involved the conveying of concepts through verbal production, writing, gesture, and drawing to enhance functional communication. This intervention is suitable for training speakers who are more severe in aphasia. According to the authors, the protocol involved six to eight hours of training and would lead to enhancement of explicit switching among verbal and non-verbal modalities among individuals with relatively intact semantic representations, thereby solidifying the use of an alternative method for them to communicate. The development of MCT was motivated by the observation that individuals with aphasia do not necessarily demonstrate spontaneous use of gestures, pointing, and/or drawing in daily communicative situations, although these forms of expression might have been trained, acquired, or used in structured situations. With the noted separation of non-verbal modality of functioning from the linguistic system, MCT aimed to promote speakers with aphasia to use non-verbal means to communicate their intended message on top of the traditionally-emphasized verbal forms of expression. It was believed that through this systematic and intense training that invoked simultaneous and focused multimodal concepts, more sophisticated integration of intermodal lexical representations would be formed that would, in turn, contribute to better communication skills. That is, more automated links between a semantic concept and its alternative means of expression would make the alternative modality more available for use in spontaneous communication. The results based on two subjects with moderate to severe aphasia suggested that MCT could improve referential communication and compensatory usage as reflected by the increase of modality-switching behaviors.

- Gestural + verbal treatment (GVT) (Raymer et al., 2006): The GVT aims to improve communication by increasing spoken word retrieval of trained nouns and verbs among speakers with aphasia and by promoting their use of gestures as an alternative means to communicate during instances of word-finding problems. The GVT was originally designed for targeting single-word level performance. A modified protocol for discourse was applied to a group of eight individuals with aphasia to examine its treatment effects on discourse content and efficiency of language production, as compared to another group of six individuals receiving conventional semantic-phonological treatment that did not involve gesture training (del Toro et al., 2008). Specifically, the modified GVT involved the following five steps:

  1. The clinician starts by presenting a picture with its verbal model and a gesture matching the picture simultaneously presented. The speaker with aphasia is required to repeat the target word and gesture three times.
  2. This is followed by the clinician performing the gesture without the word and the subject imitating the gesture model three times. Assistance on manipulation of the limbs of speakers with aphasia is given, if needed, to produce an accurate gesture.
  3. The clinician models the target word and the speaker with aphasia verbally repeats it three times.
  4. The clinician repeats the word again, syllable by syllable if necessary.
  5. After a pause of five seconds, the speaker with aphasia is asked to say the name the word again and perform the corresponding gesture one final time. A correct model will be given if the subject fails to provide a correct response.

  According to del Toro et al. (2008), each speaker with aphasia was trained on production of 20 nouns and 20 verbs for a total of ten sessions, in the frequency of three to four sessions per week. Each target item was trained at least nine times per session. The results indicated that in addition to the significant increase in noun production in post-treatment conversation samples, the use of minimal sentences decreased. The GVT was also reported to promote the production of grammatical sentences, although the change was not significant. On the other hand, information content of the conversation, as reflected by the measure of "utterances with new information (UNIs)," increased significantly as a result of the treatment, although neither the length (i.e., mean length of utterance, MLU) nor the lexical diversity (i.e., Type-Token Ratio, TTR) of the conversation changed significantly due to the GVT.

- Combined gesture therapy approach: Similar to the above-mentioned GVT that was specifically designed to enhance spoken word performance, some studies have reported positive outcomes in conversation by combining gestures with conventional language therapy. For example, the facilitative effect of combining semantic and gesture treatments for verb retrieval and use among speakers with chronic Broca's aphasia was reported by Boo and Rose (2011). These treatment effects included increased production of verbs per **correct information unit (CIU)**, increased use of substantive verbs in conversation, and increased informativeness of speech output. Rose et al. (2002) also suggested that the use of iconic gestures significantly facilitated picture naming in aphasia. The combined used of pointing, visualization, and cued articulation has led to clinical improvement of reduced frequency of phonological naming errors in conversation.

Neuromodulation of Discourse Treatment

Neuromodulation is defined by the International Neuromodulation Society as: "the alteration of nerve activity through targeted delivery of a stimulus, such as electrical stimulation or chemical agents, to specific neurological sites in the body" (www.neuromodulation.com/learn-more). Two examples of non-invasive neuromodulation strategies are the techniques of transcranial magnetic stimulation (TMS) and transcranial direct current stimulation (tDCS). They involve the delivery of magnetic (e.g., electromagnetic induction) and electrical current, respectively, through probes that sit outside the skull focusing on and/or stimulating a specific brain area. Some studies have explored their application to treatment of neuropsychiatric conditions of depression or anxiety. Language-specific benefits have also been reported; for example, anodal tDCS has been linked to improvement of word retrieval in unimpaired speakers and those with non–fluent aphasia (e.g., Fiori et al., 2011), enhanced divergent naming ability (verbal fluency in neurologically unimpaired young speakers; e.g., Pisoni et al., 2018), or reduced overall aphasia severity, as reflected by aphasia quotient of Western Aphasia Battery (e.g., Heikkinen et al., 2019).

Given the increasing popularity of neuromodulation neurorehabilitation, a small number of investigations have also studied the potential clinical application of these two techniques to discourse production. Medina et al. (2012) administered repetitive transcranial magnetic stimulation (rTMS) in ten individuals with mild to moderate non-fluent aphasia induced by left hemisphere middle cerebral artery strokes. Based on repeated measurement of their Cookie Theft picture descriptions before and after ten sessions of rTMS over two weeks at a site previously shown to improve naming, significant improvement in multiple measures of discourse productivity (e.g., production of open–class and closed–class words, or total number of verbs and unique nouns) was found. It was concluded that the improved lexical-semantic access resulting from the rTMS treatment facilitated discourse production. More recently, Matar et al. (2020) found a positive effect of anodal tDCS on discourse production (e.g., improved Correct Information Units in tasks of descriptive recount, procedural recall, and retelling the Cinderella story) in healthy older speakers. The authors concluded that it would be an effective method to counteract age-related decline in language abilities and further suggested that, with more research evidence, it could be a viable rehabilitative tool for those with higher-level language skills.

Training Discourse Using a Group Therapy Approach

The use of the group therapy approach in managing aphasia has been widely described based on its structure, client selection criteria, communicative goals and activities in relation to client characteristics, and group dynamics (e.g., Elman & Bernstein-Ellis, 1999; Ewing, 2007; Marshall, 1999). Its application has been reported in the context of social interactions or conversation for speakers with aphasia. Therapist-centered sessions are usually more structured and didactic, with the clinician primarily in charge of the group content, dynamics, and interaction. On top of planning the sessions, administering the pre-selected activities, and maintaining the focus on specific deficit areas or discourse structures of therapy, the clinician tends to control the tempo and the pace of the group. As a result of the relatively rigid framework that parallels a "teaching" paradigm, it is not uncommon to see a reduced number of and variety in speech acts demonstrated by participants. In addition, opportunities to select communication choices may be limited in this kind of group setting.

On the contrary, client-centered sessions are more socially oriented and tend to promote social interactions among the participants because this approach resembles more closely the context of natural communication (Kagan & Gailey, 1993). One of the keys to success lies in the interaction and inter-relationships with the group (Elman, 2000). The clinician can act as a facilitator, instead of a convener, to the group by providing resources to run a clinical session. Interactions within the group can also better approximate natural peer communication or conversation with families or friends. Instead of implementing defined tasks selected by the clinician, self-initiated interactions among group participants as the basis of treatment outcome should be promoted.

A qualitative study that examined successful features for discourse management in a group therapy setting for aphasia was reported by Simmons-Mackie et al. (2007). It was concluded that the following features were often present in a well-managed social group therapy session:

- Establishing the feel of discourse equality: This can be done by promoting equal opportunities for group participants to contribute to and comment on the therapy content, to show agreement as well as disagreement during the therapeutic process, to ask questions about and to evaluate the treatment, to seek opinions from others, and to negotiate as well as to share ideas about the running of subsequent intervention, irrespective of the actual length of speech or duration of production. In this sense, everyone in the group should feel encouraged to express and contribute, and be treated with respect. A symmetrical conversation between the clinician and the participants should also be established, so that the clinician is not the "center" or "boss" of the group but one of the members that can facilitate open discussion.

- Focusing on everyday communicative events and genres: The clinician should avoid the use of rigidly structured discourse in a group. Instead, natural discourse patterns or genres similar to everyday narratives or conversation can enhance the group dynamics. Overt discourse control should also be avoided. If needed, the clinician can provide appropriate reinforcement to the carrying on of a topic, advancing to the next topic, changing to a new topic, or initiating a related topic within the group.
- Employing multiple communication modes: For groups including more severe participants, use of multi-modal communicative strategies should be encouraged, especially for participants who encounter communication breakdown, need to repair, or substitute verbal means of communication by non-verbal behaviors. If necessary, the clinician can also provide models of gestures, writing, drawing, and/or pointing for group participants to interact in the training.
- Mediating communication: When one or more participants in the group have difficulties following the content of discussion or when members struggle to understand each other, the clinician may provide assistance in several ways. They include (1) reiterating a message; (2) translating the original message; (3) repeating, expanding, or extending the message; and (4) supplementing the message by additional information in other modalities (such as drawing or writing). Note that this process also marks the interest and attention of the clinician, which is a key component in keeping a social group running.
- Calibrating corrections: Instead of direct and explicit correction of participants' errors, strategies such as mediated talk or implicit correction is considered to be more accepted by group members in a social group. This approach of handling communication breakdown will not discourage the members' involvement in the group due to the loss of confidence contributed by the clinician's direct correction. In cases where a participant publicly asks for help or openly acknowledges their own errors, the clinician may also enlist the group to help solve the problem.
- Aiding turn allocation: With the aim of promoting full involvement and balanced participation across members in a social group, the clinician may apply strategies such as solicitation questions or requests, as well as silence and gaze solicitation, to provide discrete aids for turn taking.

Concerning the use of solicitation questions or requests, instead of asking for specific, known, or expected responses and/or information from one or more participants, the clinician may encourage the group to share responsibilities for allocating turns within the group or to self-select a member to mediate group dynamics. This "softer" approach would avoid the clinician's overt control of the flow of exchange. Redirecting less active participants to join the discussion with general questions or prompts, such as "Who else would like to share more?", can also be useful. Short pauses with silence and gaze within a social group or moving the gaze around a group to indicate a "next turn" opening also provide opportunities for members to adjust the turn-taking behaviors and to enter the discission as appropriate.

- Judiciously employing teachable moments: The clinician may sometimes provide educational materials, introduce new techniques, or engage specific problem-solving skills in a social group. At the same time, caution should be taken to avoid a change of the group dynamics or interpersonal patterns of the session. Ensuring a respectful orientation to the participants, with use of appropriate tone of language and body language that shows interest, respect, and attention to the members, is often welcomed by the group as a whole.

Involvement of Communication Partners

Communication partners play an important role in the rehabilitation process of aphasia. They may include familiar or usual partners, such as family members, immediate caregivers, friends, and volunteers. They tend to perform differently when responding to and managing expressive problems in people with aphasia (Laakso & Godt, 2016). A body of literature has discussed the intervention for conversational partners to induce a change in their behaviors or to enhance their skills when communicating with their significant others affected by aphasia. The majority of these studies have addressed directing coaching or training of family members (e.g., Bradley & Douglas, 2008) and volunteers (e.g., Kagan et al., 2001), which often involve the use of some outcome measures to reflect the changes of conversation aspects in both the individuals with aphasia and the communication partners (see conversational analysis in Chapter 3). The ultimate goal of involving partner training is to increase communicative access for the speakers with aphasia and reduce the psychosocial consequences of the associated language problems (Turner & Whitworth, 2006). The following components, such as educational information or materials about aphasia and its related discourse problems, behavioral observation and discussion, selection of strategies to improve verbal exchange, role play, skill practice, and systematic self-evaluation, are typically included in training of communication partners. More details can be found in the following protocols:

- Supporting Partners of People with Aphasia in Relationships and Conversation (SPPARC; Lock et al., 2001)
- Supported Conversation for Adults with Aphasia (SCA; Kagan,1998)
- Conversation Coaching (Hopper et al., 2002)
- Communication Partner Training (Simmons-Mackie et al., 2016).

Principles of Treatment to Facilitate Discourse in Traumatic Brain Injury

Compared to aphasia, individuals with traumatic brain injury (TBI) demonstrate a very different profile of language impairments (see Chapter 1). Snow and Douglas (2000) have discussed the problem of limited empirical evidence in guiding the therapeutic management of discourse deficits associated with TBI. Generally speaking, language-based interventions are suitable for addressing micro-structural or sentential impairments because they are more linguistically related (Coelho, 2007). However, deficits of discourse super-structures, such as story grammar, or pragmatic problems are more aligned with the non-linguistic and cognitive impairments associated with TBI. Hence, speakers with TBI are more apt to benefit from specific training targeting cognitive dimensions. Although various approaches of intervention have been proposed in the literature, there is still a lack of clear consensus relative to how language deficits in TBI are best treated, possibly due to the great variability in the treatment methods used and reported so far (Gindri et al., 2014). Nevertheless, since most discourse deficits associated with TBI are highly related to negative impact on social reintegration and quality of life, it is believed that addressing these problems using one or more of the following approaches, with a systematic organizational schema that can guide better discourse formulation in TBI, is beneficial to this population.

Linguistically-Based or Discourse Specific Intervention

Language is one of the major domains of cognition. Given the close relationship between linguistic and cognitive processes, Hinchliffe et al. (2001) have introduced the higher-order language approach to address the discourse problems associated with TBI. Within this framework, TBI discourse is trained with reference to two production structures, including the surface and base structures. While the surface structure represents the total output that is organized into sentences, the base structure concerns how well the meaning of the text used is represented in an organized way. The base structure of discourse can be further divided in micro-linguistic and macro-linguistic structures, where the former is related to the degree of well-formedness and the latter is related to the global semantic content of the discourse. Concerning the surface structure of discourse, targets for intervention typically include strategies to address (or improve) the productivity (e.g., number of narrative words, T-units, or number of communication units, etc.), accuracy (e.g., number of syntactic and lexical errors or **mazes**), efficiency (e.g., degree of dysflency or hesitational phenomena), and quality (e.g., syntactic complexity, ratio of subordination, etc.) of a speaker's performance at the sentential level. Intervention on cohesive ties can enhance the conjoining of meanings across sentences within a discourse, and therefore is commonly included in training of micro-linguistic skills. As for the macro-linguistic structures of TBI discourse, treatment tends to focus on the ability to provide propositions of a narrative with gist information or to provide a summary or moral of a story (see Ulatowska & Chapman, 1989). In summary, procedures mentioned in the aphasiology literature can be directly adapted or modified for use here. The major advantage of this approach is that the linguistic abilities (in terms of communicative functions, discourse skills, or specific language abilities) can be trained within the context of other cognitive skills (Coelho, 2007).

Following this approach, Whitworth (2010) investigated the efficacy of a rehabilitation protocol that combined different levels of language complexity, ranging from the word, sentence, to narrative level of oral production. This was a prototype of NARNIA (see p. 246–247) and the treatment sessions were conducted twice a week over the course of ten weeks. Training of narrative production was conducted using picture sequences as prompts and the goal was for speakers with TBI to identify the main events and to correctly name the verbs and nouns depicted in the pictures. A grammar-based narrative discourse structure was introduced for clients to create an argumentative discourse. Sentences with a beginning, a middle, and an end were formulated to narrate the story. The results revealed significant improvement of daily communication among the TBI speakers receiving this intervention. NARNIA has recently been piloted in a small group of four individuals with cognitive-communication difficulties (Whitworth et al., 2020). All participants demonstrated a significant gain in terms of output quantity, informativeness, and production efficiency; two of them also showed improved memory or working memory.

Another example is hierarchical discourse therapy (HDT; Penn et al., 1997) that addresses cognitive-communication disorders in speakers with closed head injury (CHI). This remediation protocol was developed based on the Strategies of Observed Learning Outcomes (SOLO) (Biggs & Collis, 1982) technique. The SOLO contains five levels of taxonomy describing the consistent sequence or learning cycle displayed by TBI speakers over a variety of tasks. Specifically, individuals' performance on a linguistic task is observed and rated using the following scheme:

1. SOLO level 1 (pre-structural) – there is no relation between question and answer
2. SOLO level 2 (uni-structural) – only one relevant aspect is mentioned

3. SOLO level 3 (multi-structural) – several relevant features are mentioned, but the features are not linked up
4. SOLO level 4 (relational) – general conclusions are correctly drawn from particular instances
5. SOLO level 5 (extended abstract) – there is elaboration and extrapolation beyond a given situation that incorporates all relevant data.

Two individuals with CHI received 15 SOLO therapy sessions on improving their ability to answer increasingly complex questions based on personally relevant discourse texts. According to Penn et al., a positive treatment effect was found as both CHI speakers demonstrated a higher level of text comprehension, improved ability to organize and integrate information, and better use of self-cueing and self-monitoring techniques. It was concluded that the enhanced metacognitive and metalinguistic abilities also led to improvement of the CHI speakers' discourse skills.

Targeting Story Grammar

Narrative training addressing completeness of oral narratives in a brain-injured speaker often relies on tasks such as retelling daily events. A common approach of discourse intervention focuses on speakers' use of story grammar. Coelho (2007) called this approach the "discourse abilities approach" because the training was characterized by its centering on various aspects of discourse that are noted to be impaired in speakers with TBI. In particular, Cannizzaro and Coelho (2002) introduced a treatment specific to story grammar, with a focus on treating their underlying components in spoken discourse, including (1) recognition of relationships and roles of depicted characters, (2) development of insights and making predictions of potential outcomes, (3) identification of story episodes and missing component(s) in a story, and (4) generation of stories using simple to complex pictures. This story grammar training sequence included two training conditions:

1. Story retelling condition: An individual first watched a filmstrip or looked at a picture sequence story. He or she was then asked to retell the story, with prompts such as "What were the parts of the story?" provided as necessary. The clinician would help the identification of related episodes and components if the individual had difficulty doing so. These procedures were repeated until the speaker with TBI could identify all episodes and components for a given story, with minimal or no external assistance.
2. Story generation condition: An individual was instructed to tell a story about what was happening in a picture, with the emphasis of asking him or her to use episodes as opposed to simply labelling. The telling of the story was recorded and then played back for the individual to evaluate if anything was missing and, if so, what had been omitted. The individual

was then prompted to identify the missing components and to provide with story structures as necessary to complete the story generation task. These procedures were repeated until the individual could generate at least one complete episode per picture stimulus.

This approach was applied to a male speaker with chronic TBI (post-onset of 12 years). Ten 60-minute treatment sessions were given for each treatment condition, with a frequency of three sessions per week. The results indicated a marked increase in the number of complete episodes generated over the course of treatment. However, follow-up probes, once at one month and another at three months after treatment, indicated limited carryover and poor generalization of the treatment effects. A number of factors, such as limited total duration of the treatment program, co-morbid cognitive deficits in attention, memory, and organization, and the lack of direct connection between the treatment nature and real-world consequences, might have contributed to this observed poor maintenance.

Focusing on Conversation and Social Skills

Impairment in social communication skills, or impaired pragmatics, is a common sequel to TBI and is more prevalent among those with a moderate to severe degree of brain injury (Hartley, 1995; Marsh, 1999). As a result of the cognitive deficits and personality changes secondary to the brain injury, a wide range of problems with social communication will emerge among survivors of TBI (Struchen, 2005; Ylvisaker, 1992) that can adversely affect their social well-being and social reintegration. In particular, intact social communication not only allows one to understand others and what communication partners mean to communicate, but also enables one to express thoughts and feelings to others in a way others can understand. These skills can be verbal (such as initiating and terminating a conversation, taking turns, or seeking clarifications) and non-verbal (such as using gestures, indicating feelings with facial expressions, maintaining eye contact during a conversation, or using appropriate tone of voice to express meaning and feelings) in nature. A recent interesting case study by Azios and Archer (2018) has reported the use of conversation analysis (CA) to explore the unusual instances of singing demonstrated by a TBI survivor across different therapy sessions. Although these behaviors have negatively affected this speaker's pragmatic functions, they were able to help perform facework (e.g., to project a more respected and competent image of the client) in situations of communication breakdown.

Factors such as an individual's premorbid cognitive abilities, emotional reactions to disability, and immediate environment may also complicate the pragmatic deficits of TBI (Morton & Wehman, 1995; Snow et al., 1998). Unlike the linguistically-based or discourse specific approaches mentioned above, the social skills approach focuses more on addressing problematic communicative behaviors within a specific social context, which will be crucial for subsequent employment or ultimate community reintegration. This approach employs a wider range of treatment strategies, such as role play, scripting of specific communication situations, and conversation practice with review. Establishing self-monitoring skills of targeted performance and raising awareness of own pragmatic problems are emphasized on the part of individuals with TBI. In addition, the clinician provides direct modeling and specific feedback to consolidate appropriate pragmatic functions. More detailed descriptions of some programs reported to be effective for enhancing the pragmatic skills of TBI survivors are as follows:

- Communication Awareness Training (CAT) (Snow & Douglas, 2000): This program aims to eliminate disruptive behaviors of TBI survivors. The intervention procedure involves a three-step technique that (1) increases a speaker's awareness of disrupted discourse with the use of videotaped feedback, (2) develops strategies that are mutually agreed upon by both the TBI speaker and clinician to improve discourse performance, and (3) carries out practice to apply the trained strategies to novel situations and implements a reinforcement schedule to consolidate the learning. On top of the significant treatment effect as demonstrated by the decrease of disruptive behaviors in conversation, generalization to conversation groups and socialization sessions was reported. In addition, this improvement was found to maintain in follow-up sessions nine weeks after the end of the treatment.
- Interpersonal Process Recall (IPR) (Helffenstein & Wechsler, 1982): This program requires an individual to participate in an interaction with the clinician that is videotaped. The content of the video is then structurally reviewed with feedback provided by the clinician and a conversational partner. Self-evaluation of problematic interactions from the participant is also required. This is followed by the development of alternative communication skills or strategies that will be practiced, modelled, and rehearsed. (Note that some of the components in the IPR are similar to Step 1 in the above-mentioned CAT.) Results based on the application of the IPR intervention to 16 individuals with brain injury who received 20 hours of the IPR sessions indicated that there was a significantly reduced level of anxiety and improved self-concept. The participants were also rated as having significantly greater improvement in specific interpersonal skills by professional staff and independent observer raters blinded to treatment assignment. This communication improvement was also found to maintain one month after the end of the treatment.
- Social Skills Group (SSG) (Dahlberg et al., 2007): Participants take part in a 12 intervention sessions with the initial sessions focusing on self-assessment and goal-setting. Practice of communication goals are carried

out in the next several sessions when specific feedback is provided by the clinician. The final sessions focus on practice of problem-solving in other social situations. The results, based on 52 adults with TBI, indicated that the SSG intervention could improve functional impairments. Participants also self-reported communication improvement and greater life satisfaction at the end of the program. Continued improvement or maintenance was found six months after the intervention.

- Social Skills Treatment (SST) (McDonald, Tate, Togher, Bornhofen, Long, Gertler, & Bowen, 2008): This program consists of a total of 48 treatment hours, divided into 12 weeks. Each week a client receives a one-hour individual session addressing psychological issues (e.g., social well-being, mood, or self-esteem), two hours of group therapy focusing on social behavior, and another group hour focusing on remediation of social perception. Significant improvement of social behaviors was found for those who completed the SST.

- Conversation scripting (Cherney & Halper, 2008; Cherney et al., 2008): Three routines of personalized conversational scripts were developed for participants with cognitive impairments to practice at home using a software program (AphasiaScripts™) over the course of three weeks, with 30-minutes of daily practice. These routines included both dialogues and monologues. A weekly 30-minute session was arranged for the clinician to review and assess the participants' progress. Improvements in the content and grammatical complexity of the conversation routines were found across all participants.

- Teaching compensatory strategies (Ylvisaker et al., 2001, 2008): The components in this intervention include (1) increasing a client's meta-cognitive awareness in terms of discriminating effective from ineffective language performance and becoming more aware of their current discourse strengths and weaknesses; (2) helping the client to recognize the importance of being strategic through tasks such as brainstorming, video review, or discussion with other TBI survivors; (3) assisting the client to identify and select specific procedures in overcoming personal obstacles; (4) teaching the client specific strategies selected in (3) through modeling, direct instructions, or practice; and (5) helping the client to generalize and maintain the strategic behaviors beyond the training context. As suggested by the authors, because these components may have some overlap, they can be addressed in any order depending on a client's need and performance level.

Selective Training on Cognitive Abilities (or Cognitive-Based Training)

Based on the premise that a complex interaction of linguistic, cognitive, and social abilities enable effective conversational discourse (Coelho, 1999), this approach focuses on the training on various cognitive abilities, which typically include attention, working memory, and executive functions. Therefore, customized decontextualized cognitive training (also known as cognitive rehabilitation; see Ylvisaker et al., 2008) that involves the use of cognitive exercises that target one or more specific cognition aspects in a hierarchical manner, and delivery of these exercises using massed learning trials, would improve oral output (as well as other functional cognitive skills).

For example, Youse and Coelho (2009) have demonstrated that improving attention through the use of the Attention Process Training (APT) program (Sohlberg et al., 1994), a hierarchical and multi-level treatment program, in speakers with closed head injuries could facilitate conversational performance. Specifically, the APT program defines attention as a multidimensional cognitive domain with five levels of attention. The most basic type of attention, **focused attention**, is at the bottom of the model, followed by selective attention, sustained attention, and **alternating attention**. **Divided attention** is considered to be the most difficult form of attention processing and is at the top of this model (Sohlberg & Mateer, 1987, 2005). Following this hierarchy, a particular type of attention deficit is first identified to determine the attention training tasks needed to address the specific level of attentional function(s). A criterion of 85% accuracy must be met before the next attention task in the hierarchy is presented; otherwise, the same tasks are repeated until an accuracy of 85% is achieved:

1. Focused attention: The ability to respond to or focus on specific visual, auditory, or tactile stimuli, such as the attention needed for a standard Stroop Test.
2. Selective attention: The ability to selectively attend to a target stimulus while ignoring peripheral non-target stimuli.
3. Sustained attention: The ability to maintain focus on a stimulus during continuous or repetitive activities. Examples include selection of a target stimulus from various stimuli or cancellation tasks.
4. Alternating attention: The ability to switch focus between two or more sets of stimuli during different cognitive tasks.
5. Divided attention: The ability to simultaneously focus on two or more stimuli concurrently.

It is believed that enhanced attentional skills can contribute to discourse improvement because of the better skills in comprehending complex information, more efficient organization of internal thoughts, and improved inhibition of irrelevant or tangential utterances associated with the attention training (Body et al., 1999; McDonald et al., 1999; Palmese & Raskin, 2000). This in turn can improve the sequencing of words and propositions within an oral discourse.

Coelho (2007) have also summarized how researchers in the field have hypothesized that aspects of discourse might be mediated by working memory. In particular, an increase of working memory capacity may reduce the chances that information is lost during on-line processing. This may hypothetically, in turn, ensure more efficient conveying of information, higher content accuracy, and better semantic connectivity. Knowing that impaired working memory may be associated with atypical discourse patterns in TBI, such as problems with syntax, parenthetical utterances, and mazes (Sohlberg & Mateer, 2001), management of working memory may potentially lead to some degree of discourse improvement (although the efficacy of these procedures have yet been universally agreed). In addition, a later study by Peach (2013) has suggested that sentence planning impairments in discourse after TBI are associated with deficient organization and monitoring of language representations in working memory. Therapy techniques that can address the activation, organization, and/or maintenance of language representations for sentence production should hypothetically reduce the quantity of pausing, abandoned utterances, and mazes in TBI discourse.

Apart from attention and memory skills, several studies have reported correlations between a variety of discourse tasks and measures of executive functions, such as self-awareness and goal setting, planning, self-directing or initiating, drive, self-inhibiting or response inhibition, self-monitoring, self-regulation, self-evaluation, organization, task persistence, generative thinking, and flexible problem solving (e.g., Coelho et al., 1991, 1995; Levin et al., 1979). According to Coelho (2007) and Ylvisaker et al. (2001, 2008), many communicative impairments associated with TBI are secondary to disruption of one or more executive functions mentioned previously. Similarly, discourse deficits in the presence of inadequate cohesion or cohesive ties, disorganized propositions, or impaired story grammar, may benefit from improved executive functions because of their higher level of organizational schemas for thought units across multiple utterances (Shallice, 1982). This can be done by first identifying the specific communication deficits associated with executive dysfunctions, followed by introducing related exercise(s) to target those impaired functions (Sohlberg & Mateer, 2001). Individuals with TBI should be provided with sufficient opportunities to practice these targeted skills, so that improvement in functional behaviors and raised confidences are seen before they are put to more challenging aspects of naturalistic communication contexts.

Involvement of Communication Partners

The nature of information exchange for a person with TBI varies with the communication partner (Tu et al., 2011). Individuals with TBI were found to have a tendency to provide more information when interacting with communication partners who are closer to them, as reflected by exchange structure analysis. Moreover, family members are more sensitive in perceiving the communication difficulty demonstrated by their significant others with TBI, as compared to other communication partners such as volunteers or paid caregivers. This highlights the importance of including appropriate communication partners in the remediation process of discourse among TBI survivors.

Sim et al. (2013) described the benefit of joint communication training for TBI survivors with their everyday communication partners (ECPs). Fourteen adults with severe TBI, each paired with an ECP, received ten weeks of joint group training in social communication. The joint group included 2.5 hours of group sessions and one hour of individual sessions every week, totaling 35 hours. The aim of these sessions was to maximize communicative effectiveness using several behavioral techniques, including role playing, video reviewing for specific feedback on conversation, and using of cues for self-monitoring. Participants with TBI were guided in problem solving, practicing the use of appropriate verbal and non-verbal behaviors in social situations, and troubleshooting the use of new strategies. Their ECPs were provided concurrent training on ways to support their partner with TBI to contribute more successfully in conversations. The training procedures also involved the ECPs to apply positive, collaborative, and productive strategies to provide feedback and scaffolding in everyday casual conversations. The results suggested that this joint training positively changed discourse behavior in TBI, as reflected by enhanced global ratings of quality of conversation as well as improved scores on adapted measures of participation in conversation. A follow-up study was conducted by Togher et al. (2013), who investigated the differences between this joint training and a "SOLO" training (see p. 258–259) where ECPs were not paired with the individuals with TBI. It was reported that the "SOLO" group (n=15) had a significantly lower degree of improvement in everyday interactions then the group receiving joint training with ECPs (n=14). In other words, the involvement of ECPs in the therapeutic process could successfully lead to more efficacious treatment effects that benefited the performance of TBI.

Sohlberg and Mateer (2001) have also suggested several effective skills that should be addressed in training involving communication partners. They include providing sufficient practice and home training guidelines to ensure both the client and communication partner can independently demonstrate the target communication behaviors, making sure each of them provide feedback to each other, widening the range of communication contexts or situations for practice, and establishing a plan for ongoing monitoring. When the client demonstrates communication breakdown due to difficulties in following the communication partner's speech, it has been suggested that prompting the client's own repetition strategy can be beneficial to self-monitoring (Penn & Cleary, 1988) as well as enhancing accuracy of processing conversation and recall (Kurtz, 2011).

Coelho et al. (2002) have highlighted that the nature of the interpersonal relationship between patient-partner dyads may have influenced the conversational behaviors in chronic TBI. A more recent study (Brassel et al., 2016) has further examined the conversational topics discussed by speakers with severe TBI and their communication partners during sub-acute recovery. It was suggested that most participants could better engage with familiar communication partners in appropriate conversations. Initial discussions of mutually important topics (with themes centering around the impacts of brain injury as well as connecting and re-engaging) evolved to reflection of sub-acute rehabilitation experiences. In addition, the conversational behaviors of participants with TBI were also influenced by the nature of their interpersonal relationship with the communication partners.

A Group Intervention Approach

Using a group therapy context to manage pragmatic deficits in speakers with TBI has two important clinical values. First, modeling can be provided by clinicians to target specific skills during communication exchange; second this setting has been found to promote generalization (Sohlberg & Mateer, 1989). When addressing discourse problems in this population within a group setting, the principles of therapy are consistent with those mentioned for aphasia (see p. 254–256). Use of appropriate practice exercises must be carefully considered with reference to the skill level of the clients and their needs. Scenarios resonating daily communication challenges can be role played and practiced in a group setting. Other possible activities include, but are not limited to, (1) commercially available communication games to promote interaction, conflict resolution, and teamwork, (2) perspective-taking activities to raise pragmatic skills, and (3) field trips in the community to facilitate generalization of target discourse or communication skills (Sohlberg & Mateer, 2001). Furthermore, raising clients' level of awareness of their own discourse and communication problems can be facilitated in a group format through strategies such as peer observation, group discussion, and peer appraisal.

When conducting group sessions of discourse exercises for clients with TBI, it will be a good idea to have a relatively homogenous group. In particular, an ideal group should comprise of members with similar linguistic, cognitive, and social skills (or breakdown). This way a clinician can focus on one or two carefully selected client-centered skills at a time. In reality, there may be challenges in recruiting clients at a similar skill level to form a group; hence, clear demonstration, repetition, and massive practice are critical to success. Immediate and specific feedback provided by the clinician during group activities, in addition to specific homework assignments with individual feedback, will also promote clients' generalization. On some occasions, allocating some time for the group to debrief a training exercise and brainstorm solutions to problematic behaviors identified can help members to review problems that have occurred.

Principles of Treatment to Facilitate Discourse in Right Hemisphere Damage

Use of inference generation tasks and integration tasks is the major trend for clinicians to address deficits of narratives and conversational discourse among individuals with right hemisphere damage (RHD). Inference problems can lead to difficulties in generating macrostructures or thematic inferences, problems in bridging gaps through coherence references in a discourse, and impairments of making individual inferences (Myers, 1999; Tompkins et al., 1992). Therefore, direct treatment of inference generation or indirectly addressing its underlying process, including integration and selective attention, can hypothetically enhance discourse production in RHD. In addition, due to the difficulty in suppressing unwanted meanings to allow rapid selection of the most appropriate one for a given context (Tompkins, 1995), narratives produced by speakers with RHD may benefit from treatment of suppression deficits.

Training on Macrostructures and Inference Generation

Picture or story interpretation can be used to strengthen accurate inference production. To do so, the clinician can start with presenting stories or pictured scenes for the speakers with RHD to interpret and summarize. Responses from the client can then be rated on the degree of completeness and accuracy, as well as plausibility of the interpretation. If this task is too difficult for the patient, a guided inference generation task can be conducted instead by providing him or her with a step-by-step guidance to interpret a particular stimulus. For example, guidance may include the elements (or labels) of the stories or pictured scenes, pointing to elements that are related to one another, and explaining the relationships among the characters or items in the pictorial stimuli.

To strengthen the integration skills and macrostructure of a discourse, tasks that require the speaker with RHD to provide a story headline or picture title can be implemented. Alternatively, the clinician can work with the speaker to continue an unfinished story, so that he or she can provide an ending of the story or can pick an ending from a number of choices. While responses can be evaluated based on how appropriate, related, and plausible the output is (in relation to the content presented in the first place), a systematic review of the speaker's response with immediate and specific feedback may facilitate the overall learning. Finally, the use of tasks requiring the speaker to comprehend individual inferences may also lead to more proper use of macrostructure in spontaneous narratives (Myers, 1999).

Training That Involves Integration Tasks

A number of integration tasks can also be used in parallel to the activities mentioned above. For example, to improve integration skills, a sentence or picture arrangement task can be conducted by asking an individual with RHD to arrange a random sequence of materials and provide a logical procedure discourse based on the correct order. Focus should be put on helping him or her to identify the components (e.g., individual pieces of semantic contents) and their relationships to form a correct sequence. A non-verbal version of this arrangement task can also be done by using puzzles or objects, but the ultimate goal should involve the use of verbal language to perform a narrative task. In addition, tasks that require the speaker to identify commonalities through grouping sets of written or pictured stimuli by themes can lead to better recognition of relationships and integration. For example, pictures or photos of objects, actions, or scene pictures can be presented to the speaker with RHD, who will then be required to group them by categories (Myers, 1999). The speaker is then prompted to orally describe the basis of how categorization was done.

Management of Suppression Deficits

Management of difficulties in suppressing irrelevant meanings may include a combination of activation and suppression tasks (Myers, 1999; Tompkins et al., 2000; Tompkins et al., 2002). For examples, activities aiming to help the speaker with RHD interpret alternate meanings, comprehend indirect or non-literal language (e.g., idioms or metaphors), and understand or interpret other people's points of view (e.g., Theory of Mind) can be used. In order to stimulate the activation of alternate meanings in RHD, clinicians may use language tasks such as (1) word association to group related word items by category, (2) homograph training through elicitation of two or more meanings for common homographs, or (3) a disambiguation activity to retrieve two or more meanings for ambiguous lexical entities. In order to improve the awareness and conscious control of suppressing inappropriate alternate meanings during oral discourse, tasks such as semantic relations or sentence interpretation are suitable. For example, in a sentence interpretation task, an individual with RHD is required to interpret a sentence with multiple meanings (e.g., "He is green" in the context of the movie Shrek versus the description of a fresh graduate) and subsequently to eliminate meanings unrelated to a given context. Note that treatment complexity can be modified or adjusted by manipulating the length of stimuli, number of cues or distractors in the materials, number of inter-relationships among characters in a story, or amount of relevant versus irrelevant content of the training materials.

A Group Approach to RHD Management

A commonly seen difficulty in persons with RHD is their reduced ability to generalize learned skills to real-life situations. This problematic transfer of newly acquired skills and compensatory behaviors applies to change from one treatment task to another or from a particular setting of training to a new one (Brookshire, 2003). As a result, group intervention provides a great opportunity for RHD clients to practice and facilitate their overall generalizations. Cherney and Halper (2007) described a few group treatment programs that have been proven to be clinically useful for this group of speakers in terms of promoting functional generalization as well as cognitively- and linguistically-specific processes for using narratives:

1. Orientation group: Skills to facilitate time, place, and person orientation are targeted in this group based on the premise that orientation skills can affect communication, activities of daily living, as well as social activities. Specifically, training will address sustained and selective attention, attention to the neglected space on patients' left visual view, memory of personal biographical information, perception of environmental signs, and using orientation compensatory strategies (such as watches, smartphones, or daily planners). The optimal frequency of this group is twice per day (including weekends if possible), once at the beginning and another at the end of a day, so that members can have discussions around issues to help start a day and debrief the closure of a day's events, respectively.

2. High level cognitive group: This group focuses on the common impaired processes of RHD including organization, reasoning, problem solving, and memory. To promote greater independence and functional communication, skills that are trained should include one or more of the following: (a) effectively using compensatory memory strategies in a more natural setting; (b) organizing, sequencing, and prioritizing information related to daily life events or situations; and (c) analyzing and identifying appropriate solutions to functional problems. Hourly sessions to be given twice per week are recommended.

3. Pragmatics group: This group has a focus on increasing one's awareness of extralinguistic, paralinguistic, and linguistic context. For example, appropriate awareness and proper use of non-verbal (e.g., facial expression, gestures, or proxemics) and verbal communication skills (e.g., topic initiation, maintenance, and termination, turn taking, and referencing skills) are addressed. In addition, self-monitoring and implementation of appropriate response length and completeness of spoken content can be targeted in a group situation to facilitate participants' social interactions. It is recommended that the group be arranged at least twice per week to enhance the anticipated practice effects. In terms of the sequence

of treatment procedures, activities involving structured conversations, video reviews, and discourse activities should be given prior to more complex and open tasks (such as role playing or community integration activities).

4.   Life skills group: Compared to the three groups mentioned above, this group is more oriented to apply learned compensatory skills or to extend goals of high level cognitive groups to community situations. Instead of directly or indirectly addressing narrative skills as in the above groups, a life skills group focuses on helping a client to effectively use community resources, such as planning and carrying out community activities, using self-monitoring strategies to make appropriate adaptations for life events, or applying appropriate techniques to address everyday problems. Two sessions per week and involvement of other allied health professionals in the group are recommended.

Principles of Treatment to Facilitate Discourse in Dementia

Difficulties in thinking, generating, and ordering ideas among individuals with dementia have limited their use of oral narratives. With the difficulty in comprehending linguistic information as a result of impaired inferential capabilities and difficulty accessing contents from semantic memory, their ability to use conversational speech may be further impeded. As the condition of dementia progresses, one's ability to make connections of contents within semantic memory deteriorates. The production of oral discourse then becomes an increasingly difficult task for the population. With the goals of dementia management focusing on (1) strengthening patients' knowledge and cognitive processes relying on spared cognitive systems that have the potential to improve, and (2) providing stimuli that can evoke positive fact memory, action, and emotion, several methodologies of managing discourse production have been reported as outlined below. Most of them have been designed to work around the use of spontaneous conversational language. One should note that the ultimate goal for discourse intervention in dementia is to create a naturalistic context with support for these individuals to demonstrate preserved narrative skills and to potentially slow down their rate of deterioration. This is different from targeting improvement of specific linguistic and cognitive abilities by directly stimulating the impaired systems, as in the case of aphasia, TBI, or RHD. In addition, the degenerative nature of dementia is not necessarily a barrier to its rehabilitation.

Language Intervention

Arkin and Mahendra (2001) reported the use of language training to 11 individuals with Alzheimer's disease, each of whom received two blocks of ten-week therapy with weekly language activities including the following: free and prompted descriptions of Norman Rockwell pictures, associations with evocative words, proverb completion and interpretation (Hirsch et al., 1988), 60-second category fluency exercises, and advice and opinion questions. These tasks were selected to address semantic memory deficits and difficulties in providing thematic structures among the participants. It was hypothesized that activation of concepts or nodes that constitute semantic memory could be enhanced with the above cognitive-linguistic stimulation tasks. The association between a stimulus and the retrieved information could also be strengthened by repeated activation of a particular concept, which could in turn facilitate the triggering of word and concept retrieval for spoken language. Results indicated that these memory- and language-stimulating tasks have led to a higher diversity of nouns in the participants' discourse. Furthermore, the participants who received treatment as a group also did not decline in terms of several other discourse measures, such as ratio of topic comments to total utterance and vague noun to total noun ratio.

A recent study by Taylor-Rubin et al. (2021) has revealed that when persons with primary progressive aphasia (PPA) experience lexical retrieval difficulties in everyday interactions, their verb phrase production could benefit from external cueing of noun or verb (e.g., from their communication partners). The authors speculated that "provision of verb and noun cues in these contexts could have a positive impact on verb phrase production, sentence production and potentially, conversation" (p.193). Moreover, communication partners who are familiar to individuals with dementia could significantly facilitate the patients' ability to manage topics in spoken conversations (Hall et al., 2018). Piloting the previously mentioned protocol of "Better Conversations with Aphasia" (see p. 250–251) in the PPA population has also been proposed (Volkmer et al., 2018). It was argued that the adapted "Better Conversations for PPA" would have potential to reduce barriers and increase facilitators to conversations between people with PPA and their conversation partners; this would consequently improve the confidence level in patients' communication and their quality of life.

Reading Group Activity

With the aim of promoting the highest level of functioning in speakers with dementia and maintaining their social skills as long as possible, a reading group activity using the Question Asking Reading (QAR) procedures in an adult day care center was reported by Stevens et al. (1993). The QAR was designed to increase skills of reading comprehension and recall, to decrease cognitive demands of reading, and to increase social interaction. After individually reading some carefully selected materials (passages), participants were asked to take part in a group discussion which was facilitated with the use of a structured question and answer exercise and written aid of a script. It was found that the amount of verbal interaction among group members and retention of information presented increased as a result of this intervention.

Reminiscence Therapy in the Format of an Individual or Group Session

Reminiscence therapy relies on one's memories from the remote past through the process of recalling and reflecting on own life experiences. It can be conducted in the format of either an individual or group session when participants go through a structured program to share reflections on their past experience (Hopper, 2007). With the hypothesis that remote memories tend to be more resistant to decay and better consolidated than memories that are recently acquired, this clinical therapeutic technique can be facilitated by the use of visual stimuli and props relevant to the conversation between a client and a clinician or the discussion topic of a reminiscence session. Apart from enhancing the psycho-social wellbeing of individuals with dementia, other positive discourse outcomes of reminiscence therapy include (1) increased intention to communicate, (2) higher degree of spontaneous and unaided verbal output, (3) improved overall discourse abilities, as well as (4) better cognitive functioning (Kim et al., 2006). The implementation of a group therapy will result in a more favorable outcome with the inclusion of an effective group facilitator. More successful interactions among group members are expected if the facilitator can simplify the syntax of instructions, repeat and rephrase key information during discussion, use contextual support (such as written or graphic cues) in conversation, and use more close-ended prompts or questions (Hopper, 2007).

Montessori-Based Group Intervention

The treatment technique in the Montessori-based interventions (Camp, 1999) focuses on the use of real life environments and contexts during the therapeutic process. This intervention has been applied to individuals with Alzheimer's-related dementia. The tasks involved were broken down to various levels of components and were emphasized to tap into a client's skills on discriminating auditory, visual, and tactile information. While tasks are generally presented from simple to complex and from concrete to abstract, extensive cues are also given by clinicians to ensure successful task repetition and completion. For example, in a group activity of story generation based on given pictorial stimuli, cues in the form of written words, pictures, and/or language models, etc., can be provided to facilitate a group to achieve the training goal. This manipulation of progressive complexity and concreteness of tasks can promote spared procedural and factual memory and reduce the demand of working and episodic memory that is typically impaired in dementia. According to the review by Mahendra et al.

(2006), Montessori-based treatments could enhance cognitive-communication impairments in Alzheimer's patients, in terms of a better engagement and participation in (non-)communicative activities and improved ability to engage in treatment groups.

Use of External Memory Aids to Reduce Demands on Memory

Bourgeois and Hickey (2009) have suggested that the increasing difficulties in retrieving factual, conceptual, and procedural information from the long-term memory has proved to be a marked challenge for dementia. Use of external memory aids and graphic cueing strategies, therefore, is another approach to address discourse problems in speakers with dementia. For example, use of a memory wallet which remained visible in a conversation was found to significantly increase the number of statements and, at the same time, significantly decrease the use of ambiguous utterances in conversation by speakers with dementia (Bourgeois, 1990). In addition, these individuals benefited from the use of memory aids in terms of producing statements that are novel and more on-topic (Bourgeois, 1992). It was concluded that the application of these aids could alleviate the demands that conversation places on a speaker's episodic and working memory. Personalized memory books, with pictures or photos about people or place familiar to the speaker, also promoted positive reminiscence and emotion, and subsequently his or her conservational behaviors and performance. Advances in computer technology in the past decade have led to a more sophisticated use of computer-based devices to support communication clinically (e.g., see Kong, 2020). Appendix 7.2 shows a sample questionnaire to assess the readiness of elderly patients in using computer-based technology, modified from Kong (2015).

Indirect Intervention of Environmental Modification

A number of **indirect intervention** strategies that modify the physical and/or linguistic environment around speakers with dementia have been found to support communication (Bayles & Yomoeda, 2007). Some common techniques include reducing distraction (e.g., auditory distractors such as noise from the environment as well as visual distractors from a client's background or irrelevant objects on a therapy table) and modifying and setting the output target for individual clients. Specifically when clinicians are targeting conversational responses from speakers with dementia, providing a "tangible" topic (such as talking about the here and now) or a "visible" topic (such as a common point of reference between the speaker and listener) may stimulate spoken language. Use of pleasurable stimuli for socialization, such as food, cooking, gardening, or movies, can trigger more spontaneous interaction through conversations. When an individual with dementia forgets a particular topic of conversation, the clinician may provide a brief summary of what has been said to facilitate the ongoing flow of exchange and eliminate embarrassment. Use of the non-verbal modality to express ideas, such as gestures or writing, should not be discouraged. Constant and repeated corrections of the patients' erroneous statement should also be avoided.

Conclusions

This chapter reviewed a variety of language- and/or cognition-enhancing interventions that either directly address deficits of discourse or indirectly target prerequisite or lower-level skills to facilitate discourse production for speakers with acquired neurogenic communication disorders. Although there is a large body of literature on intervention studies with encouraging outcomes, there is still a need for evidence that documents the efficacy of these various treatment approaches. This is especially true for the information extracted from case studies summarized in this chapter, for which future investigations on their generalizability are warranted. Given that the primary goal of discourse intervention is to help clients become functional in communicating with others using oral narratives and to maintain their independent use of discourse skills, clinicians should carefully select appropriate intervention protocols and strategies after considering their remediation principles in relation to clients' needs, breakdown levels, and corresponding functional goals. When choosing a topic for language training, it is always a good idea that the clients' own interests and personal experiences be considered for eliciting production (Law et al., 2018) because this can increase relevancy to the clients and their level of motivation. Furthermore, appropriate supports (e.g., clinicians' assistance or scaffolding strategies, as well as external artifacts of whiteboards, papers and pencils, etc.) and attitudes (e.g., good engagement and facilitative behaviors of clients) can likely lead to more meaningful client participation in complex communicative activities (Archer et al., 2018). With greater understanding and awareness of the strengths and limitations of the therapy options described in this chapter, clinicians are encouraged to modify the treatment content and/or cueing methods, as needed, so that the therapeutic process will better fit the specific needs of clients. This may subsequently lead to more desirable treatment outcomes of discourse rehabilitation.

References

Antonucci, S. M. (2009). Use of semantic feature analysis in group aphasia treatment. *Aphasiology*, *23*, 854–866.

Archer, B., Tetnowski, J., Freer, J. C., Schmadeke, S., & Christou-Franklin, E. (2018). Topic selection sequences in aphasia conversation groups. *Aphasiology*, *32*(4), 394–416.

Arkin, S., & Mahendra, N. (2001). Discourse analysis of Alzheimer patients before and after intervention: Methodology and outcomes. *Aphasiology, 15*, 533–569.

Azios, J. H., & Archer, B. (2018). Singing behaviour in a client with traumatic brain injury: A conversation analysis investigation. *Aphasiology, 32*(8), 944–966.

Balardin, J. B., & Miotto, E. C. (2009). A review of Constraint-Induced Therapy applied to aphasia rehabilitation in stroke patients. *Dementia & Neuropsychologia, 3*(4), 275–282.

Bayles, K. & Yomoeda, C. (2007). *Cognitive-communication disorders of dementia*. San Diego, CA: Plural Publishing.

Beeke, S., Maxim, J., & Wilkinson, R. (2007). Using conversation analysis to assess and treat people with aphasia. *Seminars in Speech and Language, 28*, 136–147.

Beeke, S., Sirman, N., Beckley, F., Maxim, J., Edwards, S. & Best, W. (2018) The impact of Better Conversations with Aphasia on current practice by UK speech and language therapists. *Aphasiology, 32*(sup1), 16–17.

Bernstein-Ellis, E., & Elman, R. E. (2007). Aphasia group treatment: The Aphasia Center of California approach. In R. E. Elman (Ed.), *Group treatment of neurogenic communication disorders: The expert clinician's approach* (pp. 71–94). San Diego, CA: Plural.

Best, W., Maxim, J., Heilemann, C., Beckley, F., Johnson, F., Edwards, S. I., Howard, D., & Beeke, S. (2016). Conversation therapy with people with aphasia and conversation partners using video feedback: A group and case series investigation of changes in interaction. *Frontiers in Human Neuroscience, 10*, 562.

Bhogal, S. K., Teasell, R. W., Foley, N. C., & Speechley, M. R. (2003). Rehabilitation of aphasia: More is better. *Topics in Stroke Rehabilitation, 10*(2), 66–76.

Biggs, J. B., & Collis, K. F. (1982). *Evaluating the quality of learning: The SOLO taxonomy*. New York: Academic Press.

Body, R., Perkins, M., & McDonald, S. (1999). Pragmatics, cognition, and communication in traumatic brain injury. In S. McDonald, L. Togher, & C. Code (Eds.), *Communication disorders following traumatic brain injury* (pp. 81–112). Hove, UK: Psychology Press.

Boles, L. (1997). Conversation analysis as a dependent measure in communication therapy with four individuals with aphasia. *Asia Pacific Journal of Speech, Language and Hearing, 2*, 43–61.

Boles, L. (1998). Conversational discourse analysis as a method for evaluating progress in aphasia: A case report. *Journal of Communication Disorders, 31*, 261–278.

Boles, L., & Lewis, M. (2003). Working with couples: Solution focused aphasia therapy. *Asia Pacific Journal of Speech, Language and Hearing, 8*, 153–159.

Boo, M., & Rose, M. L. (2011). The efficacy of repetition, semantic, and gesture treatments for verb retrieval and use in Broca's aphasia. *Aphasiology, 25*, 154–175.

Bourgeois, M. S. (1990). Enhancing conversation skills in patients with Alzheimer's disease using a prosthetic memory aid. *Journal of Applied Behavior Analysis, 23*(1), 29–42.

Bourgeois, M. S. (1992). Evaluating memory wallets in conversations with persons with dementia. *Journal of Speech and Hearing Research, 35*(6), 1344–1357.

Bourgeois, M. S., & Hickey, E. M. (2009). *Dementia: From diagnosis to management – A functional approach*. New York, NY: Psychology Press.

Boyle, M. (2004). Semantic feature analysis treatment for anomia in two fluent aphasia syndromes. *American Journal of Speech-Language Pathology, 13*, 236–249.

Boyle, M. (2011). Discourse treatment for word retrieval impairment in aphasia: The story so far. *Aphasiology, 25*(11), 1308–26.

Boyle, M., & Coelho, C. A. (1995). Application of semantic feature analysis as a treatment for aphasia dysnomia. *American Journal of Speech-Language Pathology, 4,* 94–98.

Bradley, M., & Douglas, J. (2008). Conversation partner training – its role in aphasia: A review of the literature. *Acquiring Knowledge in Speech, Language and Hearing, 10,* 18–21.

Brady, M. C., Kelly, H., Godwin, J., & Enderby, P. (2012). Speech and language therapy for aphasia following stroke. *Cochrane Database of Systematic Review, 16*(5), CD000425.

Brassel, S., Kenny, B., Power, E., Elbourn, E., McDonald, S., Tate, R., MacWhinney, B., Turkstra, L., Holland, A., & Togher, L. (2016). Conversational topics discussed by individuals with severe traumatic brain injury and their communication partners during sub-acute recovery. *Brain Injury, 30*(11), 1329–1342.

Brookshire, R. H. (2003). *Introduction to neurogenic communication disorders.* St Louis, MO: Mosby.

Byng, S., & Duchan, J. (2005). Social model philosophies and principles: Their applications to therapies for aphasia. *Aphasiology, 19,* 906–922.

Camp, C. J. (1999). *Montessori-based activities for persons with dementia.* Beachwood, OK: Menorah Park Center for the Aging.

Cannizzaro, M. S., & Coelho, C. A. (2002). Treatment of story grammar following traumatic brain injury: a pilot study. *Brain Injury, 16,* 1065–1073.

Carragher, M., Conroy, P., Sage, K. & Wilkinson, R. (2012), Can impairment-focused therapy change the everyday conversations of people with aphasia? A review of the literature and future directions, *Aphasiology, 26*(7), 895–916.

Chapey, R., Duchan, J. F., Elman, R. J., Garcia, L. J., Kagan, A., Lyon, J. G., & Simmons-Mackie, N. (2000). Life Participation Approach to Aphasia: A statement of values for the future. *The ASHA Leader, 5*(3), 4–6).

Cherney, L. R., & Halper, A. S. (2007). Group treatment for patients with right hemisphere damage. In R. J. Elman (Ed.), *Group treatment of neurogenic communication disorders: The expert clinician's approach* (pp. 269–296). San Diego, CA: Plural Publishing Inc.

Cherney, L. R., & Halper, A. S. (2008). Novel technology for treating individuals with aphasia and concomitant cognitive deficits. *Topics in Stroke Rehabilitation,* 15(6), 542–554.

Cherney, L. R., Halper, A. S., Holland, A. L, & Cole, R. (2008). Computerized script training for aphasia: Preliminary results. *American Journal of Speech- Language Pathology,* 17, 19–34.

Cicerone, K., Langenbahn, D., Braden, C., Malec, J., Kalmar, K., Fraas, M., Felicetti, T., Laatsch, L., Harley, J. P., Bergquist, T., Azulay, J., Cantor, J., & Ashman, T. (2011). Evidence-based cognitive rehabilitation: Updated review of the literature from 2003 through 2008. *Archives of Physical Medicine and Rehabilitation,* 92(4), 519–530.

Coelho, C. A. (1999). Discourse analysis in traumatic brain injury. In S. McDonald, L. Togher, & C. Code (Eds.), *Communication disorders following traumatic brain injury* (pp. 55–79). Hove, UK: Psychology Press.

Coelho, C. A. (2007). Management of discourse deficits following traumatic brain injury: Progress, caveats, and needs. *Seminars in Speech and Language, 28*(2), 122–135.

Coelho, C. A., Liles, B. Z., & Duffy, R. J. (1991). Discourse analyses with closed head injured adults: Evidence for differing patterns of deficits. *Archives of Physical Medicine and Rehabilitation, 72,* 465–468.

Coelho, C. A., Liles, B. Z., & Duffy, R. J. (1995). Impairments of discourse abilities and executive functions in traumatically brain-injured adults. *Brain Injury, 9*(5), 471–477.

Coelho, C. A., Youse, K., & Le, K. (2002). Conversational discourse in closed head-injured and non-brain-injured adults. *Aphasiology, 16,* 659–672.

Conroy, P., Sage, K., & Ralph, M. L. (2009). Improved vocabulary production after naming therapy in aphasia: Can gains in picture naming generalize to connected speech? *International Journal of Language & Communication Disorders, 44*(6), 1036–1062.

Dahlberg, C., Cusick, C. P., Hawley, L. A. Newman, J. K., Morey, C. E., Harrison-Felix, C. L., & Whiteneck, G. G. (2007). Treatment efficacy of social communication skills training after traumatic brain injury: A randomized treatment and deferred treatment controlled trial. *Archives of Physical Medicine and Rehabilitation, 88,* 1561–1573.

Davis, L. A., & Stanton, S. T. (2005). Semantic Feature Analysis as a functional therapy tool. *Contemporary Issues in Communication Sciences and Disorders, 32,* 85–92.

del Toro, C. M., Raymer, A. M., Leon, S., Blonder, L. X., Rothi, L. J. G., & Altmann, L. (2008). Changes in aphasic discourse after contrasting treatments for anomia. *Aphasiology, 22,* 881–892.

Dipper, L., Marshall, J., Boyle, M., Botting, N., Hersh, D., Pritchard, M. & Cruice, M. (2020). Treatment for improving discourse in aphasia: A systematic review and synthesis of the evidence base. *Aphasiology, 35*(9), 1125–1167. https://doi.org/10.1080/02687038.2020.1765305

Elman, R. E. (2000). Working with groups: Neurogenic communication disorders [Videotape]. Rockville, MD: American Speech-Language-Hearing Association.

Elman, R. E. & Bernstein-Ellis, E. (1999). The efficacy of group communication treatment in adults with chronic aphasia. *Journal of Speech, Language, and Hearing Research, 42*(2), 411–419.

Ewing, S. E. A. (2007). Group process, group dynamics, and group techniques with neurogenic communication disorders. In R. E. Elman (Ed.), *Group treatment of neurogenic communication disorders: The expert clinician's approach* (pp. 15–31). San Diego, CA: Plural.

Fiori, V., Coccia, M., Marinelli, C. V., Vecchi, V., Bonifazi, S., Ceravolo, M. G., Provinciali, L., Tomaiuolo, F., & Marangolo, P. (2011). Transcranial direct current stimulation improves word retrieval in healthy and nonfluent aphasic subjects. *Journal of Cognitive Neuroscience, 23*(9), 2309–2323.

Gindri, G., Pagliarin, K. C., Casarin, F. S., Branco, L. D., Ferré, P., Joanette, Y., & Fonseca, R. P. (2014). Rehabilitation of discourse impairments after acquired brain injury. *Dementia & Neuropsychologia, 8*(1), 58–65.

Goodwin, C., & Heritage, J. (1990). Conversation analysis. *Annual Reviews of Anthropology, 19,* 283–307.

Goral, M., & Kempler, D. (2009). Training verb production in communicative context: Evidence from a person with chronic non-fluent aphasia. *Aphasiology*, *23*, 1383–1397.

Green, G. (1984). Communication in aphasia therapy: Some of the procedures and issues involved. *British Journal of Disorders of Communication*, *19*(1), 35–46.

Greenwood, A., Grassly, J., Hickin, J., & Best, W. (2010). Phonological and orthographic cueing therapy: A case of generalised improvement. *Aphasiology*, *24*, 991–1016.

Grice, H. P. (1975). Logic and conversation. In P. Cole & J. L. Morgan (Eds.), *Speech acts, syntax and semantics* (Vol. 3, pp. 41–58). New York, NY: Academic Press.

Haarbauer-Krupa, J., Moser, L., Smith, G., Sullivan, D. M., & Szekeres, S. F. (1985). Cognitive–rehabilitative therapy: Middle stages of recovery. In M. Ylvisaker (Ed.), *Head injury rehabilitation: Children and adolescents* (pp. 287–310). San Diego, CA: College-Hill Press.

Hall, K., Lind, C., Young, J. A., Okell, E., & Steenbrugge, W. (2018). Familiar communication partners' facilitation of topic management in conversations with individuals with dementia. *International Journal of Language & Communication Disorders*, *53*(3), 564–575.

Hartley, L. L. (1995). *Cognitive-communicative abilities following brain injury*. San Diego, CA: Singular Publishing Group, Inc.

Heikkinen, P. H., Pulvermüller, F., Mäkelä, J. P., Ilmoniemi, R. J., Lioumis, P., Kujala, T., Manninen, R.-L., Ahvenainen, A., & Klippi, A. (2019). Combining rTMS with intensive language-action therapy in chronic aphasia: A randomized controlled trial. *Frontiers in Neuroscience*, *12*, 1036.

Helffenstein, D. A., & Wechsler, F. S. (1982). The use of interpersonal process recall (IPR) in the remediation of interpersonal and communication skill deficits in the newly brain-injured. *Clinical Neuropsychology*, *4*, 139–142.

Hengst, J. A., Duff, M. C., & Dettmer, A. (2010). Rethinking repetition in therapy: Repeated engagement as the social ground of learning. *Aphasiology*, *24*, 887–901.

Hengst, J. A., Duff, M. C., & Prior, P. A. (2008). Multiple voices in clinical discourse and as clinical intervention. *International Journal of Language & Communication Disorders*, *43*, 58–68.

Herbert, R., Best, W., Hickin, J., Howard, D., & Osborne, F. (2003). Combining lexical and interactional approaches to therapy for word finding deficits in aphasia. *Aphasiology*, *17*, 1163–1186.

Hickin, J., Best, W., Herbert, R., Howard, D., & Osborne, F. (2001). Treatment of word retrieval in aphasia: Generalization to conversational speech. *International Journal of Language and Communication Disorders*, *36*, 13–18.

Hinchliffe, F. J., Murdoch, B. E., & Theodoros, D. G. (2001). Discourse production in traumatic brain injury. In: B. E. Murdoch & D. G. Theodoros (Eds.), *Traumatic brain injury: Associated speech, language and swallowing disorders* (pp. 223–246). Clifton Park, NY: Thomson Delmar.

Hirsch, E. D., Kett, J. F., & Trefil, J. (1988). *Dictionary of cultural literacy: What every American needs to know*. Boston, MA: Houghton Mifflin.

Hopper, T. (2007). Group cognitive-communication treatment for people with dementia. In R. J. Elman (Ed.), *Group treatment of neurogenic communication disorders: The expert clinician's approach* (pp. 341–354). San Diego, CA: Plural Publishing Inc.

Hopper, T., Holland, A., & Rewega, M. (2002). Conversational coaching: treatment outcomes and future directions. *Aphasiology, 16*, 745–761.

Howard, D., & Hatfied, F. M. (1987). *Aphasia therapy: Historical and contemporary issues.* Hove, East Sussex, UK: Lawrence Erlbaum Associates.

Kagan, A. (1998). Supported conversation for adults with aphasia: Methods and resources for training conversation partners. *Aphasiology, 12*, 816–830.

Kagan, A., Black, S., Duchan, J., Simmons-Mackie, N., & Square, P. (2001). Training volunteers as conversation partners using 'Supported Conversation for Adults with Aphasia' (SCA): A controlled trial. *Journal of Speech, Language, and Hearing Research, 44*, 624–638.

Kagan, A., & Gailey, G. (1993). Functional is not enough: Training conversation partners in aphasia. In Holland, A. & Forbes, M (Eds.), *Aphasia treatment: World perspectives* (pp.199–226). San Diego, CA: Singular.

Kempler, D. (2005). *Neurocognitive disorders in aging.* Thousand Oaks, CA: Sage Publications.

Kempler, D. & Goral, M. (2011). A comparison of drill- and communication-based treatment for aphasia. Aphasiology, 25(11), 1327–1346.

Kendall, D. L., Oelke, M., Brookshire, C. E., & Nadeau, S. E. (2015). The influence of phonomotor treatment on word retrieval abilities in 26 individuals with chronic aphasia: An open trial. *Journal of Speech Language and Hearing Research, 58*, 798–812.

Kim, E. S., Cleary, S. J., Hopper, T., Bayles, K. A., Mahendra, N., Azuma, T., & Rackley, A. (2006). Evidence-based practice recommendations for working with individuals with dementia: Group reminiscence therapy. *Journal of Medical Speech-Language Pathology, 14*(3), xxiii–xxxiv.

Kong, A. P. H. (2015). Conducting cognitive exercises for early dementia with the use of apps on iPads. *Communication Disorders Quarterly, 36*(2), 102–106.

Kong, A. P. H. (2020). The use of free non-dementia-specific apps on iPad to conduct group communication exercises for individuals with Alzheimer's disease (Innovative Practice). *Dementia, 19*(4), 1252–1264

Kurtz, M. M. (2011). *Encyclopedia of clinical neuropsychology.* New York, NY: Springer.

Laakso, M., & Godt, S. (2016). Recipient participation in conversations involving participants with fluent or non-fluent aphasia. *Clinical Linguistics & Phonetics, 30*(10), 770–789.

Law, S.-P., Kong, A. P.-H., & Lai, C. (2018). An analysis of topics and vocabulary in Chinese oral narratives by normal speakers and speakers with fluent aphasia. *Clinical Linguistics and Phonetics, 32,* 88–99.

Levin, H. S., O'Donnell, V. M., & Grossman, R. G. (1979). The Galveston orientation and amnesia test: A practical scale to assess cognition after head injury. *Journal of Nervous and Mental Disease, 167*, 675–684.

Lock, S., Wilkinson, R., & Bryan, K. (2001). *Supporting partners of people with aphasia in relationships and conversation (SPPARC): Resource pack.* Bicester, UK: Speechmark Publishing Ltd.

LPAA Project Group (in alphabetical order: Chapey, R., Duchan, J. F., Elman, R. J., Garcia, L. J., Kagan, A., Lyon, J., & Simmons Mackie, N.) (2000). Life participation approaches to aphasia: A statement of values for the future. *ASHA Leader, 5*(3), 4–6.

Mahendra, N., Hopper, T., Bayles, K. A., Azuma, T., Cleary, S., & Kim, E. (2006). Evidence-based practice recommendations for working with individuals with dementia: Montessori-based interventions. *Journal of Medical Speech-Language Pathology, 14*(1), xv–xxv.

Manheim, L. M., Halper, A. S., & Cherney, L. R. (2009). Patient-reported changes in communication after computer-based script training for aphasia. *Archives of Physical Medicine and Rehabilitation, 90,* 623–627.

Marsh, N.V. (1999). Social skill deficits following traumatic brain injury: Assessment and treatment. In: S. McDonald, L. Togher, & C. Code (Eds.). *Communication disorders following traumatic brain injury* (pp. 175–210). Hove, UK: Psychology Press Limited.

Marshall, R. C. (1999). *Introduction to group treatment for aphasia: Design and management.* Boston, MA: Butterworth-Heinemann.

Massaro, M., & Tompkins, C. A. (1992). Feature analysis for treatment of communication disorders in traumatically brain injured patients: An efficacy study. *Clinical Aphasiology, 22,* 245–256.

Matar, S. J., Sorinola, I. O., Newton, C., & Pavlou, M. (2020). Transcranial direct-current stimulation may improve discourse production in healthy older adults. *Frontiers in Neurology, 11,* 935

McDonald, S., Tate, R,. Togher, L,. Bornhofen, C., Long, E., Gertler, P., & Bowen, R. (2008). Social skills treatment for people with severe, chronic acquired brain injuries: A multicenter trial. *Archives of Physical Medicine and Rehabilitation, 89,* 1648–1659.

McDonald, S., Togher, L., & Code, C. (1999). The nature of traumatic brain injury: Basic features and neuropsychological consequences. In S. McDonald, L. Togher, & C. Code (Eds.), *Communication disorders following traumatic brain injury* (pp. 19–54). Hove, UK: Psychology Press.

Medina, J., Norise, C., Faseyitan, O., Coslett, H. B., Turkeltaub, P. E., & Hamilton, R. H. (2012). Finding the right words: Transcranial magnetic stimulation improves discourse productivity in non-fluent aphasia after stroke. *Aphasiology, 26*(9), 1153–1168.

Morton, M.V., & Wehman, P. (1995). Psychosocial and emotional sequelae of individuals with traumatic brain injury: A literature review and recommendations. *Brain Injury, 9*(1), 81–92.

Myers, P. (1999). *Right hemisphere damage: Disorders of communication and cognition.* San Diego: Singular Publishing Group, Inc.

Palmese, C. A., & Raskin, S. A. (2000). The rehabilitation of attention in individuals with mild traumatic brain injury using the APT II programme. *Brain Injury, 14,* 535–548.

Peach, R. K. (2013). The cognitive basis for sentence planning difficulties in discourse after traumatic brain injury. *American Journal of Speech-Language Pathology, 22,* S285–S297.

Peach, R. K., & Reuter, K. A. (2010). A discourse-based approach to semantic feature analysis for the treatment of aphasic word retrieval failures. *Aphasiology, 24,* 971–990.

Penn, C., & Cleary, J. (1988). Compensatory strategies in the language of closed head injured patients. *Brain Injury, 2*(1), 3–17.

Penn, C., Jones, D., & Joffe, V. (1997). Hierarchical discourse therapy: A method for the mild patient. *Aphasiology, 11*, 601–632.

Pisoni, A., Mattavelli, G., Papagno, C., Rosanova, M., Casali, A. G., & Romero Lauro, L. J. (2018). Cognitive enhancement induced by anodal tDCS drives circuit-specific cortical plasticity. *Cerebral Cortex, 28*(4), 1132–1140.

Purdy, M., & Cocchiola, K. (2006, February 1–4). *Training cognitive flexibility in aphasia* [Paper presentation]. Thirty-fourth annual International Neuropsychological Society Conference, Boston, MA, United States.

Purdy, M., & Van Dyke, J. A. (2011). Multimodal communication training in aphasia: A pilot study. *Journal of Medical Speech-Language Pathology, 19*(3), 45–53.

Rautakoski, P. (2011). Training total communication. *Aphasiology, 25*, 344–365.

Raymer, A. M., Singletary, F., Rodriguez, A., Ciampitti, M., Heilman, K. M., & Rothi, L. J. G. (2006). Effects of gestural + verbal treatment for noun and verb retrieval in aphasia. *Journal of the International Neuropsychological Society, 12*, 867–882.

Rose, M., Douglas, J., & Matyas, T. (2002). The comparative effectiveness of gesture and verbal treatments for a specific phonologic naming impairment. *Aphasiology, 16*, 1001–1030.

Shallice, T. (1982). Specific impairments of planning. *Philosophical Transactions of Royal Society of London, 298*, 199–209.

Silkes, J. P., Fergadiotis, G., Graue, K., & Kendall, D. L. (2021). Effects of phonomotor therapy and semantic feature analysis on discourse production. American Journal of Speech-Language Pathology, 30(1S), 441–454.

Silkes, J. P., Fergadiotis, G., Pompon, R. H., Torrence, J., & Kendall, D. L. (2019). Effects of phonomotor treatment on discourse production. *Aphasiology, 33*(2), 125–139.

Sim, P., Power, E., & Togher, L. (2013). Describing conversations between individuals with traumatic brain injury (TBI) and communication partners following communication partner training: Using exchange structure analysis. *Brain Injury, 27*, 717–742.

Simmons-Mackie, N. (1998). In support of supported communication for adults with aphasia: Clinical forum. *Aphasiology, 12*, 831–838.

Simmons-Mackie, N. (2000). Social approaches to the management of aphasia. In L. Worrall & C. Frattali (Eds), *Neurogenic communication disorders: A functional approach* (pp. 162–187). New York, NY: Thieme.

Simmons-Mackie, N. (2008). Social approaches to aphasia intervention. In R. Chapey (Ed.), *Language intervention strategies in adult aphasia and related disorders* (pp. 162–187). Baltimore, MD: Williams & Wilkins.

Simmons-Mackie, N., Elman, R. J., Holland, A. L., & Damico, J. S. (2007). Management of discourse in group therapy for aphasia. *Topics in Language Disorders, 27*(1), 5–23.

Simmons-Mackie, N., Raymer, A., & Cherney, L. R. (2016). Communication Partner Training in aphasia: An updated systematic review. *Archives of Physical Medicine and Rehabilitation, 97*(12), 2202–2221.

Simmons-Mackie, N., Savage, M. C., & Worrall, L. (2014). Conversation therapy for aphasia: A qualitative review of the literature. *International Journal of Language & Communication Disorders, 49*(5), 511–526.

Snow, P. C., & Douglas, J. M. (2000). Conceptual and methodological challenges in discourse assessment with TBI speakers: Towards an understanding. *Brain Injury*, *14*, 397–415.

Snow, P., Douglas, J., & Ponsford, J. (1998). Conversational discourse abilities following severe traumatic brain injury: A follow-up study. *Brain Injury*, 12(11), 911–935.

Sohlberg, M. M., Johnson, L., Paule, L., Raskin, S. A. & Mateer, C. A. (1994). *Attention Process Training II: A program to address attentional deficits for persons with mild cognitive dysfunction*. Puyallup, WA: Association for Neuropsychological Research and Development.

Sohlberg, M. M., & Mateer, C. (1987). Effectiveness of an attention-training program. *Journal of Clinical and Experimental Neuropsychology*, *9*, 117–130.

Sohlberg, M. M., & Mateer, C. A. (1989). *Introduction to cognitive rehabilitation: Theory and practice*. New York, NY: Guilford Press.

Sohlberg, M. M., & Mateer, C. A. (2001). *Cognitive rehabilitation: An integrative neuropsychological approach*. New York, NY: Guilford Press.

Sohlberg, M. M., & Mateer, C. (2005). *Attention Process Training: A program for cognitive rehabilitation to address persons with attentional deficits ranging from mild to severe*. Wake Forest, NC: Lash & Associates Publishing/Training Inc.

Springer, L., Huber, W., Schlenck, K. J., & Schlenck, C. (2000). Agrammatism: Deficit or compensation? Consequences for aphasia therapy. *Neuropsychological Rehabilitation*, *10*, 279–309.

Stevens, A. B., King, C. A., & Camp, C. J. (1993). Improving prose memory and social interaction using question asking reading with adult day care clients. *Educational Gerontology*, *19*, 651–662.

Struchen, M. A. (2005). Social communication interventions for persons with traumatic brain injury. In W. M. High, A. M. Sander, M. A. Struchen, & K. A. Hart (Eds.). *Rehabilitation of traumatic brain injury* (pp. 88–117). New York: Oxford University Press.

Szaflarski, J. P., Ball, A. L., Grether, S., Al-fwaress, F., Griffith, N. M., Neils-Strunjas, J., Newmeyer, A., & Reichhardt, R. (2008). Constraint-induced aphasia therapy stimulates language recovery in patients with chronic aphasia after ischemic stroke. *Medical Science Monitor*, 14(5), CR243–CR250.

Taylor-Rubin, C., Croot, K., & Nickels, L. (2021). Is word learning enough? Improved verb phrase production following cueing of verbs and nouns in primary progressive aphasia. *Cortex*, *139*, 178–197.

Teasell, R. W., Foley, N. C., & Salter, K. (2011). Evidence-based review of stroke rehabilitation. www.ebrsr.com.

Togher, L., McDonald, S., Tate, R., Power, E., & Rietdijk, R. (2013). Training communication partners of people with severe traumatic brain injury improves everyday conversations: A multicenter single blind clinical trial. *Journal of Rehabilitation Medicine*, *45*, 637–645.

Tompkins, C. A. (1995). *Right hemisphere communication disorders: Theory and management*. San Diego, CA: Singular.

Tompkins, C. A., Baumgaertner, A., Lehman, M. T., & Fassbinder, W. (2000). Mechanisms of discourse comprehension impairment after right hemisphere brain damage: Suppression and enhancement in lexical ambiguity resolution. *Journal of Speech, Language and Hearing Research, 43*, 62–78.

Tompkins, C. A., Boada, R., McGarry, K., Jones, J., Rahn, A. E., & Ranier, S. (1992). Connected speech characteristics of right-hemisphere-damaged adults: A re-examination. *Clinical Aphasiology Conference, 21*, 113–112.

Tompkins, C. A., Lehman-Blake, M. T., Baumgaertner, A., & Fassbinder, W. (2002). Characterizing comprehension difficulties after right brain damage: Attentional demands of suppression function. *Aphasiology, 16*, 559–572.

Tu, L. V., Togher, L., & Power, E. (2011). The impact of communication partner and discourse task on a person with traumatic brain injury: The use of multiple perspectives. *Brain Injury,* 25(6), 560–580.

Turner, S., & Whitworth, A. (2006). Conversational partner training programmes in aphasia: A review of key themes and participants' roles. *Aphasiology, 20*(6), 483–510.

Ulatowska, H. K., & Chapman, S. B. (1989). Discourse considerations for aphasia management. *Seminars in Speech and Language, 10*, 298–314.

Volkmer, A., Spector, A., Warren, J. D., & Beeke, S. (2018). The "Better Conversations with Primary Progressive Aphasia (BCPPA)" program for people with PPA (Primary Progressive Aphasia): Protocol for a randomised controlled pilot study. *Pilot and Feasibility Studies, 4*, 158.

Whitworth, A. (2010). Using narrative as a bridge: Linking language processing models with real-life communication. *Seminars in Speech and Language, 31*, 64–75.

Whitworth, A., Leitão, S., Cartwright, J., Webster, J., Hankey, G. J., Zach, J., Howard, D., & Wolz, V. (2015). NARNIA: A new twist to an old tale. A pilot RCT to evaluate a multilevel approach to improving discourse in aphasia. *Aphasiology,* 29(11), 1345–1382.

Whitworth, A., Ng, N., Timms, L., & Power, E. (2020). Exploring the viability of NARNIA with cognitive-communication difficulties: A pilot study. *Seminars in Speech and Language, 41*(1), 83–98.

Wilkinson, R. (1995). Aphasia: Conversation analysis of a non-fluent aphasic person. In M. Perkins, & S. Howard (Eds.), *Case Studies in clinical linguistics* (pp. 271–292). London: Whurr.

Ylvisaker, M. (1992). Communication outcome following traumatic brain injury. *Seminars in Speech and Language, 13*, 239–251.

Ylvisaker, M., Szekeres, S. F., & Feeney, T. (2001). Communication disorders associated with traumatic brain injury. In R. Chapey (Ed.), *Language intervention strategies in aphasia and related neurogenic communication disorders* (pp. 745–800). Philadelphia, PA: Lippincott, Williams & Wilkins.

Ylvisaker, M., Szekeres, S. F., & Feeney, T. (2008). Communication disorders associated with traumatic brain injury. In R. Chapey (Ed.), *Language intervention strategies in aphasia and related neurogenic communication disorders* (pp. 879–962). Philadelphia, PA: Lippincott, Williams & Wilkins.

Youse, K. M., & Coelho, C. A. (2009). Treating underlying attention deficits as a means for improving conversational discourse in individuals with closed head injury: A preliminary study. *NeuroRehabilitation, 24*, 355–364.

Appendix 7.1

Suggested Training Exercises for Discourse Treatment

Picture description: A client turns over one picture card at a time and describes it with pre-rehearsed sentences or with spontaneous speech. The picture stimuli can be of increasing levels of difficulty, in terms of the number of target elements (e.g., noun and verbs) and inter-relations of characters within the picture.

Picture sequence: A clinician and a client are positioned on either side of a barrier to ensure only verbal communication is used. The client and the clinician have the same stack of four or five unrelated picture cards in front of them in a random order. The client is asked to arrange the cards in a particular sequence and to describe each picture in the order arranged so that the clinician can mirror the sequence. At the end of each series, both parties reveal their picture cards to see if they match.

Map task: A clinician and a client are positioned on either side of a barrier to ensure only verbal communication is used. The client and the clinician each has a map in front of them. A sheet of paper with multiple action pictures associated with various locations on the map, displayed in a random spatial pattern, is also given. The goal is for the client to describe the route to the clinician so that the clinician can trace the identical route on the map. At the end of each turn, the client and clinician reveal their maps to see if they have matching patterns.

Procedural description: A client is asked to describe the procedures of doing an everyday task with spontaneous speech or pre-rehearsed sentences. For example, a client may be asked to describe the steps to make a sandwich or fix a broken window. Topics around daily routines or with a higher degree of personal relevancy will likely enhance the motivation and facilitate the performance level of the client.

"What will you do?": A clinician describes a situation or a problem to be solved and a client is asked to provide a solution(s) with spontaneous speech. Presentation of these situations or problems can also be done using video clips. The content selected can be based on the hobbies or interests of the client. Generally speaking, starting this task with familiar events will likely facilitate the client's responses. Events that are less probable or more complicated will pose more challenges for the client but will work better for those who are functioning at a higher level.

Story telling: A client reads a story book with all words covered. After removing the book from the client's view, he or she then tells the story using spontaneous speech. Spontaneous speech can be targeted but pre-rehearsed sentences may also be used in this activity.

Story construction: A client and a clinician take turns saying sentences to form a short story based on a single picture. Alternatively, two pictures with one depicting the beginning and another depicting the end of a story are used for the client and clinician to take turns to produce suitable sentences to complete the story. Specific sentence structures and story grammar can be targeted in this activity.

Event recall: With the help of the primary caregiver, a client is asked to bring in photo albums, family video clips, and/or memorable object items to a clinical session. The client is asked to recall and describe one or more events related to the materials. Spontaneous speech or pre-rehearsed sentences may be used in this activity.

Structured conversation: A clinician selects a topic that is interesting or personally relevant to a client. The client and clinician then carry on the conversation for a pre-set duration of time, say three minutes or more. Inclusion of one or more communication partners may be considered depending on how the client is responding to the therapy. Specific conversation strategies can be targeted. In addition, sharing of feedback provided by communication partners can also be done. Video review, ideally immediately after each treatment trial, can be conducted.

Appendix 7.2

A Sample Questionnaire to Determine Participants' Use of Technology

1. Do you use technology, such as a computer, tablet device, or smartphone?
   ☐ Yes   ☐ No

2. What type of technology do you use at home?
   a. Desktop computer   ☐ Yes   ☐ No
   b. Laptop or Netbook   ☐ Yes   ☐ No
   c. Tablet device, e.g., iPad   ☐ Yes   ☐ No
   d. Smartphone   ☐ Yes   ☐ No
   e. Others (please specify:_____)

3. How frequently do you use each of the technology listed in Question 2?
   1 [Less than once per month] --- 2 [Once per month] --- 3 [Once per week] --- 4 [A few time per week] --- 5 [Everyday]
   a. Desktop computer   1 --- 2 --- 3 --- 4 --- 5
   b. Laptop or Netbook   1 --- 2 --- 3 --- 4 --- 5
   c. Tablet device, e.g., iPad   1 --- 2 --- 3 --- 4 --- 5
   d. Smartphone   1 --- 2 --- 3 --- 4 --- 5
   e. Others (please specify:_____)   1 --- 2 --- 3 --- 4 --- 5

4. Overall, do you enjoy using technology at home?
   1 [Do not enjoy] --- 2 [Somewhat dislike] --- 3 [Neutral] --- 4 [Somewhat enjoy] --- 5 [Love it]

5. What do you use technology for?
   _____
   _____

6. Would you like to see more technology used in clinic?
   ☐ Yes   ☐ No

7. Do you think you could benefit from using technology in clinic?
   ☐ Yes   ☐ No

8. How do you think you can benefit from using technology in clinic?
   _____
   _____

9. How optimistic do you fell about using technology in clinic?
   1 [Very pessimistic] --- 2 [Pessimistic] --- 3 [Neutral] --- 4 [Optimistic]
   --- 5 [Very optimistic]
   1 --- 2 --- 3 --- 4 --- 5

10. What would you like to work on with technology? (Check all that apply)
    ☐ Memory
    ☐ Attention
    ☐ Numbers
    ☐ Language
    ☐ Others (please specify:_____)

11. What types of games would you be interested in?
    ☐ Memory
    ☐ Word Scrambles
    ☐ Trivia
    ☐ Brain stimulation
    ☐ Naming
    ☐ Others (please specify:_____)

12. Would you prefer to use technology in a group or individual setting?
    ☐ Group
    ☐ Individual
    ☐ Both

Source: Adapted from Kong (2015)

Chapter 8

Considerations for Multilingual and Culturally Diverse Populations

Chapter Objectives

The reader will be able to:

1. provide existing definitions of bilingualism and/or multilingualism in the literature
2. compare and contrast Pitres' law and Ribot's law on bilingual language recovery
3. describe the various patterns of recovery in bilingual aphasia
4. describe the factors that are related to early stages of language recovery among bilingual or multilingual speakers with aphasia
5. explain and justify the components of examining multilingual history
6. explain how acculturation affects manifestation of bilingual aphasia symptoms
7. discuss the clinical application of the Bilingual Aphasia Test (BAT) and the Multilingual Aphasia Examination (MAE)
8. differentiate between (pathological) **code switching** and **code mixing** in bilingual aphasia
9. discuss factors to be considered when including interpreters versus laypersons in the process of assessing and managing bilingual or multilingual speakers
10. describe the principles of adopting and modifying existing English-based discourse quantification systems for use in multilingual or multicultural speakers
11. discuss important factors to be considered when conducting language intervention for bilingual or multilingual speakers with acquired language impairments.

DOI: 10.4324/9781003254775-8

Introduction

A majority of the world's population speaks more than one language (de Bot, 1992). The era of globalization has directly contributed to the promotion of bilingualism worldwide. A report by Kiran et al. (2011) estimated that 60% of the world is bilingual or multilingual; suggesting that this mode of communication, involving the use of two or more languages, is very common in contemporary society. According to census reports (U.S. Bureau of the Census, 2010, 2013), the number of multilingual speakers is expected to grow in the nation. Based on the 2018 U.S. Census Bureau data, the Center for Immigration Studies (https://cis.org/) estimated that 67.3 million residents in the nation speak a language other than English at home.

In the United States alone, it has been estimated there are at least 45,000 new cases of bilingual aphasia every year (Paradis, 2001). A review by Ansaldo and Saidi (2014) further suggested that the prevalence of bilingual aphasia is increasing and this growing bilingual (or multilingual) population worldwide is large. Aphasia among multilingual speakers has, therefore, become an increasingly important topic of research (Lorenzen & Murray, 2008). More critically, the complex behavioral patterns observed clinically among speakers with bilingual aphasia pose challenges for clinicians to assess and manage this unique clientele. This is because the condition concerns at least two languages, whose language symptoms and pattern of recovery in each language do not necessarily follow the same profile.

Despite the above, research in aphasia, and particularly discourse production, has focused primarily on monolingual speakers of Indo-European languages. At present, very limited investigations that examine the discourse disruptions and their associated linguistic behaviors have been reported. Given that there are almost endless possible combinations of language and/or dialect pairs in bilingual (or multilingual) aphasia, the aim of this chapter is to discuss the existing definitions of bilingualism in the literature, the reported recovery patterns and affecting factors of bilingual aphasia, and issues around assessment as well as therapy of bilingual and/or multilingual speakers with acquired language impairments.

Definitions of Bilingualism and Multilingualism in Typical Speakers

Various definitions of bilingualism have been proposed in the literature. For example, Pearce (2005) suggested that bilingualism was the use of at least two languages in a speaker's everyday life. However, this does not necessarily mean that the "bilingual speaker" knows the two or more languages equally well as most laypersons think. Instead, the term "dual monolingual" has been used to refer to bilingual speakers who master two languages equally well as if they are native monolingual speakers in both the first or native language (L1) and second or non-native language (L2). Fabbro (2001) defined bilingual speakers as those who acquire and use two languages for various purposes, in various domains of life, and with various communication partners. More than half the population of the world would fulfil this definition and can, therefore, be classified as bilingual speakers. Among other descriptions, Grosjean (1989) used functional criteria to characterize bilingual (or multilingual) speakers as those who speak two (or more) languages in daily life for different purposes and consequently have different proficiency levels within their languages across various domains. With this definition, over half the world's population can also be considered as multilingual speakers.

Note that some researchers have also suggested that bilingualism is not a dichotomy but a continuum. There is, therefore, not an arbitrary point that can readily discriminate individuals who are bilingual from unilingual speakers. Roberts et al. (2002) have proposed a set of inclusive criteria for selecting functionally unilingual adult speakers as listed below. To be specific, a speaker can be considered as functionally monolingual only when all the four criteria are fulfilled:

- being unable to understand the news on the radio in any other languages except one's L1
- being unable to explain his or her occupation to someone in a two- to three-minute monologue in any other languages except for L1
- use of other language(s) is not more than 10% of the time in each of four domains: at work, at home, reading, and watching TV or movies
- the verbal expression of the L2 is rated "3" or below on a self-rating scale of 1 to 10, with "10" being "native speaker level of ability" and "1" being "no knowledge."

Based on the information presented above, it is fair to say that defining bilingualism is still a controversial issue due to its multidimensional aspects (also see the review in Hoffmann, 1991). To have more hands-on experience for facilitating interactions with the multilingual and culturally diverse population, professional practitioners or student clinicians may consider the suggestions by Owens (2014) listed in Box 8.1.

Box 8.1 Possible Options to Enhance Interactions With the Culturally Diverse Population Who Are Bilingual or Multilingual

Speech-and-language pathologists, student clinicians, and other related professionals who would like to become more familiar with another culture or language may consider the following options:

- volunteering in or joining community cultural organizations
- attending cultural festivals
- joining other ethnical church groups
- taking a foreign language course or a course in cultural diversity
- shadowing a bilingual speech–and–language pathologist

Source: Owens (2014)

Bilingualism and Multilingualism in Speakers with Aphasia and Its Recovery

Pitres' law versus Ribot's law

The topic of recovery from acquired multilingual aphasia has been debated since the late 19th century. Two major principles have been proposed, which have laid an important foundation for subsequent investigations of bilingual aphasia:

- Pitres' law (Pitres, 1895): This principle claims that recovery of linguistic skills comes first and most completely in the language that is used most premorbidly just before the injury, irrespective of whether or not it is the mother tongue of the speaker.
- Ribot's law (Ribot, 1883): This principle states that in a multilingual patient with aphasia, the person's native language should recover first and the degree of its recovery tends to be higher. In other words, the mother tongue gets better recovery.

As one may expect, because of the various personal and linguistic factors (as well as their combined interactive effects) across bilingual speakers with aphasia, it is reasonable to expect different patterns of recovery. Specifically, Fabbro (1995) has reported that about 40% of bilingual speakers with aphasia exhibited recovery where both the L1 and L2 tended to recover to the same degree relative to their pre-morbid levels. Another 32% of speakers had a tendency to show a better recovery of L1 than L2 and vice versa for the remaining 28%. According to Paradis (1977, 2004), there are six basic recovery patterns of bilingual aphasia, as listed in Table 8.1. A recent systematic review of factors influencing language impairment in bilingual aphasia (Kuzmina et al., 2019) suggested that the language one acquired earlier is more resistant to brain damage, i.e., lexical items learned early in life tend to be better preserved in aphasia. However, the status of late versus early bilingual (i.e., one who learned an L2 after or before the age of 7 years, respectively) could affect the magnitude of this difference; late bilingual speakers with aphasia were found to show a better

Table 8.1 Six major patterns of recovery in bilingual aphasia

Pattern	Characteristics	Clinical prevalence rate
Parallel recovery	It occurs when both languages are impaired and restored at the same rate.	61%
Differential recovery	It occurs when languages recover differentially relative to their pre-morbid levels.	18%
Successive recovery	It occurs when two languages recover but recovery of the second language may only begin after the first language has recovered.	9%
Antagonistic recovery	It occurs when one language recovers to a certain extent first and starts to regress. At the same time, another language begins to recover.	
Selective recovery	It occurs when at least one language is not recovered at all.	5%
Blended recovery	It occurs when patients demonstrate a mixed (and/or inappropriate) pattern of language changes, possibly due to mutual interference of both languages.	7%

performance in their L1 compared to L2. Early bilinguals, on the other hand, were comparable in terms of performance in their two languages. Concerning the factor of premorbid language proficiency, individuals with higher L1 proficiency and those with equal proficiency in both languages showed better overall performance in L1. There was also a significantly greater magnitude of L1 advantage in speakers who used L1 more frequently (as compared with those who had a more frequent use of L2), highlighting the role language use plays in defining patterns of language impairment in bilingual aphasia.

Linguistic Improvement in the Period of Spontaneous Recovery

While the majority of studies in the literature of bilingual aphasia tend to report language recovery in the sub-acute or chronic stage of aphasia, a small number of investigations have been researched on how post-morbid use of L1 and L2 would affect the recovery of bilingual aphasia at the early onset period of stroke, i.e., at the stage of spontaneous recovery. For individuals with a relatively severe degree of aphasia (such as global aphasia), auditory comprehension and repetition tended to show the greatest recovery during the first year (Nagaratnam, 1996; Smania et al., 2010). Improvement in naming only emerged between one to three years post-onset. Narrative performance such as spontaneous speech did not demonstrate changes until in the chronic stage of aphasia (Smania et al., 2010).

On the other hand, based on a case study of a 75-year-old multilingual female speaker with better initial discourse skills and relatively higher-level linguistic functioning during the early onset period of aphasia, a different recovery pattern has been reported by Kong and Whiteside (2014). The speaker in this case study was reported to have comparable pre-morbid percentage use and proficiency of her L1 and L2. However, at the early recovery period, results of standardized aphasia batteries indicated that, without any language intervention in L1, the recovery of her native language was greater in extent, more rapid, and more complete than her L2 (which received intervention). In particular, spontaneous speech and oral narrative abilities were found to be the parameters that displayed the most rapid recovery. Naming and auditory comprehension were the next best parameters that demonstrated changes. This was followed by the improvement in reading and writing, which was found to be more important in reflecting the overall improvement than oral repetition skills. Extending Goral's (2012) findings, Kong and Whiteside (2014) further suggested the positive impact of the use of a language post-morbidly on a multilingual speaker's language recovery. That is, the immediate post-morbid language proficiency was reported to play a critical role in the later language outcome involving two or more languages in acute recovery or during early onset of aphasia. The conclusion by Kong and Whiteside also further supported previous findings about the facilitative effect of the language status of bilingual aphasia (L1) on its recovery patterns (Weekes, 2010).

It should also be noted that similar languages tend to be coincidentally more impaired and also recover more equally in bilingual aphasia (Paradis, 1993) because the cognitive neuropsychological language substrata may be shared to a greater extent in these cases. Most studies found that speakers with bilingual aphasia are better at naming in L1 than L2. Moreover, object naming tends to be better preserved than action naming although the reverse pattern has also been reported (Hernández et al., 2008; Kambanaros & van Steenbrugge, 2006; Poncelet et al., 2007; Weekes & Raman, 2008).

Cross-Linguistic Difference, Generalization, or Transfer

Studies from the past two decades, such as Edmonds and Kiran (2006) and Miertsch et al. (2009), have reported the cross-linguistic generalization or transfer of therapy effect from a treated to an untreated language among bilingual speakers with aphasia. The transfer effect was also reported to happen in cases when the treated language was the second language (and presumably less proficient than the L1) to the untreated and better preserved mother tongue (see Kiran & Iakupova, 2011; Kurland & Falcon, 2011). Goral (2012), on the other hand, believed that post-morbid language proficiency plays a more critical role in determining the extent of cross-linguistic therapy transfer. In a later review article by Ansaldo and Saidi (2014), it was concluded that many factors can affect the overall linguistic transfer effects from the treated to untreated language, including:

- the word types in L1 versus L2 (e.g., **cognates** and non-cognates) – a tendency of higher transfer effects if the two languages contain more cognate pairs
- the degree of structural overlap between languages (i.e., language distance between L1 and L2) – a tendency of higher transfer effects for similar language pairs
- the type of therapy treating L1 or L2 – patients who are responsive to language intervention tend to demonstrate a better transfer in general
- the language proficiency profiles before and after a brain injury – higher language proficiency generally leads to better transfer
- the status of cognitive control circuit for language switching – a tendency of better transfer for speakers with more preserved control units.

Use of Culturally Appropriate Assessment Materials

One of the greatest challenges for clinicians who provide speech and language services to bilingual or multilingual speakers is the lack of culturally and linguistically appropriate diagnostic batteries (Centeno, 2009). This is especially evident for practitioners who work with languages that are linguistically unique and different from English, or languages that are poorly understood or scarcely researched in the field of aphasiology.

When working with clients who have culturally diverse backgrounds, it is important to distinguish language differences from language disorders. There is a critical need to use language assessment measures that are appropriate for the language background of the multilingual clients. Assessment (and subsequently treatment) in only one of the two or more languages spoken by the multilingual patients may easily lead to under-rating of their overall language abilities. Given that multilingual speakers with aphasia do not necessarily manifest the same language disorders with the same degree of severity across their spoken languages, it is not considered to be ethically acceptable for clinicians to assess patients in only one language (Paradis, 1995). Some common components of assessing bilingual or multilingual speakers with acquired language disorders that should be addressed by clinicians when working with this clientele are outlined below.

Multilingual History

Clinicians should establish a client's language dominance in the initial testing of language, so that the most appropriate language to be used in extended language evaluation (and subsequently language intervention) can be determined. Before the administration of formal assessment, it is helpful to obtain a detailed summary of a speaker's multilingual history as well as pre- and post-morbid language use. This can be done by a self-report from the client, with verification by family members, significant others, primary caregivers, spouses, and/or friends, if needed. The application of formal interviewing, self-rating scales, and questionnaires of language use is also common in daily practice. A sample intake form for obtaining the linguistic background and history of bilingual adult speakers can be found in Appendix 8.1. Major components in this form include a speaker's demographic information (Part A), social information (Part B), and language history, experience, and use (Part C). In many cases of persons with aphasia, as a result of changed daily routine and/or language proficiency, the pattern of using language on a daily basis may be altered. Capturing the change of this pattern of language use is clinically important for a healthcare professional to understand how a speaker's pre- and post-morbid language profile is related to the corresponding deficits in these languages.

An example of summary chart to report the approximate percentage daily language use in a multilingual speaker (three languages in the example including English, Spanish, and French) is given in Table 8.2. Remarks on the context of how a client uses various languages and significant life events that relate to the client's language acquisition and/or use can be added. More details about relevant information to be collected regarding language history in bilingual or multilingual speakers is given in Box 8.2.

Table 8.2 Sample summary detailing approximate percentage daily language use before and after stroke in a trilingual speaker with aphasia

Client's age	Approximate % daily use		
	L1 (English)	L2 (Spanish)	L3 (French)
Before stroke 0 to 18 years	80% [at home & in school]	15% [in school & with friends]	5% [in school]
19 to 40 years	50% [at home]	40% [at work and with friends]	10% [at work]
41 to 53 years	50% [at home]	30% [at work and with friends]	20% [at work and with friends]
After stroke > 53 years	90% [at home and in support group]	10% [with friends]	0%

Remarks: Pre-morbidly, the client's work required him to use Spanish in different modalities (speaking, hearing, writing, and reading). After his stroke, he retired from work and has been using English predominantly at home with his family and in community support groups which he attends up to four days weekly.

Box 8.2 Important Information to be Collected When Assessing Language History in Bilingual or Multilingual Speakers

When a speech-and-language pathologist works with a bilingual or multilingual client, the following information related to language history should be gathered:

- age and manner of how each of the languages was acquired
- age and manner of how a dialect(s) of each language was spoken
- length of exposure to each language spoken
- characteristics of using each of the languages at home, in schools, at work, and/or in community
- language(s) used within the family versus language of choice with peers
- contact with native speakers of the primary language
- language of academic instruction and academic performance in each language spoken
- age of immigration and exposure to the non-native language.

Source: Rimikis et al. (2013)

Acculturation and Language Use

Acculturation refers to the process in which a member of a cultural group adopts the beliefs and behaviors of another group. The process of acculturation often involves the acquisition and usage of a new (second and non-native) language. For example, new immigrants to a foreign country (or new language environment) are put into an acculturation scenario where they may or may not maintain their preference for using their native language. Depending on the age when an individual is introduced to the new environment, the learning of a second language may take place formally in a classroom, or informally through interactions with peers or new friends in the community, as well as exposure to various mediums of culture such as television, music, reading materials (newspapers or magazines), and social media (or a combination of the above). This group of speakers are often named "late bilinguals" and are characterized by the different language proficiency levels between their L1 and L2. Those who do not assimilate into (or even reject) the dominant culture may only have minimal functional use of the L2. In contrast, those who assimilate well into the dominant culture may gradually and eventually take the L2 for their own. Clinicians who work with this population will need to pay considerable amount of attention to the speaker's values of their native culture.

For individuals coming from a minority cultural background, such as the second generation of immigrants from foreign countries, one interesting but relatively less researched area is the factors that influence their language acculturation as they relate to the dominant culture. This group of speakers are often called "childhood bilinguals" who usually demonstrate comparable proficiency of their mother tongue (or the language directly related to their race and ethnicity) and the language in their dominant culture of the residing country. Determination of the "native language" of these speakers is not as straightforward, mainly because of the fact that many of them are exposed to, and therefore use and acquire, both languages at the same time when they are young, i.e., in the critical period of language acquisition. It is also not uncommon to find childhood bilinguals being less proficient in using the language of origin, i.e., the language of the country these speakers or their parents come from. Choice of and exposure to language for communication would significantly affect their performance in each spoken language. Clinicians who need to conduct linguistically-based assessment and/ or treatment for this bilingual population should carefully determine the clients' language profiles and preference.

Celenk and Van de Vijver (2011) reported a review of publicly available acculturation measures in the literature, focusing on the scale descriptors, psychometric properties, and conceptual and theoretical structure (such as acculturation conditions, orientations, and outcomes, as well as life domains) of these measures. It was concluded that the majority of these tools were useful for assessing behavioral acculturation outcomes. In this section, two examples of acculturation scales will be illustrated: the Abbreviated Multidimensional Acculturation Scale (AMAS) (Zea et al., 2003), which has been validated for use in the American and Latino/Latina populations, and the Asian American Multidimensional Acculturation Scale (AAMAS) (Chung et al., 2004), which has been validated for use in the Asian and American populations. Note that if someone comes from a multicultural family, it is recommended to conduct an acculturation evaluation for all the corresponding cultures, or at least for the culture(s) the client relates to the most.

The AMAS contains 42 question items to assess a person's acculturation in the United States and in the country of origin in terms of three factors: identity, language competence, and cultural competence. An examinee is required to uses a 4-point Likert-type scale to respond to questions related to each of the three factors, such as:

- Identity: "I feel that I am part of U.S. American culture" or "I have a strong sense of being Latino/Latina"; 1 – "Strongly disagree", 2 – "Disagree somewhat," 3 – "Agree somewhat," 4 – "Strongly agree."
- Language competence: "How well do you speak English with American friends?" or "How well do you understand your native language

words in songs?"; 1 – "Not at all," 2 – "A little," 3 – "Pretty well," 4 – "Extremely well."

- Cultural competence: "How well do you know American national heroes?" or "How well do you know about popular newspapers and magazines in your native language?"; 1 – "Not at all," 2 – "A little," 3 – "Pretty well," 4 – "Extremely well."

The AAMAS consists of 15 items to measure four acculturation domains, cultural identity, language, cultural knowledge, and food consumption, which then allow a more complex assessment of the acculturation level of Asian Americans and its relationship to a person's psychological functioning. An examinee is required to uses a 6-point Likert-type scale (from 1 – "Not very much," 3 – "Moderately," to 6 – "Very much) to respond to questions related to each domain, such as:

- Cultural identity: "How much do you interact and associate with people from the United States?" or "How proud are you to be a part of the culture of origin?"
- Language: "How well do you read and write in the language of English?" or "How often do you listen to music or watch movies and read magazines from your country of origin?"
- Cultural knowledge: "How knowledgeable are you about American history?" or "How much do you actually practice the traditions and keep the holidays of your country of origin?"
- Food consumption: "How often do you actually eat American food?" or "How much do you like the food of the country of origin?"

The Bilingual Aphasia Test (BAT)

There is a lack of appropriate assessment tools for clients with culturally diverse backgrounds because most existing tests widely used by speech-and-language pathologists are English-based and are normed on a sample population comprised of monolingual English speakers. Therefore, using a formal and standardized English language battery to assess bilingual or multilingual clients can be problematic (and in some cases, misleading).

The Bilingual Aphasia Test (BAT) was designed to assess each of the languages of a bilingual or multilingual individuals with aphasia in an equivalent way (Paradis & Libben, 1987). It has been developed for use in speakers of more than 59 languages but different versions of the BAT are not mere translations of each other. Instead, each version has been culturally and linguistically validated and the criteria of cross-language equivalence vary with each task. The e-BAT of all available language versions are downloadable from www.mcgill.ca/linguistics/research/bat#ebat. There are three main sections in the BAT:

- Part A is a questionnaire on the history of bilingualism that includes 50 questions. Information on a speaker's pre-morbid state of bilingualism and contexts of language acquisition and use can be obtained.
- Part B is the major part of the test and consists of 428 items to evaluate a speaker's proficiency and impairment across various modalities within the language being tested. Table 8.3 details all language subtests, three of which contain measures specific to sentential and discourse level performance. For example, the "Spontaneous speech" section elicits conversational samples using topics around the client's own illness, work, foreign travel experience, and family. The sample is then analyzed with reference to the micro-linguistic features, including output quantity, fluency, pronunciation, grammar, and use of vocabulary. The "Description" section of telling a story, with the use of pictures of a cartoon strip, addresses the macrostructures of the output, such as its story structure and degree of connectedness. Both sets of language samples can also be analyzed using additional quantitative measures, such as mean length of utterance (MLU), Type-Token Ratio (TTR), numbers of neologisms, paraphasias and perseverations, and numbers of omitted obligatory grammatical morphemes (Paradis, 2011).
- Part C consists of 85 items that specifically examine a speaker's ability to recognize, produce, and provide grammatical judgment of translated language pairs. The aim of this section is to determine if one language is recovered better than the other.

According to Paradis (2011), although the scores of the BAT do not provide a clear-cut classification of patients' syndromes or aphasia types, clinicians are encouraged "to use taxonomy that fits their theoretical framework and infer syndromes on the basis of a patient's relative scores on some specific tasks considered to be characteristic of a specific aphasia type" (p.428). In other words, by administering the relevant language version of the BAT, the important procedure of classifying aphasic syndromes can be done to assess specific language domains to guide speech therapy (Goodglass et al., 2001). The BAT profile may provide clinicians with indications regarding which language is best suited for verbal communication and allow intervention to precisely focus on aspects in each of the client's languages that are in need of remediation. Since the full BAT may require up to 2.5 hours to complete, a BAT screening test that comprises subtests and items from the full BAT becomes an option for assessing clients who potentially cannot finish the whole test (see details in Table 8.3).

Table 8.3 Language subtests and their item numbers in Part B of the Bilingual Aphasia Test (English version)

Section	BAT full version		BAT screening test+	
	Item number	Maximum achievable score	Example (Item number)	Remarks for scoring
Spontaneous speech *	18–22	20	18–22	Add a rating on borrowing or code-switching behaviors: from '1' being very frequent to '5' being absent
Verbal comprehension				
Pointing	23–32	10	23–26, 31	Select five items other than the ones chosen for naming
Single and semi-complex commands	33–42	10	34–36, 39, 41, 42	Select three simple and three semi-complex commands
Complex commands	43–47	20	43	Select one complex command
Verbal auditory comprehension	48–65	18	48, 53, 55, 57, 60, 62, 65	Select six among the best stimuli and one with X as an answer
Syntactic comprehension	66–152	87	66	Select ten of the best stimuli, including:
				- one standard sentence (S)
			69	- one pronominal reference sentence (P)
			84	- one non-standard 1 sentence (NS1)
			87, 94	- two non-standard 2 sentences (NS2): one subject-topicalized and one object-topicalized
			121	- one standard negative (SN) sentence
			140, 143, 150	- three reversible noun-phrase constructions
Semantic categories	153–172	20		
Grammaticality judgment	173–182	10		

Semantic acceptability	183–192	10		
Repetition				
Words	193–252	20	193, 207, 237, 243, 245, 249, 251	Choose seven of the best word stimuli. Make sure the list contains stimuli of increasing phonological complexity
Non-sense words	193–252	10	199, 209, 219, 231, 247	Choose five of the best non-sense word stimuli. Make sure the list contains stimuli of increasing phonological complexity
Sentences	253–259	7	253, 254, 259	Choose three of the best sentences, including one standard sentence (S), one pronominal reference sentence (P) and one standard negation (SN) sentence
Lexical decision				
Words	193–252	20		
Non-sense words	193–252	10		
Series	260–262	3	260, 261	From 1 to 15
Verbal fluency (phonological)	263–268	3	263, 264	Use "animals" if culturally appropriate
Naming	269–288	20	269–271, 282, 286, 288	Select six among the best-suited stimuli
Sentence construction *				
Response obtained	289–313	5		
Correct sentence	289–313	5		
Sentence make sense	289–313	5		
Number of stimulus words used	289–313	16		

(continued)

Table 8.3 Cont.

Section	BAT full version		BAT screening test+	
	Item number	Maximum achievable score	Example (Item number)	Remarks for scoring
Total number of words	289–313	total count		
Semantic opposites	314–323	10	314, 317, 320–322	Choose five of the best stimuli
Derivational morphology	324–333	10		
Morphological opposites	334–343	10		
Description *	344–346	6		
Mental arithmetic	347–361	15		
Listening comprehension	362–366	5		
Reading				
Words	367–376	10	367–371 △	Choose five of the best word stimuli
Sentences	377–386	10	377–380 △	Choose four of the best sentence stimuli sentences including one standard sentence (S), one pronominal reference sentence (P), one non-standard 1 sentence (NS1), and one non-standard 2 sentence (NS2 – subject topicalization)
Paragraph	387–392	6		
Copying	393–397	5	393, 397 △	Choose two of the best items
Dictation				
Words	398–402	5	399, 400, 402 △	Choose three of the best word stimuli
Sentences	403–407	5	406 △	Choose one of the sentence stimuli involving standard negation (SN)

Reading comprehension				
Words	408–417	10	410, 413, 414, 417 △	Choose four of the best items
Sentences	418–427	10	419, 421, 422, 427 △	Choose four of the best items among the more complex, including one pronominal reference sentence (P), one non-standard 2 sentence (NS2), one standard negation (SN) sentence, and one passive negation sentence
Writing	Unnumbered	Open-ended analysis with reference to criteria of tasks with * and other quantitative measures, including MLU, TTR, # of neologisms, paraphasias, and perseverations, or # of omitted obligatory grammatical morphemes (Paradis, 2011)		

Note: *: Subtests with an asterisk denotes testing tapping performance at the sentence or narrative level. +: The BAT screening tests comprises subtests and items from the full BAT. Ready-made versions are available for the following languages (in alphabetical order): Arabic, Castilian, English, French, German, Italian, Korean, Portuguese, and Russian. The remarks and examples given here are specific to the English screener. △: Subtests for literate patients only.

Source: Bilingual Aphasia Test (BAT) by Paradis & Libben (1987).

Preferably, each of the BAT evaluations is carried out by different examiners who are native and fluent speakers of the language being assessed (e.g., Dronkers et al., 1995; Goral et al., 2010). If such an arrangement is not possible, the sections may be conducted by a bilingual clinician (e.g., Dai et al., 2012; Roberts & Deslauriers, 1999) or a combination of monolingual and bilingual examiners. To eliminate any practice effects, two (or more) language versions of the BAT should be conducted a few days to no more than two weeks apart from one another. Arranging two versions to be done on the same day is not encouraged because it will more likely cause interaction and/or interference effects of the two languages being examined.

A special issue in Clinical Linguistics & Phonetics (2011, vol. 25, issue 6–7) was published to illustrate the application of the BAT in cases of bilingual or multilingual aphasia and bilingual primary progressive aphasia, to examine the construct validity of the test, as well as to discuss the development of a BAT for less-researched languages (Paradis, 2011). The fact that these reported studies included bilingual or multilingual speakers from four continents (Asia, Australia, Europe, and North American) and concerned a total of 16 languages would be of interest to researchers and/or clinical professionals who want to learn more about the clinical values and application of the BAT.

Multilingual Aphasia Examination (MAE)

The Multilingual Multilingual Aphasia Examination (MAE) was first designed by Benton (1969) to examine the presence and evaluate the severity of disorders in two or more languages. The MAE Third Edition (Benton et al., 1994) is the most current version with 11 tests and rating scales that provide ample sampling of the performance of spoken language production, verbal comprehension, reading comprehension, and writing. These tests and rating scales are as follows:

1. visual naming
2. sentence repetition
3. controlled word association
4. oral spelling
5. written spelling
6. block spelling
7. MAE token test
8. aural comprehension of words and phrases
9. reading comprehension of words and phrases
10. rating of articulation
11. rating of praxic features of writing.

For the English version of the MAE, normative data based on 360 native English speakers, ranging in age between 16 and 69 years, stratified by age, education, and gender are available. Corrections for age, education, and gender were also established for each of the 11 sections, which allowed users to clinically compare an examinee's performance with corresponding controls based on his or her demographic characteristics. A Spanish version of the MAE was published in 1992 (Rey & Benton, 1992). Test users interested in this version are advised to contact the authors for additional information. An additional five language versions (Chinese, French, German, Italian, and Portuguese) are being prepared which will allow direct research or clinical cross-language comparisons of multilingual speakers (Spreen & Risser, 2003). A more detailed review of the assessment battery was given by McNeil (1989), including information on test items, standardization, and administration as well as how the construct and **content validity** was established.

Standardized Language Batteries Translated, Normalized, and Validated in Languages Other Than English

With the use of two language versions of the same standardized language battery, speech-and-language pathologists can directly measure, compare, and describe the aphasic symptoms of the two corresponding languages in bilingual speakers with aphasia. Many non-English aphasia batteries are adaptations of the classical tests developed for English speakers, such as the Boston Diagnostic Aphasia Examination (BDAE; Goodglass et al. , 2001), Western Aphasia Battery (WAB; Kertesz, 1982), or Comprehensive Aphasia Test (CAT; Swinburn et al., 2004) (see Chapter 1 for more details on standardized assessment batteries for acquired communication disorders). When used appropriately, these adapted and translated tests can allow clinicians to conduct a linguistically valid assessment of bilingual aphasia (Ansaldo & Saidi, 2014).

According to a recent review by Ivanova and Hallowell (2013), a critical limitation for some of these adapted and translated versions of existing assessment batteries is their lack of normative data based on native speakers of the target languages other than English. While only a small proportion of these novel assessment tools are formally published (with norms and linguistically specific scoring criteria), the majority of them have very limited circulation. Clinicians who would like to take advantage of these resources for daily practice often have little or even no access to the full set of assessment materials. Box 8.3 summarizes reported translations of some well-known and widely used aphasia batteries in English.

Box 8.3 A Summary of Some Well-Known and Widely Used Aphasia Assessment Batteries in English with Translation Into Other Languages

Original tests in English	Available versions in other languages (in alphabetical order)
Boston Diagnostic Aphasia Examination (Goodglass et al., 2001)	• Chinese – Mainland China Mandarin/Putonghua (Naeser & Chan, 1980) • Chinese – Taiwan Mandarin (Tseng, 1993) • Finnish (Laine et al., 1993) • French (Mazaux & Orgogozo, 1982) • Hindi (Kacker et al., 1991) • Portuguese (Goodglass et al., 2000) • Spanish (Garcia-Albea et al., 1986)
Boston Naming Test (Goodglass & Kaplan, 2001)	• Chinese – Hong Kong Cantonese (Tsang, 2000) • Finnish (Laine et al., 1993) • French – Quebec (Roberts & Doucet, 2011) • French – Switzerland (Thuillard-Colombo & Assal, 1992) • Italian (D'Agostino, 1985) • Korean (Kim & Na, 1997, 1999) • Spanish (Kaplan et al., 1986)
Western Aphasia Battery (Kertesz, 1982) or Western Aphasia Battery – Revised (Kertesz, 2006)	• Bengali (Keshree et al., 2013) • Chinese – Hong Kong Cantonese (Yiu, 1992) • Japanese (Sugishita, 1986) • Korean (Kim & Na, 2004) • Brazilian Portuguese (Neves et al., 2014) • Tagalog (Ozaeta & Kong, 2012; Ozaeta et al., 2013) • Spanish (Kertesz et al., 1990)
Comprehensive Aphasia Test (Swinburn et al., 2004)	• Arabic (Abou El-Ella et al., 2013) • Danish (Swinburn et al., 2014) • Dutch (Visch-Brink et al., 2014) • Hungarian (Zakariás & Lukács, 2021)

The development of almost all of these adapted versions of the BDAE, BNT, WAB (or WAB-R), and CAT was motivated by the lack of formal language assessment tools in the target languages. Most of the reports of these translated batteries contain descriptions about the properties of the specific language version of a test, as well as normative data from unimpaired native speakers and pathological data from individuals with aphasia. As further mentioned by Fyndanis et al. (2017), one major, important, and critical advantage of establishing an international network of multidisciplinary aphasia researchers to systematically develop different language versions of a language battery is the potential to "pave the way for collecting and pooling large amounts of comparable data with different versions of the same outcome measure and facilitate more robust research on aphasia rehabilitation" (p.698). For example, at present, adaptations of the CAT in 11 different languages spoken in Europe are underway: Basque, Catalan, Croatian, Cypriot Greek, French, (Standard Modern) Greek, Norwegian, Serbian, Spanish, Swedish, and Turkish.

Specific Factors to Consider for Assessment and Management of Discourse Problems in Bilingual or Multilingual Speakers

Code-Switching and Code-Mixing Behaviors

Code-switching and code-mixing mechanisms first described by Paradis (1993, 2008) are part of a behavior selection system involved in the frontal lobe system. Following the definition by Ritchie and Bhatia (1996, 2005), while "code switching" in bilingual speakers refers to the inter-phrasal language switching behaviors, "code mixing" refers to switching at the intra-phrasal level. In healthy adults, voluntary language switching is considered an instance of task switching as it involves, at a minimum, a switch between different stimulus-response sets (Kong et al., 2014).

Pathological language switching and mixing is likely to reflect a deficit in **executive function** that is controlled by the frontal cortex (Heaton et al., 1993). Bilingual speakers with aphasia may demonstrate (1) "pathological switching behaviors" by alternating their languages across different utterances, and/or (2) "pathological mixing behaviors" by intermingling different languages within a single utterance (Fabbro et al., 2000). In other words, pathological language switching is characterized by the alternation of utterances from one language to the other across sentence boundaries. For example, Excerpt 1 below is part of a dialog between the examiner (INV) and a bilingual English-Spanish person with aphasia (PAR) in a testing session. The narrative task involved the PAR providing a procedural discourse of making a peanut butter and jelly sandwich. Pathological language switching behaviors can be found from sentence 11 to 12 and from 13 to 14. Pathological language mixing, on the other hand, involves the mixing of elements of two or more languages in a single utterance (Aglioti et al., 1996; Aglioti & Fabbro, 1993; Fabbro et al., 1997). This involuntary and uncontrolled language switching and mixing is a distinctive and unique feature of multilingual aphasia (Paradis, 1993). An example can be found in sentences 09 and 15 of Excerpt 1, when the speaker was mixing the lexical item of "bread" and used the Spanish word "pan" in the utterances. This pattern can also be seen in sentences 01, 04, and 06 of Excerpt 2, which is the transcript of a bilingual Chinese-English speaker with aphasia describing a set of sequential pictures in Cantonese Chinese. Both pathological switching phenomena can happen, in combination or isolation, even if the interlocutor does not understand one of the two languages being used by the speaker with aphasia. In other words, unlike typical speakers who would voluntarily control the use of L1 versus L2 with consideration of the language knowledge of an interlocutor, speakers with pathological switching and/or mixing fail to appropriately adjust their code-switching behaviors.

EXCERPT (1)

01	INV:	we're gonna do somethin(g) a little bit different now .
02	PAR:	okay.
03	INV:	I want you to tell me how you would make a peanut butter and jelly sandwich.
04	PAR:	how I would make one.
05	INV:	how would you make a peanut butter and jelly sandwich?
06	PAR:	assuming we have all the stuff?
07	INV:	yes.
08	PAR:	okay.
09	PAR:	then &um we'd take out the loaf of el pan (*the bread*).
10	PAR:	open it.
11	PAR:	take a couple of two slices.
12	PAR:	uh tomar un poco de mantequilla de maní (*take some peanut butter*).
13	PAR:	sí (*yes*).
14	PAR:	yes.
15	PAR:	um and um spread the peanut butter on one side of the pan (*bread*).
16	PAR:	and then I'd get jelly.
17	PAR:	open that.
18	PAR:	spread that on the other piece.
19	PAR:	and then put (th)em together.
20	INV:	okay.

Note: All verbal responses in Spanish are underlined. Glosses and/or remarks in English are *italicized* and given in (parentheses).

EXCERPT (2)

01	PAR:	哩 個 老人家 喺度 喺度 整緊 carrot carrot.
	gloss:	This old person is preparing some carrot(s) carrot(s).
02	PAR:	就 喺度 切緊 啲 菜 .
	gloss:	She is cutting some vegetables.

03	PAR:	<u>okay</u>.
	gloss:	okay.
04	PAR:	哩 個 呢 又 係 有 啲 <u>carrot</u> 喺度.
	gloss:	Here are some carrot(s) too.
05	PAR:	但係 一 切 就 切到 隻 手 .
	gloss:	But (she) cuts her hands.
06	PAR:	佢 切到 隻 手 嘞 就 走 去 攞 依 個 依 個 咩 啊 去 依 個 <u>station</u>.
	gloss:	She cuts her hands and goes to this this go to this station.
07	PAR:	<u>they want take the pen</u>.
08	PAR:	<u>they go out the door</u>.

Note: All verbal responses in English were <u>underlined</u>. Glosses and/or remarks in English are given in the "gloss" tier.

Earlier studies have suggested that pathological language switching and mixing is present in about 7% of speakers with bilingual aphasia (Albert & Obler, 1978). Language switching and mixing are considered pathological if they occur involuntarily and are beyond the control of the speaker as in bilingual aphasia (Abutalebi & Green, 2007). One explanation of these phenomena is that language switching and mixing is a result of the malfunctioning of a "language control" device that separates the languages of a multilingual speaker during production (Green & Abutalebi, 2008). A key question in bilingual language production relates to the specificity of the language control device that is used by multilingual individuals. Failures in language control may lead to unwanted language switching as observed in some cases of bilingual aphasia (Goral et al., 2006).

Munoz et al. (1999) have demonstrated the use of a modified Matrix Language Frame (MLF) model (Myers-Scotton, 1993) to examine intra-sentential code switching in four bilingual speakers of English and Spanish with aphasia and their controls. The analysis involved coding of switching behaviors using seven categories. The categorization was done based on the hierarchical relationship between the Matrix Language (ML), which was defined as the base language of the conversation that contributed the most system morphemes to the interaction and set the morphosyntactic structure of the utterance, and the Embedded Language (EL), defined as the less active language inserted into the structure established by the ML. Four of the categories were drawn directly from Myers-Scotton (1993), including ML islands, ML shifts, EL islands, and ML + EL. Three additional categories were added by Munoz et al. (1999) to reflect the linguistic characteristics unique to speakers with aphasia: Borrowed Forms, EL insertions, and Revisions.

Table 8.4 Description of constituent categories in Matrix Language Frame
(MLF) model

MLF category	Description
ML Islands	Well-formed constituents consisting entirely of ML morphemes demonstrating syntactic structure
ML Shift	Change in the ML in consecutive utterances or clausal structures
EL Islands	Well-formed constituents consisting of at least two EL morphemes showing syntactic structure which have been inserted into the ML
ML + EL	A single EL lexeme (not a borrowed form) inserted into the syntactic frame of any number of ML morphemes
Borrowed form	A lexeme from one language incorporated into the morpho-syntactic structure of a second language and judged to be widely accepted by monolingual speakers of the second (non-native) language
EL insertions	Multiple EL lexemes demonstrating no syntactic structure inserted into the syntactic frame of any number of ML morphemes
Revisions	Lexical insertions that do not contribute to the meaning of an utterance, including speech errors, restatements, circumlocutions, and indicators of word finding problems

Note: Matrix Language (ML) is the base language of the conversation; Embedded Language (EL) is the less active language inserted into the structure established by the ML.

Source: Munoz et al. (1999)

According to Munoz et al., the MLF model can "identify grammatical relationships and constraints related to the dominant and subordinate role of each language" (p.250) and the revised model can "provide a useful coding scheme to organize a comparison and discussion of code switching patterns" (p.251). Table 8.4 provides more detailed information for each of the seven coding categories.

Including Interpreters and/or Family Members in the Assessment and Rehabilitation Process

Speech-and-language pathologists frequently receive referrals of speakers with bilingual aphasia or clients who speak languages of which they have little or even no knowledge. Penn and Beecham (1992) have reported their experience in using trained first-language speakers as raters to assess the oral discourse produced by a multilingual speaker with aphasia. It was concluded that with appropriate training, judgements by these raters could be reliable. Hence, in situations when qualified bilingual speech-and-language pathologists with competence in the languages concerned are not available, this approach of using trained raters may be a solution to assessment of multilingual aphasia.

Alternatively, when a clinician is not proficient in the language spoken by the person with aphasia, a trained and qualified interpreter who has knowledge of the specific requirements for speech pathology can be used. The American Speech-Language-Hearing Association has provided some guidelines on proficiency requirements for interpreters in a Relevant Paper (www.asha.org/practice-portal/professional-issues/bilingual-service-delivery/). In addition, clinical professionals are encouraged to consider the language demands of a client (and his or her own family members) and their own language proficiency in the target language being remediated. There are important advantages of using professionally trained interpreters who are familiar with both the culture and language of speakers with aphasia. This is because this mechanism can improve the quality of care, reduce potential errors or breakdown of communication, and lead to a higher patient satisfaction (Flores, 2005; Karliner et al., 2007), all of which are clinically critical.

It was suggested that interpreter-mediated assessments of aphasia are inherently limited, in terms of compromised content validity of test items in the process of administration (Roger & Code, 2011). More specifically, the content validity was more vulnerable at the point when the test was administered by the interpreter or when a patient's responses were reported back to the clinician by the interpreter. There are three critical factors that clinicians should carefully consider when choosing to use an interpreter in the clinical assessment and intervention procedures (Owens, 2014). They include selection, relationship to the family and community, and training:

- When selecting the right interpreter, clinicians may want to select candidates who demonstrate high linguistic, ethical, and professional competency. An interpreter who possesses a high level of proficiency in understanding, speaking, paraphrasing of, and switching between the two (or more) languages spoken by the bilingual speakers with aphasia can probably better ensure the content validity of the translation. In addition, those who have some background in communication sciences or related fields will likely to be more knowledgeable in communication terminology and aphasiology.

- In addition to the above, interpreters who can maintain a positive and professional relationship with the clients and their caregivers can facilitate the ongoing of any diagnostic and intervention sessions. This positive rapport also promotes the participation level on the part of the speakers with language deficits. It is more preferable to match a given client speaking a minority language with an interpreter with a similar cultural background. Using the same interpreter(s), instead of using different personnel on a random basis, is also important.

- While finding the "perfect" interpreter usually sounds easier said than done and can often be out of a clinician's control, components of the training to be given to the interpreter by the clinician become more critical. Specifically, good training should include clear explanation of the purpose, procedures, and methods of conducting various standardized and non-standardized assessment instruments, as well as implementing published or tailor-made informal treatment protocols. Specific needs when interacting with a bilingual client in terms of (1) exact translations from one language to another and vice versa; (2) providing clear instructions that are consistent with those given by the clinician; (3) effective questioning, cueing, and prompting strategies; and (4) rapport-building techniques must be explained. Emphasis on the need to avoid adding or omitting words or ideas in the translation process is of particular importance. This can be achieved by clinician directly demonstrating and teaching the required skills as a part of the training and requiring the interpreter to observe the clinician to reflect how these skills are implemented with real clients. Of course, sharing of professional knowledge and experiences with the interpreter on typical responses and behaviors of clients with acquired communication disorders that are indicative and essential for diagnosis can also be useful (Kambanaros & van Steenbrugge, 2004).

When involving an interpreter in a clinical session, Roger and Code (2011) have identified several areas that are more at risk of weakening the content validity of aphasia assessment. For example, since most standardized tests contain items that have been carefully designed, it is possible that the nature of some test items is changed in the process of interpretation. Ensuring that the interpreter understands the content to be used within a particular assessment tool and the purpose of including various items in the battery is crucial. Another common issue that can be harmful to the interpretation of a client's performance is the consistency in repeating test items (such as repeating verbatim versus reformulating a command or prompt) by the interpreter during formal evaluation. When examining the discourse abilities through tasks such as picture descriptions, spontaneous speech, or social conversational interactions that often occurred at the beginning of a session, it is not uncommon to find that interpreters may have a tendency to expand a client's utterances in the process of interpretation. How well an interpreter can preserve the form of the original utterances when translating the oral production will also critically affect how a clinician determines the clients' adequacy on various linguistic aspects. Therefore, thorough and comprehensive training may avoid any potential errors or misdiagnosis of performance. In addition, if the interpreter is on the same page with the clinician by knowing what linguistic (and/or paralinguistic and non-linguistic) elements are being targeted and examined, responses from the clients may be more accurately and sensitively recorded. Pre-session briefings to agree on the details of test administration may also facilitate the collaboration and translation process.

When a professional interpreter is not available, untrained interpreters such as family members, friends, or co-workers may provide help to the clinician but, at the same time, can potentially give rise to ethical issues of privacy and confidentiality (Brisset et al., 2013). As these laypersons tend to lack professional knowledge about the conditions of the language impairment, their reliability and accuracy of interpreting specific linguistic symptoms may sometimes be questionable; more caution is necessary when a clinician is incorporating their input into the diagnostic process. Nevertheless, one should note that when a client chooses to use a family member or a friend to act as an interpreter, the clinician should still take this preference into consideration and explain any possible anticipated pitfalls.

Adoption and Modification of Existing Systems Aimed at Unilingual Speakers

Earlier cross-linguistic studies have reported evidence to support manifestations of language-specific symptoms in aphasia, many of which were discussed in the context of agrammatism. Some examples, in alphabetical order, include Basque (Laka & Korostola, 2001), Catalan (Peña-Casanova et al., 2001), Chinese (Cantonese) (Yiu & Worrall, 1996), Chinese (Mandarin) (Packard, 1993), Czech (Leheckova, 2001), Dutch (Kolk et al., 1990), Finnish (Helasvuo et al., 2001), French (Nespoulous et al., 1990), Friulian (Fabbro & Frau, 2001), German (Stark & Dressler, 1990), Greek (Tsapkini et al., 2001), Hebrew (Goral, 2001), Hindi (Bhatnagar, 1990), Hungarian (Kertesz & Osman-Sagi, 2001), Italian (Miceli & Mazzucchi, 1990), Japanese (Sasanuma et al., 1990), Persian (Nilipour & Raghibdoust, 2001), Polish (Ulatowska et al., 2001), Spanish (Centeno & Obler, 2001), and Swedish (Månsson & Ahlsén, 2001). However, only scattered reports specific to the impaired discourse production among monolingual and/or multilingual speakers of these languages are published. More recently, a small number of studies focusing on cross-linguistic differences and manifestations of related symptoms at the discourse level have become available (e.g., Grasso et al., 2019; Mazumdar et al., 2020; Sung et al., 2016).

Given the great paucity of linguistically appropriate and specific tools to address narrative-level performance among bilingual or multilingual speakers with aphasia, clinical practitioners, such as speech-and-language pathologists, have modified existing systems geared for evaluating discourse production in English to assess discourse abilities in non-English speakers. For example, Dai et al. (2012) described the adaptation of Conversation Analysis Profile for People with Aphasia (CAPPA) (Whitworth et al., 1997; see Chapter 3 for more details) to assess the conversational narrative skills of a trilingual speaker of Chinese (Cantonese), Chinese (Mandarin), and English with aphasia. More specifically, apart from using the original CAPPA indices, additional measures were newly included to capture the client's code-switching behaviors, off-topic content, and repetition deficits. Appendix 8.2 details the modified CAPPA and the clinical implications of the new indices suggested. Clinicians may refer to this kind of report and consider if the same approach works for their clientele.

Using Multiple Language Versions of the Same Discourse Analytic Systems for Direct Comparison of Narrative Skills

Another useful approach to compare discourse performance of the languages spoken by a bilingual speaker is through the use of different language versions of the same discourse analytic systems. This, of course, requires the availability of these versions of the assessment in the first place. The following two examples are described here to illustrate how this approach can be implemented clinically:

- Ramsberger et al. (2014) and Hilger et al. (2014) have reported the use of the Linguistic Communication Measure (LCM) (Menn et al., 1994; see Chapter 3 for more details) and its modified Chinese version (Kong & Law, 2004) to reflect deterioration in an English-Shanghainese speaker with logopenic variant primary progressive aphasia. The discourse skills and speech characteristics in describing the Cookie Theft picture were found to decline differently between the two languages.
- Kong and Whiteside (2014) used the Main Concept Analysis in English (MCA; Kong et al., 2016) and its Chinese (Cantonese) version (Kong, 2009; see Chapter 3 for more details) to systematically monitor the improvement of discourse in both languages exhibited by a multilingual speaker during the period of spontaneous recovery. In addition, changes of aphasia syndrome fluency rating, and grammaticality (as reflected by the Western Aphasia Battery and its Cantonese version), were monitored in parallel with the MCA. It was revealed that improvement in oral discourse between Chinese and English over time could be differentiated.

What perhaps is unique to this approach is the advantage of direct comparison of two (or more) languages using objective quantifications of discourse performance. Note that most existing narrative analyses are not necessarily universal and can sometimes be ethnically context-bound (Van Dijk, 1985), i.e., they are more suitable for use in the Western culture. For this particular reason, if geographically sensitive analysis guidelines, scoring criteria that include geographically specific examples, and/or culturally specific norms are available for individual language versions of an existing English-based discourse measure, clinicians are advised to follow the corresponding scoring procedures to ensure scoring consistency and test validity.

Implications for Therapy

In a recent article discussing international practice of speech and language services (Davis-McFarland, 2020), it was emphasized that successful clinical services to the non-U.S. mainstream clientele (e.g., people from "minority world countries") would require clinicians' cultural knowledge as well as clinical skills and competencies. In addition, careful planning and community input is needed to ensure that services provided are relevant, accessible, sustainable, and responsive to the needs of those being served. It was also specified that using available human and cultural resources would ensure a more culturally sensitive clinical practice. Examples of how to achieve this include paying respects to and embracing local culture of the clients, and building on successful services and/or programs that already exist in the client's local community.

As a result of an aging population and the overall high incidence of cardiovascular diseases in older individuals in many countries in the world, the global effect of high rates of stroke and other neurogenic conditions interact with local health care realities in terms of the services provided by rehabilitation specialists, including speech-and-language pathologists, in each country worldwide (Norrving & Kissela, 2013). A number of factors are intertwined with language rehabilitation and affect the dynamics of service delivery, including domestic social factors in each nation (such as diversity trends) and the availability of the qualified personnel and the research evidence needed to support clinical management (Centeno, 2009; Harris, 2011; World Health Organization, 2011).

Considerations of Linguistic, Cognitive, Cultural, and Sociocultural Variables in Bilingual or Multilingual Speakers

Based on the U.S. census results in 2000, about 47 million people aged five or above were reported to be speakers of a language other than English at home. According to the Center for Immigration Studies (https://cis.org/), this number has grown dramatically to an estimated 67.3 million residents in the nation in 2018. While English-Spanish bilingualism is the most frequent, sizable numbers of residents speak Chinese, French, or other languages apart from English. According to Lorenzen and Murray (2008), sufficient research-based evidence and empirical supports regarding language remediation of bilingual aphasia is currently lacking. Based on reported investigations of various aspects of multilingual aphasia in the existing literature, a number of factors have been found to influence the outcome of bilingual aphasia therapy. Although most of the same intervention designs and principles for monolingual aphasia should apply to bilingual or multilingual language-impaired speakers, selectively using one or more treatment strategies summarized below with careful consideration of the relevant linguistic, cognitive, sociocultural, and/or psychosocial variables would likely increase therapy effectiveness:

- Careful assessment of speech, language, and communication deficits in each of the languages spoken by a client, with identification of specific linguistic and cultural aspects that may affect a client's functional need.
- The capability of discourse production in monolingual speakers with aphasia cannot be fully assessed using only one technique (Capiluoto et al., 2006). It is reasonable to assume the same notion applies to bilingual or multilingual speakers. The use of a combination of a wide range of elicitation and investigation procedures (including, but not limited to, single or sequential picture description, story-telling, monologic recounts, and conversations) is therefore recommended for making a more informed diagnostic decision of discourse skills (Davis & Coelho, 2004).
- Set appropriate intervention goals based on a client's pre-morbid as well as post-morbid language proficiency and usage patterns. Relevant psycholinguistic variables including age of onset, literacy level, and emotional valence should also be considered.
- Choose accessible targets in a language or dialect that a client demonstrates with a higher degree of fluency.
- Consider factors such as a client's preference and immediate language environment.
- Use concrete, rather than abstract, words to potentially facilitate direct translation between two language systems. This is motivated by previous findings on the beneficial effect of concreteness effects on lexical retrieval in bilingual speakers.
- Use cognates, or words in two languages that have a common etymological origin with shared meaning, morphology, and/or pronunciation (e.g., "pan" in Spanish and "pain" in French for "bread" or '學生' / hok6sang1/ in Cantonese Chinese and '学生' /gakusei/ がくせい in Japanese for "student"), in bilingual intervention. This is based on the positive influence cognates have on the lexical access speed, accuracy, and recovery in bilingual speakers with aphasia. More specifically, during language production, cognates share the same phonological-sublexical base that allow overlapped phonological activation of a lexical item in one language and its translated form in another language (Costa et al., 2005). This facilitative effect has been shown to be more evident for words with dense neighborhoods (i.e., words with higher number of

phonologically similar units), which can lead to better priming effects to a similar extent as that found with morphologically related words in monolingual language-impaired speakers (Napps & Fowler, 1987).

- With reference to the pre- and post-morbid linguistic profile, determine rehabilitation components (e.g., verbal versus written language across different languages) that can met the language-specific wants and needs of a client.
- Understand the similarities between languages, as well as the contexts and purposes of how a client is using different languages, to decide which language is trained. This principle also applies to determining the order of addressing two or more languages during intervention.
- Consider the effect of cross-linguistic (or cross-language) generalization or transfer (i.e., from one language to another) when addressing specific deficits in one or more languages (Faroqi-Shah et al., 2010; Penn, 2012). Specifically, according to the systematic review by Faroqi-Shah et al. (2010), positive receptive and expressive outcomes in bilingual aphasia can be yielded following language therapy provided in a non-native language. This facilitative effect is not limited to acute patients, but also applies to individuals who are in the chronic stage of aphasia.
- Include cognitive treatments for a client who demonstrates concomitant cognitive deficits because appropriate activation and inhibition of language use and switching (as well as a combination of both) affects how different languages are successfully used by a bilingual client.
- Consider the use of compensatory strategies in addition to or in place of traditional behavioral interventions. These strategies may include use of appropriate code-switching technique, digitized speech device, and communication apps on tablet or mobile devices in one or more languages spoken by a client. Cautions may be necessary when selecting the appropriate augmentative and alternative communication (AAC) devices with bilingual and multilingual speakers because some of them may present cultural barriers to non-English clients (Lorenzen & Murray, 2008).
- Involve a client's family members, caregivers, and other significant others by teaching vocabulary commonly used within the language spoken by the client which they are unfamiliar with. Other relevant factors clinicians should consider include family structure, communication styles, and their attitude towards intervention using the native language.
- Properly document improvements in all languages to determine how the overall language treatment influences therapy efficiency and effectiveness.

Readers who are interested in getting additional information about the resources for managing acquired communication disorders or specific guidelines in managing language rehabilitation in the multicultural and/or international populations may refer to Appendix 8.3.

Patterns of Recovery in Bilingual or Multilingual Aphasia

Depending on the initial overall aphasia severity, it is not uncommon to find different aspects of oral and written language improving in different time windows. Pre- and post-morbid performance level between a particular client's native and non-native language can be important prognostic factors to consider when determining the recovery of bilingual aphasia (Kong & Whiteside, 2014).

Faroqi-Shah et al. (2010) have emphasized the need to pay attention to the combined influence of various variables on outcomes of bilingual aphasia treatment. They include:

- bilingual variables, such as a client's age of acquisition and level of proficiency for each spoken language
- aphasiological variables, such as the initial severities and deficit patterns of multiple languages, the characteristics and patterns of pathological switching and mixing, and the degree of comorbid cognitive complications
- linguistic variables, such as semantic and phonological relatedness of vocabulary as well as morphological and syntactic similarities between languages, anticipated or unanticipated cross-language generalizations, etc.
- neurological variables, such as the site and extension of brain lesions, focal versus diffused brain damage with or without subcortical or white matter involvement, presence of co-existing neurological conditions, single versus multiple strokes, etc.
- sociocultural variables, such as a client's immediate language environment in different communication contexts (home, school, work, or community) and acceptability of code-mixing behaviors among unimpaired bilinguals in various life situations.

Knowing that the trajectory of language recovery in a multilingual speaker with aphasia does not necessarily parallel with the improvement patterns reported for classical monolingual aphasic syndromes, the above information about language changes over time may act as additional planning guidelines especially when a clinician attempts to prioritize the remediation of different languages in multilingual individuals.

Conclusions

This chapter has focused on the considerations for assessing and managing discourse-level impairments in the multilingual and culturally diverse populations. One should note that there is still a great paucity of information in the literature of aphasiology and communication disorders on specific diagnostic and treatment protocols for bilingual or multilingual speakers. Although it is believed that the various methodologies presented in this chapter are appropriate means to address the clinical needs of these individuals, some of them are discussed based on clinical experience with only limited supporting efficacy data. More empirical research studies are still needed to provide evidence in guiding practitioners in terms of clinical evaluation, goal setting, and delivery of intervention.

Readers who need additional information about practice resources related to culturally and linguistically diverse populations may visit the online directory by The Office of Multicultural Affairs of the American Speech-Language-Hearing Association at www.asha.org/practice/multicultural. Readers are also encouraged to refer to newer guidelines and recommendations on practices of discourse analysis in clinical management that are specific to the non-U.S. clinical populations (e.g., Cruice et al., 2020) for additional insights and practical advice.

References

Abou El-Ella, M.Y., Alloush, T. K., El-Shobary, A. M., El-Dien Hafez, N. G., Abd EL-Halim, A. I., & El-Rouby, I. M. (2013). Modification and standardisation of Arabic version of the Comprehensive Aphasia Test. *Aphasiology, 27*(5), 599–614.

Abutalebi, J., & Green, D. (2007). Bilingual language production: The neurocognition of language representation and control. *Journal of Neurolinguistics, 20*(3), 242–275.

Aglioti, S., Beltramello, A., Girardi, F., & Fabbro, F. (1996). Neurolinguistic and follow-up study of an unusual pattern of recovery from bilingual subcortical aphasia. *Brain, 119*(5), 1551–1564.

Aglioti, S., & Fabbro, F. (1993). Paradoxical selective recovery in a bilingual aphasic following subcortical lesion. *NeuroReport, 4*, 1359–1362.

Albert, M., & Obler, L. (1978). *The bilingual brain: Neuropsychological and neurolinguistic aspects of bilingualism.* New York, NY: Academic Press.

Ansaldo, A. I. & Saidi, L. G. (2014). Aphasia therapy in the age of globalization: Cross-linguistic therapy effects in bilingual aphasia. *Behavioural Neurology, 2014*, 1–10.

Benton, A. L. (1969). Development of a multilingual aphasia battery: Progress and problems. *Journal of the Neurological Sciences, 9*, 39–48.

Benton, A. L., Hamsher, K. S., & Sivan, A.B. (1994). *Multilingual Aphasia Examination.* San Antonio, TX. Psychological Corporation.

Bhatnagar, S. C. (1990). Crossed agrammatism in Hindi: A case study. In L. Menn, & L. K. Obler (Eds.). *Agrammatic aphasia: A cross-language narrative sourcebook* (pp. 975–11). Amsterdam: John Benjamins.

Brisset, C., Leanza, Y., & Laforest, K. (2013). Working with interpreters in health care: A systematic review and meta-ethnography of qualitative studies. *Patient education and counseling, 91*(2), 131–140.

Capiluoto, G. J., Wright, H. H., & Wagovich, S. A. (2006). Reliability of main event measurement in the discourse of individuals with aphasia. *Aphasiology, 20*, 205–216.

Celenk, O. & Van de Vijver, F. (2011). Assessment of acculturation: Issues and overview of measures. *Online Readings in Psychology and Culture, 8*(1). Doi:10.9707/2307-0919.1105

Centeno, J. G. (2009). Issues and principles in service delivery to communicatively impaired minority bilingual adults in neurorehabilitation. *Seminars in Speech and Language, 30*(3), 139–152.

Centeno, J. G. & Obler, L. K. (2001). Agrammatic verb errors in Spanish speakers and their normal discourse correlates. *Journal of Neurolinguistics, 14,* 349–363.

Chung, R. H., Kim, B. S. & Abreu, J. M. (2004). Asian American Multidimensional Acculturation Scale: Development, factor analysis, reliability, and validity. *Cultural Diversity & Ethnic Minority Psychology, 10*(1), 66–80.

Costa, A., Santesteban, M., & Caño, A. (2005). On the facilitatory effects of cognate words in bilingual speech production. *Brain and Language, 94*(1), 94–103.

Cruice, M., Botting, N., Marshall, J., Boyle, M., Hersh, D., Pritchard, M., & Dipper, L. (2020). UK speech and language therapists' views and reported practices of discourse analysis in aphasia rehabilitation. *International Journal of Language & Communication Disorders, 55*(3), 417–442.

D'Agostino, L. (1985). Taratura su soggetti normali di prove di denominazione per l'afasia [Unpublished thesis]. Istituto di Clinica Neurologica, Universita` degli studi di Modena, Modena, Italy.

Dai, E., Kong, A. P. H., & Weekes, B. S. (2012). Recovery of naming and discourse production: A bilingual anomic case study. *Aphasiology, 26*(6), 737–756.

Davis, G. A., & Coelho, C. A. (2004). Referential cohesion and logical coherence of narration after closed-head injury. *Brain and Language, 89,* 508–523.

Davis-McFarland, E. (2020). Ethics in international practice. *Perspectives of the ASHA Special Interest Groups, 5*(6), 1779–1784.

De Bot, K. (1992). A bilingual processing model: Levelt's speaking model adapted. *Applied Linguistics, 13,* 1–24.

Dronkers, N., Yamasaki, Y., Ross, G. W., & White, L. (1995). Assessment of bilinguality in aphasia: Issues and examples from multicultural Hawaii. In M. Paradis (Ed.), *Aspects of bilingual aphasia* (pp. 57–66). Oxford: Elsevier Science.

Edmonds, L. A. & Kiran, S. (2006). Effect of semantic naming treatment on crosslinguistic generalization in bilingual. *Journal of Speech, Language, and Hearing Research, 49,* 729–748.

Fabbro, F. (1995). *Destra e sinistra nella Bibbia: Uno studio neuropsicologico* [Right and left in the bible: A neuropsychological study]. Rimini: Guaraldi.

Fabbro, F. (1999). *The neurolinguistics of bilingualism: An introduction.* Aylesbury: Psychology Press.

Fabbro, F. (2001). The bilingual brain: bilingual aphasia. *Brain and Language, 79,* 201–210.

Fabbro, F. & Frau, G. (2001). Manifestations of aphasia in Friulian. *Journal of Neurolinguistics, 14,* 255–279.

Fabbro, F., Peru, A., & Skrap, M. (1997). Language disorders in bilingual patients after thalamic lesions. *Journal of Neurolinguistics, 10,* 347–367.

Fabbro, F., Skrap, M., & Aglioti, S. (2000). Pathological switching between languages after frontal lesions in a bilingual patient. *Journal of Neurology, Neurosurgery, and Psychiatry, 68*(5), 650–652.

Faroqi-Shah, Y., Frymark, T., Mullen, R., & Wang, B. (2010). Effect of treatment for bilingual individuals with aphasia: A systematic review of the evidence. *Journal of Neurolinguistics, 23*, 319–341.

Flores, G. (2005). The impact of medical interpreter services on the quality of health care: A systematic review. *Medical Care Research and Review, 62*(3), 255–299.

Fyndanis, V., Lind, M., Varlokosta, S., Kambanaros, M., Soroli, E., Ceder, K., Grohmann, K. K., Rofes, A., Simonsen, H. G., Bjekić, J., Gavarró, A., Kuvač Kraljević, J., Martínez-Ferreiro, S., Munarriz, A., Pourquie, M., Vuksanović, J., Zakariás, L., & Howard, D. (2017). Cross-linguistic adaptations of the Comprehensive Aphasia Test: Challenges and solutions. *Clinical Linguistics & Phonetics, 31*(7–9), 697–710.

Garcia-Albea, J. E., Sanchez-Bernardos, M. L., del Viso-Pabon, S., & Wenicke, Carlos. (1986). Test de Boston parallel enominati de la afasia: Adaptacion Espagnola. In H. Goodglass, & E. Kaplan (eds.). *La evolacion de la afasio y de transtornos relacionados* (pp. 15–58). Madrid: Editorial Medical Panamericana.

Goodglass, H., Kaplan, E., & Barresi, B. (2000). *Boston Diagnostic Aphasia Examination.* Philadelphia, PA: Lea & Febinger.

Goodglass, H., Kaplan, E., & Barresi, B. (2001). *The assessment of aphasia and related disorders.* Austin, TX: Pro-Ed.

Goral, M. (2001). Aphasia in Hebrew speakers. *Journal of Neurolinguistics, 14*, 297–312.

Goral, M. (2012). Cross-language treatment effects in multilingual aphasia. In M. R. Gitterman, M. Goral, & L. K. Obler (Eds.), *Aspects of multilingual aphasia* (pp. 106–121). Bristol, UK: Multilingual Matters.

Goral, M., Levy, E. S., & Kastl, R. (2010). Cross-language treatment enominationn: A case of trilingual aphasia. *Aphasiology, 24*, 170–187.

Goral, M., Levy, E. S., Obler, L. K., & Cohen, E. (2006). Cross-language lexical connections in the mental lexicon: Evidence from a case of trilingual aphasia. *Brain and Language, 98*, 235–247.

Grasso, S. M., Cruz, D. F., Benavidez, R., Peña, E. D., & Henry, M. L. (2019). Video-implemented script training in a bilingual Spanish-English speaker with aphasia. *Journal of Speech, Language, and Hearing Research, 62*(7), 2295–2316.

Green, D. W., & Abutalebi, J. (2008). Understanding the link between bilingual aphasia and language control. *Journal of Neurolinguistics, 21*(6), 558–576.

Grosjean, F. (1989). Neurolinguists, beware! The bilingual is not two monolingual speakers in one person. *Brain and Language, 36*, 3–15.

Harris, J. L. (2011). Multicultural and multilinguistic issues. In L. L. LaPointe (Ed.), *Aphasia and related neurogenic language disorders* (pp. 69–80). New York: Thieme.

Heaton, R. K., Chelune, G. J., Talley, J. L., Kay, G. G., & Curtiss, G. (1993). *Wisconsin Card Sorting Test manual revised and expanded.* Odessa, FL: Psychological Assessment Resources, Inc.

Helasvuo, M. L., Klippi, A., & Laakso M. (2001). Grammatical structuring in Broca's and Wernicke's aphasia in Finnish. *Journal of Neurolinguistics, 14*, 231–254.

Hernández, M., Cano, A., Costa, A., Sebastian-Galles, N., Juncadella, M., & Gascon-Bayarri, J. (2008). Grammatical category-specific deficits in bilingual aphasia. *Brain and Language, 107* (1), 68–80.

Hilger, A., Ramsberger, G., Gilley, P., Menn, L., & Kong, A. P. H. (2014). Analysing speech problems in a longitudinal case study of logopenic variant PPA. *Aphasiology, 28*(7), 840–861.

Hoffmann, C. (1991). *An introduction to bilingualism*. UK: Longman.

Ivanova, M. V. & Hallowell, B. (2013). A tutorial on aphasia test development in any language: Key substantive and psychometric considerations. *Aphasiology, 27*(8), 891–920.

Kacker, S. K., Pandit, R., & Dua, D. (1991). Reliability and validity studies of examination for aphasia test in Hindi. *Indian Journal of Disability and Rehabilitation, 5*, 13–19.

Kambanaros, M., & van Steenbrugge, W. (2004). Interpreters and language assessment: Confrontation naming and interpreting. *Advances in Speech Language Pathology, 6*(4), 247–252.

Kambanaros, M., & van Steenbrugge, W. (2006). Noun and verb processing in Greek-English bilingual individuals with anomic aphasia and the effect of instrumentality and verb-noun name relation. *Brain and Language, 97*(2), 162–177.

Kaplan, E. F., Goodglass, H., & Weintraub, S. (1986). *Test de Vocabulario de Boston*. Madrid: Panamerican.

Karliner, L. S., Jacobs, E. A., Chen, A. H., & Mutha, S. (2007). Do professional interpreters improve clinical care for patients with limited English proficiency? A systematic review of the literature. *Health Services Research, 42*(2), 727–754.

Kertesz, A. (1982). *Western Aphasia Battery*. New York, NY: Grune & Stratton.

Kertesz, A. (2006). *The Western Aphasia Battery – Revised*. San Antonio, TX: Harcourt Assessments.

Kertesz, A., & Osman-Sagi, J. (2001). Manifestations of aphasic symptoms in Hungarian. *Journal of Neurolinguistics, 14*, 312–319.

Kertesz, A., Pascual-Leone, P., & Pascual-Leone, G. (1990). *Western Aphasia Battery en enomin y adaptación castellana [Western Aphasia Battery – Spanish version]*. Valencia: Nau Libres.

Keshree, N. K., Kumar, S., Basu, S., Chakrabarty, M. & Kishore, T. (2013). Adaptation of the Western Aphasia Battery in Bangla. *Psychology of Language and Communication, 17*(2), 189–201.

Kim, H., & Na, D. L. (1997). *Korean version – Boston Naming Test*. Seoul: Hak Ji Sa.

Kim, H., & Na, D. L. (1999). Normative data on a Korean version of the Boston Naming Test. *Journal of Clinical and Experimental Neuropsychology, 21*, 127–133.

Kim, H. & Na, D. L. (2004). Normative data on the Korean version of the Western Aphasia Battery. *Journal of Clinical and Experimental Neuropsychology, 26*(8), 1011–1020.

Kiran, S., & Iakupova, R. (2011). Understanding the relationship between language proficiency, language impairment and rehabilitation: Evidence from a case study. *Clinical Linguistics and Phonetics, 25*(6–7), 565–583.

Kiran, S., Obler, L., Ansaldo, A., Goral, M., Tainturier, M. J., & Roberts, P. (2011). What do we know about impairment and recovery of language in bi-multilingual aphasia? *Procedia Social and Behavioral Sciences, 23*, 10–11.

Kolk, H., Heling, G., & Keyser, A. (1990). Arammatism in Dutch: Two case studies. In L. Menn, & L. K. Obler (Eds.). *Agrammatic aphasia: A cross-language narrative sourcebook* (pp. 179–280). Amsterdam: John Benjamins.

Kong, A. P. H. (2009). The use of main concept analysis to measure discourse production in Cantonese-speaking persons with aphasia: A preliminary report. *Journal of Communication Disorders, 42*, 442–464.

Kong, A. P. H., Abutalebi, J., Lam, K. S. Y., & Weekes, W. (2014). Executive and language control in the multilingual brain. *Behavioural Neurology, 2014*, 1– 7.

Kong, A. P. H., & Law, S. P. (2004). A Cantonese linguistic communication measure for evaluating aphasic narrative production: Normative and preliminary aphasic data. *Journal of Multilingual Communication Disorders, 2*(2), 124–146.

Kong, A. P. H., & Whiteside, J. (2014). Early recovery of a multi-lingual speaker with aphasia using Cantonese and English. *Speech, Language and Hearing, 18*(3), 133–139.

Kong, A. P. H., Whiteside, J., & Bargmann, P. (2016). The Main Concept Analysis: Validation and sensitivity in differentiating discourse produced by unimpaired English speakers from individuals with aphasia and dementia of Alzheimer type. *Logopedics Phoniatrics Vocology, 41*(3), 129–141.

Kurland, J. & Falcon, M. (2011). Effects of cognate status and language of therapy during intensive semantic naming treatment in a case of severe nonfluent bilingual aphasia. *Clinical Linguistics and Phonetics, 25*(6–7), 584–600.

Kuzmina, E., Goral, M., Norvik, M., & Weekes, B. S. (2019). What influences language impairment in bilingual aphasia? A meta-analytic review. *Frontiers in Psychology, 10*, 445.

Laine, M., Goodglass, H., Niemi, J., Koivuselka-Sallinen, P., Toumainen, J., & Martilla, R. (1993). Adaptation of the Boston diagnostic aphasia examination and the Boston naming test into Finnish. *Scandinavian Journal of Logopedics and Phoniatrics, 18*(2–3), 83–92.

Laka, I. & Korostola, L. E. (2001). Aphasia manifestations in Basque. *Journal of Neurolinguistics, 14*, 133–157.

Leheckova, H. (2001). Manifestation of aphasic symptoms in Czech. *Journal of Neurolinguistics, 14*, 179–208.

Lorenzen, B., & Murray, L. L. (2008). Bilingual aphasia: A theoretical and clinical review. *American Journal of Speech-Language Pathology, 17*, 299–317.

Månsson, A. C. & Ahlsén, E. (2001). Grammatical features of aphasia in Swedish. *Journal of Neurolinguistics, 14*, 365–380.

Mazaux, J. M. & Orgogozo, J. M. (1982). *Echelle d'évaluation de l'aphasie. Adaptation Française du Boston Diagnostic Aphasia Examination* [*Assessment of aphasia scale. French adaptation of the Boston Diagnostic Aphasia Examination*]. Paris: Editions Scientifiques et Psychologiques.

Mazumdar, B., Donovan, N. J., & Sultana, A. (2020). Comparing language samples of Bangla speakers using a colour photograph and a black-and-white line drawing. *International Journal of Language & Communication Disorders, 55*(5), 793–805.

McNeil, M. R. (1989). Review of the assessment of aphasia and related disorders. In J. C. Conoley & J. J. Kramer (Eds.), *The tenth mental measurements yearbook* (pp. 37–43). Lincoln, NE: Buros Institute of Mental Measurements.

Menn, L., Ramsberger, G., & Helm-Estabrooks, N. (1994). A linguistic communication measure for aphasic narratives. *Aphasiology, 8*(4), 343–359.

Miceli, G. & Mazzucchi, A. (1990). Crossed agrammatism in Italian: Two case studies. In L. Menn, & L. K. Obler (Eds.). *Agrammatic aphasia: A cross-language narrative sourcebook* (pp. 717–764). Amsterdam: John Benjamins.

Miertsch, B., Meisel, J. M., & Isel, F. (2009). Non-treated languages in aphasia therapy of polyglots benefit from improvement in the treated language. *Journal of Neurolinguistics, 22*(2), 135–150.

Munoz, M. L., Marquardt, T. P., & Copeland, G. (1999). A Comparison of the codeswitching patterns of aphasic and neurologically normal bilingual speakers of English and Spanish. *Brain and Language, 66*, 249–274.

Myers-Scotton, C. (1993). *Duelling languages: Grammatical structure in codeswitching.* Oxford: Clarendon Press.

Naeser, M. A. & Chan, S. W. (1980). Case study of a Chinese aphasic with the Boston Diagnostic Aphasia Exam. *Neuropsychologia, 18*, 389–410.

Nagaratnam, N. (1996). Speech recovery following global aphasia without hemiparesis. *Neurorehabilitation and Neural Repair, 10*, 115–119.

Napps, S. E. &Fowler, C. A. (1987). Formal relationships among words and the organization of the mental lexicon. *Journal of Psycholinguistic Research, 16*, 257–272.

Nespoulous, J. L., Dordain, M., Perron, C., Jarema, G., & Chazal, M. (1990). Crossed agrammatism in French: Two case studies. In L. Menn, & L. K. Obler (Eds.), *Agrammatic aphasia: A cross-language narrative sourcebook* (pp. 623–716). Amsterdam: John Benjamins.

Neves, M. B., Borsel, J. V., Pereira, M. B., & Paradela, E. M. P. (2014). Cross-cultural adaptation of the Western Aphasia Battery – Revised screening test to Brazilian Portuguese: A preliminary study. *CoDAS, 26*, 38–45.

Nilipour, R. & Raghibdoust, S. (2001). Manifestations of aphasia in Persian. *Journal of Neurolinguistics, 14*, 209–230.

Norrving, B., & Kissela, B. (2013). The global burden of stroke and need for a continuum of care. *Neurology, 80*, S5–S12.

Owens, R. E. (2014). *Language disorders: A functional approach to assessment and intervention.* Boston, MA: Allyn & Bacon.

Ozaeta, C., & Kong, A. P. H. (2012). Development of the Tagalog version of the Western Aphasia Battery-Revised: A preliminary report. *Procedia Social and Behavioral Sciences, 61*, 174–176.

Ozaeta, C., Kong, A. P. H., & Ranoa-Javier, M. B. (2013). A pilot study of using the Tagalog version of the Western Aphasia Battery-Revised in the Philippines. *Procedia Social and Behavioral Sciences, 94*, 232–233.

Packard, J. L. (1993). *A linguistic investigation of aphasic Chinese speech.* Dordrecht: Kluwer Academic Publishers.

Paradis, M. (1977). Bilingualism and aphasia. In H. Whitaker, & H. Whitaker (Eds.), *Studies in neurolinguistics* (pp. 65–121). New York: Academic Press.

Paradis, M. (1993). Bilingual aphasia rehabilitation. In M. Paradis (Ed.), *Foundations of aphasia rehabilitation* (pp. 413–419). Oxford, UK: Pergamon Press.

Paradis, M. (1995). *Aspects of bilingual aphasia.* Oxford, UK: Pergamon Press.

Paradis, M. (2001). Bilingual and polyglot aphasia. In R. S. Berndt (Ed.), *Language and aphasia* (pp. 69–91). Amsterdam: Elsevier Science.

Paradis, M. (2004). *A neurolinguistic theory of bilingualism.* Amsterdam: John Benjamins.

Paradis, M. (2008). Language and communication disorders in multilinguals. In B. Stemmer, & H. A. Whitaker (Eds.), *Handbook of the neuroscience of language* (pp. 341–350). London, UK: Academic press.

Paradis, M. (2011). Principles underlying the Bilingual Aphasia Test (BAT) and its uses. *Clinical Linguistics & Phonetics, 25*(6/7), 427–443.

Paradis, M., & Libben, G. (1987). *The assessment of bilingual aphasia.* Hillsdale, NJ: Lawrence Erlbaum Associates.

Pearce, J. (2005). A note on aphasia in bilingual patients: Pitres' and Ribot's law. *European Neurology, 54*, 127–131.

Peña-Casanova, J., Diéguez-Vide, F., Lluent, R., & Böhm, P. (2001). On manifestations of aphasia in Catalan: a case study of Broca's aphasia. *Journal of Neurolinguistics, 14*, 159–177.

Penn, C. (2012). Towards cultural aphasiology: Cultural models of service delivery in aphasia. In M. Gitterman, M. Goral, & L. K Obler (Eds.), *Aspects of multilingual aphasia* (pp. 292–306). Clevedon, UK: Multilingual Matters.

Penn, C., & Beecham, R. (1992). Discourse therapy in multilingual aphasia: A case study. *Clinical Linguistics and Phonetics, 6*, 11–25.

Pitres, A. (1895). Etudes sur l'aphasie chez les polyglottes. *Revue de medicine, 15*, 873–99.

Poncelet, M., Majerus, S., Raman, I., Warginaire, S., & Weekes, B. S. (2007). Naming actions and objects in bilingual aphasia: a multiple case study. *Brain and Language, 103*, 158–159.

Ramsberger, G., Kong, A. P. H., & Menn, L. (2014, October 5–7). Speech deterioration in an English-Shanghainese Speaker with Logopenic Variant Primary Progressive Aphasia [Poster presentation]. Fifty-second annual meeting of Academy of Aphasia, Miami, FL, USA. doi: 10.3389/conf.fpsyg.2014.64.00019

Rey, G. J., & Benton, A. L. (1992). *Examen de Afasia Multilingue.* Iowa City, IW: AJA Associates.

Ribot, T. (1883). *Les maladies de la mémoire.* Paris: Librairie Germer Balliere.

Rimikis, S., Smiljanic, R., & Calandruccio, L. (2013). Nonnative English speaker performance on the basic English lexicon (BEL) sentences. *Journal of Speech, Language, and Hearing Research, 56*, 792–804.

Ritchie, W. C., & Bhatia, T. K. (1996). *Handbook of second language acquisition.* San Diego, CA: Academic Press.

Ritchie, W. C., & Bhatia, T. K. (2005). *Handbook of bilingualism: Psycholinguistic approaches.* Oxford, UK: Oxford University Press.

Roberts, P. M., & Deslauriers, L. (1999). Picture naming of cognate and non-cognate nouns in bilingual aphasia. *Journal of Communication Disorders, 32*, 1–23.

Roberts, P. M. & Doucet, N. (2011). Performance on French-speaking Quebec adults on the Boston Naming Test. *Canadian Journal of Speech-Language Pathology and Audiology, 35*, 254–267.

Roberts, P. M., Garcia, L. J., Desrochers, A., & Hernandez, D. (2002). English performance of proficient bilingual adults on the Boston Naming Test. *Aphasiology, 16*, 635–645.

Roger, P., & Code, C. (2011). Lost in translation? Issues of content validity in interpreter-mediated aphasia assessments. *International Journal of Speech and Language Pathology, 13*(1), 61–73.

Sasanuma, S., Kamio, A., & Kubota, M. (1990). Crossed agrammatism in Japanese: A case study. In L. Menn, & L. K. Obler (Eds.). *Agrammatic aphasia: A cross-language narrative sourcebook* (pp. 1309–1356). Amsterdam: John Benjamins.

Smania, N., Gandolfi, M., Aglioti, S.M., Girardi, P., Fiaschi, A., & Girardi, F. (2010). How long is the recovery of global aphasia? Twenty-five years of follow-up in a patient with left hemisphere stroke. *Neurorehabilitation and Neural Repair, 24*, 871–875.

Spreen, O. & Risser, A. H. (2003). *Assessment of aphasia*. New York, NY: Oxford University Press.

Stark, J. A., & Dressler, W. U. (1990). Arammatism in German: Two case studies. In L. Menn, & L. K. Obler (Eds.), *Agrammatic aphasia: A cross-language narrative sourcebook*. Amsterdam: John Benjamins.

Sugishita, M. (1986). *Japanese edition of Western Aphasia Battery*. Tokyo: Igaku-Shoin.

Sung, J. E., DeDe, G., & Lee, S. E. (2016). Cross-linguistic differences in a picture-description task between Korean- and English-speaking individuals with aphasia. *American Journal of Speech-Language Pathology, 25*(4S), S813–S822.

Swinburn, K., Porter, G., & Howard, D. (2004). *Comprehensive Aphasia Test*. Hove, UK: Psychology Press.

Swinburn, K., Porter, G., & Howard, D. (2014). *Comprehensive Aphasia Test* (L. Haaber Hansen & M. Kaae Frederiksen, adaptation). Copenhagen, Denmark: Dansk Psykologisk Forlag. (Originally published 2005).

Thuillard-Colombo, F. & Assal, G. (1992). Adaptation française du test de enomination de Boston: Versions abrégées [French adaptation of the Boston naming test: Abbreviated Versions]. *Revue Européene de Psychologie Appliquée, 42*, 67–71.

Tsang, H. L. (2000). Confrontation naming abilities of the young, the elderly, and people with aphasia [Unpublished thesis]. University of Hong Kong, Hong Kong, China.

Tsapkini, K., Jarema, G., & Kehayia, E. (2001). Manifestations of morphological impairments in Greek aphasia: A case study. *Journal of Neurolinguistics, 14*, 281–296.

Tseng, O. J. L. (1993). *A Chinese version of the Boston Diagnostic Aphasia Examination* [Unpublished manuscript].

Ulatowska, H. K., Sadowska, M., & Kądzielawa, D. (2001). A longitudinal study of agrammatism in Polish: A case study. *Journal of Neurolinguistics, 14*, 321–336.

U.S. Bureau of the Census. (2010). Language use in the United States: 2007. American Community Survey Reports. Retrieved from www.census.gov/library/publications/2010/acs/acs-12.html

U.S. Bureau of the Census. (2013). Language use in the United States: 2011. American Community Survey Reports. Retrieved from www.census.gov/library/publications/2013/acs/acs-22.html

Van Dijk, T. A. (1985). *Handbook of discourse analysis: Dimensions of discourse*. London: Academic Press.

Visch-Brink, E., Vandenborre, D., de Smet, H. J., & Mariën, P. (2014). *Comprehensive Aphasia Test – Nederlandse bewerking – Handleiding*. Amsterdam: Pearson.

Weekes, B. S. (2010). Issues in bilingual aphasia: An introduction. *Aphasiology, 24*, 123–25.

Weekes, B. S., & Raman, I. (2008). Bilingual deep dysphasia. *Cognitive Neuropsychology, 25*(3), 411–436.

Whitworth, A., Perkins, L., & Lesser, R. (1997). *Conversation analysis profile for people with aphasia*. London: Whurr.

World Health Organization. (2011). *World report on disability*. Available from www.who.int/disabilities/world_report/2011/report.pdf

Yiu, E. M. L. (1992). Linguistic assessment of Chinese-speaking aphasics: Development of a Cantonese aphasia battery. *Journal of Neurolinguistics, 7*, 379–424.

Yiu, E. M. L., & Worrall, L. E. (1996). Patterns of grammatical disruption in Cantonese aphasic subjects. *Asia Pacific Journal of Speech, Language and Hearing, 1*, 105–126.

Zakariás, L., & Lukács, Á. (2021). The Comprehensive Aphasia Test–Hungarian: Adaptation and psychometric properties. *Aphasiology*. Epub ahead. https://doi.org/10.1080/02687038.2021.1937921

Zea, M. C., Asner-Self, K. K., Birman, D., & Buki, L. P. (2003). The Abbreviated Multidimentional Acculturation Scale: Empirical validation with two Latino/Latina samples. *Cultural Diversity & Ethnic Minority Psychology, 9*, 107–126.

Appendix 8.1

Bilingual Adult Intake Form of Linguistic Background and History

2) General information:

Name: _____ I.D. #: _____   Date of interview: _____
Address: _____
Home/cell phone: _____   E-mail address: _____
Marital Status: _____ Age: _____   Date of birth: _____
Education level: _____ Gender: _____   Handedness: _____

2. What is your current living arrangement?
    Alone ____   With family ____
    With significant other ____   With friends ____

2. Do you work currently? Yes or No
    • If yes, what do you do? _____

3. Are you retired? Yes or No
    • If yes, when did you last work? _____
    • If yes, what did you do? _____

4. What is your native country? _____

5. What was your year of arrival in the USA? _____

6. What was your age of arrival? _____

B) Leisure time activities:

1. How frequently are you engaged in the following social activities?

Activity	Frequently	Occasionally	Seldom	Never
Listening to music				
Watching movies/television				
Attending recreation events, such as concerts, plays, or dramas				
Attending social events, such as parties, friends or family gatherings				

Activity	Frequently	Occasionally	Seldom	Never
Talking on phone to family members and/or friends				
Visiting/Traveling with family members and/or friends				
Caring for grandchildren				
Attending a place of worship				
Participating in senior centers				
Volunteering				
Participating in a choir				

2.   How frequently are you engaged in the following physical activities?

Activity	Frequently	Occasionally	Seldom	Never
Walking				
Jogging				
Running				
Cycling				
Individual sports, such as table tennis or badminton				
Team sports, such as soccer, basketball, or baseball				
Swimming				
Dancing				
Tai Chi				
Yoga				
Gym, recreation class, or sports club				

3.   How frequently are you engaged in the following cognitive activities?

Activity	Frequently	Occasionally	Seldom	Never
Reading (books, newspapers, magazines)				
Crossword puzzles				
Sudoko				
Board games				

Activity	Frequently	Occasionally	Seldom	Never
Computer games (on desktop, laptop, tablets or mobile devices)				
Taking a class				
Driving				

C) Language information on history, experience, and use:

1.   a)   What is your native language (or dialect)? _____
     b)   At what age did you acquire this language (or dialect)? _____

2.   a)   What is your secondary language (or dialect)? _____
     b)   At what age did you acquire this language (or dialect)? _____

3.   Do you speak any other languages (or dialects)? Yes or No
     •   If yes, what are they? _____
     •   At what age did you acquire these languages (or dialects)? _____
     _____

4.   What is your educational history?

Highest level achieved	In what country?	In what language (or dialects)?
Illiterate ____		
Elementary school ____		
Middle school ____		
High school ____		
College ____		
Post college ____		

5. How would you estimate the amount of language (or dialect) use in your daily routines?

Modality	Language (Dialect)	Estimated percentage
Listening		
Speaking		
Reading		
Writing		

6. Have you ever worked in your native country? Yes or No

Job title/Duties	Company and location	Dates	Language (or dialect) spoken
		From to	
		From to	
		From to	
		From to	
		From to	
		From to	

2. Have you ever worked in the United States? Yes or No

Job title/Duties	Company and location	Dates	Language (or dialect) spoken
		From to	
		From to	
		From to	
		From to	

Job title/Duties	Company and location	Dates		Language (or dialect) spoken
		From	to	
		From	to	

2.   How would you estimate the amount of language (or dialect) use in each situation?

Activity	Percentage in native language (or dialect)	Percentage in secondary language (or dialect)	Percentage in other languages (or dialects)
Talking to spouse			
Talking to children			
Talking to immediate family members			
Talking to friends			
Talking to co-workers or colleagues			
Caring for grandchildren			
Watching television			
Reading newspapers			
Listening to radio			
Grocery shopping			
Banking			
Other important and/ or personally relevant communication contexts (please specify: _____)			

Appendix 8.2

Modified Conversation Analysis Profile for People with Aphasia (CAPPA) Indices for Bilingual or Multilingual Speakers

Area addressed:	Clinical Implications
SECTION ONE: LINGUISTIC ABILITIES	
Failure in word retrieval in native language (LI)*	To inform the degree of struggle and give up during word finding using native language
Failure in word retrieval in non-native language*	To inform the degree of struggle and give up during word finding using non-native language
Production of circumlocutions	
Production of uncorrected semantic paraphasias in LI*	To inform the degree of using wrong words without correcting in native language
Production of uncorrected semantic paraphasias in non-native language *	To inform the degree of using wrong words without correcting in non-native language
Production of phonemic paraphasias in LI*	To inform the degree of phonemic errors for a target in native language
Production of phonemic paraphasias in non-native language*	To inform the degree of phonemic errors for a target in non-native language
Production of apraxic errors in LI*	To inform the degree of struggle to get the sounds out in a word of the native language
Production of apraxic errors in non-native language*	To inform the degree of struggle to get the sounds out in a word of the non-native language
Overuse of pronouns	
Difficulty indicating yes and no reliably	
Production of agrammatic speech	
Production of neologisms	
Production of jargon	
Failure in comprehension	
(Repetition of words)	To inform the degree of repeated propositions in output

Area addressed:	Clinical Implications
SECTION TWO: REPAIR	
Ability to initiate repair on conversational partner's turn in LI*	To determine the ability to indicate difficulty in following a conversation using native language
Ability to initiate repair on conversational partner's turn in non-native language*	To determine the ability to indicate difficulty in following a conversation using non-native language
Ability to initiate repairs on own errors	
Ability after self initiation to repair own errors without help	
Ability to repair own turn when initiated by conversational partner	
Ability to repair own pathological code switching*	To determine the degree of self-awareness of own errors and ability to correct them
SECTION THREE: INITIATION AND TURN TAKING	
Ability to initiate conversations in LI*	To determine the appropriateness of pragmatics using native language
Ability to initiate conversations in non-native language*	To determine the appropriateness of pragmatics using non-native language
Delay in responding when selected as next speaker	
Production of long pauses in the middle of turns	
Violation of conversational partner's turns	
SECTION FOUR: TOPIC MANAGEMENT	
Ability to initiate new topics in LI*	To inform the ability to provide new information with appropriate timing of conversation using native language
Ability to initiate new topics in non-native language*	To inform the ability to provide new information with appropriate timing of conversation using non-native language
Failure to orient conversational partner to new topics	
Ability to maintain topics in LI*	To determine the ability to stay on a topic using native language
Ability to maintain topics in non-native language*	To determine the ability to stay on a topic using non-native language

Area addressed:	Clinical Implications
Repeated initiations of "favorite" topics in L1*	To determine the ability to initiate and provide self-related information using native language
Repeated initiations of "favorite" topics in non-native language*	To determine the ability to initiate and provide self-related information using non-native language
(Off-topics) in L1*	To determine the degree of irrelevant content when using native language
(Off-topics) in non-native language*	To determine the degree of irrelevant content when using non-native language
(Code-switching patterns)	
(Use of non-native words within a L1 utterance)	To determine the degree of code switching
(Use of non-native words, with self-repair to L1, in a L1 utterance)	To determine the degree of self-awareness of switching behaviors
(Presence of inappropriate combination of foreign words)	To determine the degree of pathological code mixing

Note: Indices in parenthesis are additional indices reported in Dai et al. (2012), indices with an asterisk are suggested new indices modified from Dai et al. (2012) and Whitworth et al. (1997) for specific use in the bilingual or multilingual population.

Source: Adapted from: Dai et al. (2012); Whitworth et al. (1997)

Appendix 8.3

Additional Resources for Management of Acquired Communication Disorders in the Multicultural and/or International Populations

Professional organizations in the U.S.:

- Academy of Aphasia: www2.academyofaphasia.org/
- Academy of Neurologic Communication Disorders and Sciences (ANCDS): www.ancds.org/
- Alzheimer's Association: www.alz.org/
- American Speech-Language-Hearing Association (ASHA): www.asha.org/
- Brain Injury Association of America (BIAA): www.biausa.org/
- National Aphasia Association (NAA): www.aphasia.org/
- The National Institute on Deafness and Other Communication Disorders (NIDCD): www.nidcd.nih.gov/

Professional organizations with an international perspective:

- Alzheimer's Disease International (ADI): www.alzint.org/
- Aphasia United: www.aphasiaunited.org/
- International Association of Logopedics and Phoniatrics: https://ialpasoc.info/
- Asian Indian Caucus (AIC): www.sites.google.com/site/asianindiancaucusasha1/
- Asian Pacific Islander Speech-Language-Hearing Caucus (APISLH Caucus): www.apislhc.com/
- Haitian Caucus: www.hcasha.org/
- Hispanic Caucus: http://ashahc.org/
- International Brain Injury Association: www.internationalbrain.org/
- National Black Association for Speech-Language and Hearing (NBASLH): www.nbaslh.org/
- Native American Caucus: https://sites.google.com/view/nacslpa-org/home
- The International Clinical Phonetics and Linguistics Association (ICPLA): www.icpla.info/

Relevant publications:

American Speech-Language-Hearing Association. (2010). Cultural competence checklist: Personal reflection. Available from www.asha.org/siteassets/uploadedFiles/Cultural-Competence-Checklist-Personal-Reflection.pdf

American Speech-Language-Hearing Association. (2010). Cultural competence checklist: Service delivery. Available from www.asha.org/siteassets/uploadedFiles/Cultural-Competence-Checklist-Service-Delivery.pdf

American Speech-Language-Hearing Association. (2014). Cultural competence. Available from www.asha.org/Practice-Portal/Professional-Issues/Cultural-Competence/

American Speech-Language-Hearing Association. (2017). Issues in ethics: Cultural and linguistic competence. Available from www.asha.org/practice/ethics/cultural-and-linguistic-competence/

American Speech-Language-Hearing Association. (2020). Multicultural affairs and resources. Available from www.asha.org/practice/multicultural/

American Speech-Language-Hearing Association. (2021). Cultural competence check-in: Culturally responsive practice. Available from www.asha.org/siteassets/uploadedfiles/multicultural/culturally-responsive-practice-checklist.pdf

American Speech-Language-Hearing Association. (2021). Cultural competence check-in: Policies and procedures. Available from www.asha.org/siteassets/uploadedfiles/multicultural/policies-and-procedures-checklist.pdf

American Speech-Language-Hearing Association. (2021). Cultural competence check-in: Self-reflection. Available from www.asha.org/siteassets/uploadedfiles/multicultural/self-reflection-checklist.pdf

Holland, A. L. & Forbes, M. M. (1993). Aphasia treatment: World perspectives. San Diego, CA: Singular Pub. Group.

Qualls, C. D. (2012). Neurogenic disorders of speech, language, cognition-communication, and swallowing. In D. E. Battle, (Ed.), Communication disorders in multicultural and international populations (pp. 148–163). St. Louis, MO: Mosby.

The Institute of Medicine. (2011). Cognitive rehabilitation therapy for traumatic brain injury: Evaluating the evidence. Washington, DC: The National Academies Press. https://doi.org/10.17226/13220

World Health Organization. (2011). World report on disability. Available from www.who.int/disabilities/world_report/2011/report.pdf

Chapter 9

Further Directions of Clinical Discourse Analysis

Discourse Analysis: The Story So Far?

There is a long history of discourse analysis but its application in the field of communication sciences or related language disorders is relatively less established. Schiffrin et al. (2001) provides a good overview of how different linguistic theories are demonstrated by conducting careful discourse analyses in native unimpaired speakers of a language. Specifically, whether and how oral and written discourse varied across language contexts, such as in the field of anthropology, communication, computer sciences, education, law, media (radio and television broadcasting and publishing), medicines, politics, psychology, and social sciences, were systematically discussed. Generally speaking, one major problem is that discipline-specific information on discourse analysis tends to have limited generalization to the clinical population, i.e., speakers with language deficits specific to different types of brain damages and/or neurological conditions. One of the very few textbooks that addresses clinical utility of discourse analysis in different adult clinical populations was presented by Bloom et al. (1994). Theoretical issues on different models of discourse production were examined and the relationships between discourse production and linguistic, cognitive, as well as social deficits across various clinical populations were summarized.

One major reason for the lack of regular use of discourse analyses among speech-and-language pathologists is that the relevant content behind their theories and clinical significance are often not covered extensively in the academic curriculum and clinical practicum. The relatively restricted amount of research done in this area, compared to other aspects of communication disorders, as well as the lack of appropriate and readily-useable teaching materials, further hindered its development in the field of speech pathology. With the coverage of content about neurogenic discourse production in this textbook, it is hoped that readers will be presented with a more thorough discussion of various relevant topics, which hopefully will

DOI: 10.4324/9781003254775-9

lead to better understanding of the nature, assessment, and remediation of discourse deficits in aphasia and related disorders.

There are several specific goals in writing this text. They include the aims (1) to provide a systematic summary of existing assessment options of oral discourse for the purpose of clinical evaluation and research studies; (2) to review various elicitation methods of discourse samples and to promote the use of multi-level, multi-modal, and multi-faceted analyses of oral narratives; (3) to equip students in the field of communication sciences and disorders, linguistics, neuro-linguistics, psychology, and related disciplines with fundamental and relevant knowledge about impaired discourse with different etiologies; and (4) to provide clinical practitioners with a refreshment of acquired knowledge on discourse production, an update about contemporary issues of discourse annotations and analyses, and some important insights in applying evidence-based practice in the management of acquired neurogenic communication disorders. Attempting to bridge the gap between research on neurogenic disordered discourse and the clinical assessment and intervention of patients with this condition, it is crucial to highlight that much more work is still needed to further extend our knowledge about the mechanism of oral impairment at the discourse level.

Extension of Current Work on Discourse Analysis

In this concluding chapter, I consider the future of researching and clinically applying discourse analyses. Many of the following areas have not been systematically examined, partly because they were neglected in the past and also partly because insufficient knowledge has been gained to motivate their studying (and hence their advancement) in the literature. Hence, the discussion provided here will provide a glimpse of where these individual topics may be headed. Specifically, two relevant questions are considered for each of the major issues warranting future investigations:

1. What has been examined and reported in the literature so far?
2. What future development can benefit our understanding of discourse analysis?

In other words, apart from highlighting issues around disordered discourse production that are most likely to be addressed in the near future, readers will gain a "heads-up" to follow the upcoming development of these topic areas. Consequently, it is believed that individuals with acquired deficits of discourse production will benefit from future research that indicates the importance of evidence-based and accurate evaluations as well as the most appropriate and suitable therapeutic options.

Neural Correlates of Verbal and Non-Verbal Discourse

Compared to our current understanding of neural correlates of human language development and its impairment in children (e.g., Friederici, 2006), phonological processing in adult individuals (Hickok, 2009), or naming (e.g., Gorno-Tempini & Price, 2001; Grabowski et al., 2000; Vigliocco et al., 2011) and sentence processing in adult speakers (e.g., Keller et al., 2001; Peelle et al., 2010), very little is known about the neural basis of oral discourse production. A multitude of lesion and neuroimaging studies of word and sentence production of unimpaired individuals and speakers with aphasia are available (see Caplan, 2009; Cato et al., 2001; Damasio et al,, 2004; Dogil et al., 2002), but a comparable number of reports on discourse deficits is still currently lacking.

Given that discourse production always involves complex organization and expression of events and relevant propositions, understanding how the process is mediated by various brain regions is not straightforward. The neural systems associated with different linguistic characteristics of connected speech are also complicated. However, reports identifying relationships between brain regions and discourse production only began to emerge about two decades ago. For example:

- Borovsky et al. (2007) were among the first who analyzed conversation production of speakers with aphasia using the mean length of utterance (MLU), Type-Token Ratio (TTR), and overall tokens taking the approach of voxel-based lesion-symptom mapping (VLSM; Bates et al., 2003). It was found that damage to the anterior insula, inferior frontal gyrus, sensorimotor, and anterior temporal areas was associated with poor performance of MLU and tokens, while lesions to posterior temporal regions were linked to reduced TTR.
- Working with individuals with primary progressive aphasia, Wilson et al. (2010) analyzed speech samples elicited from a picture description task in terms of speech rate, fluency disruption, lexical content, and syntactic structure and complexity, following the framework of Quantitative Production Analysis (QPA; Saffran et al. 1989) (see Chapter 4 for more details). The results of a voxel-based morphometry analysis showed that atrophy in the frontal regions was associated with deterioration in syntactic processes. The anterior and inferior temporal regions were also found to be related to lexical retrieval, and the posterior temporal regions were found to link to phonological errors and fluency disruptions. Interestingly, it was also suggested that lesions in any part of the above-mentioned regions were associated with reduced speech rate.

A potential limitation of the above two studies is their focus on analyses at the word and sentence levels, leaving linguistic devices that reflect the cohesion and coherence of speech (i.e., macro-structural level analyses) largely unattended. Troiani et al. (2008) have reported the employment of functional magnetic resonance imaging (fMRI) to monitor brain activities during narrative production of a story-telling task among 15 healthy, young English-speaking adults. It was found that activations in the area of bilateral prefrontal and left temporal-parietal regions were significantly related to the participants' performance in the description task. Further conclusion about the role of the inferior frontal cortex plays in narrative production was also given.

Since the first edition of this book was released, a growing number of structural (e.g., Schumacher et al., 2020; Wilmskoetter et al., 2019) as well as functional neuroimaging studies have addressed issues around a neural basis of discourse, prompting a revision that updates this literature. For example, Alyahya et al. (2020) in a recent VLSM study examined a wider range of discourse genres (including a simple description of the BDAE "Cookie Theft" picture, and two naturalistic forms of connected speech: a "Dinner Story" telling narrative using an eight-panel sequential picture set and an unsupported procedural discourse of preparing a cup of tea) in 46 speakers with aphasia (25 fluent + 21 non-fluent) and 20 neurotypical older adults. The results suggested a more widespread involvement of cortical regions and their white matter connections in these discourse tasks. Specifically, there was evidence that the quantity and quality of fluent connected speech production was engaged by our left frontal regions and the underlying white matter tracts corresponding to the frontal aslant tract and the anterior segment of the arcuate fasciculus. Alyahya et al. (2020) also highlighted the roles cognitive functions play in spoken discourse, by discussing the association between executive functions involved in discourse production and the left frontal regions, as well as the association between verbal quality and widespread frontal region involvement related to higher cognitive functions of working memory, monitoring, attention, and executive semantic control. In another study, Ding et al. (2020) examined if and how impaired content production in spoken discourse and its related structural deficits were related to different patterns of focal brain damage. It was the first reported investigation that focused on the acute stage of left hemisphere stroke and the relationship between brain damage and impaired content and structure of spontaneous connected speech. Results of a multivariate lesion behavior mapping, based on 52 acute stroke patients, revealed that damage to the left temporal-parietal regions had the most impact on the patients' ability to retrieve words and their subsequent production within increasingly complex combinations. In addition, patients' production of syntactically accurate structures in spoken discourse was found to deteriorate by damage to the inferior frontal cortex. Readers interested in this topic may refer to the following related studies, including den Ouden et al., 2019; Schumacher et al., 2019, or a recent review article by Wilson and Hula (2019) for additional details. Note that Crosson et al. (2019) have also reviewed and discussed a series of publications around neuroplasticity and aphasia treatments, with a focus on how contemporary aphasia treatments have allowed the recruitment of both residual and new neural mechanisms to improve language functions (some of which are fundamental skills to discourse production) and how neuroimaging techniques would hold promise in predicting treatment outcomes.

Also worth mentioning is the investigations of functional and anatomical correlates in discourse-level sign language. For example, Inubushi and Sakai (2013) performed analyses of cortical activity of deaf signers during discourse-level decision tasks using MRI and voxel-based morphometry. It was found that a larger region in the frontal language areas was activated for discourse-level, compared to word- and sentence-level, processing. Braun et al. (2001) also compared brain regions essential for the production of discourse in generating autobiographical narratives, using PET, in spoken English and in American Sign Language (ASL) by hearing individuals who were native users of both languages. Common activations detected in the brain for both languages included left hemisphere language areas as well as the left and right extrasylvian. The posterior perisylvian and basal temporal regions were also found to serve the process of self-generated formulation and language production.

Of the few studies in the current imaging literature that examined a neural basis of discourse production, evidence suggested so far has been inconclusive. It is hoped that further studies will address not only the anatomical correlates of post-sentential level verbal production, but will also focus as well on the functional, behavioural, and neural integrations between frontal language areas and other corresponding regions mediating oral narratives. By doing so, clinical practitioners such as speech-and-language pathologists will be empowered to make more accurate predictions about outcomes of language abilities at the discourse level with reference to individual patients' neurological profiles.

Assessment and Treatment Challenges for Individuals With Disabilities of Under-Represented Racial or Ethnic Groups

According to the National Institutes of Health (2011), the definition of individuals with disabilities is "those with a physical or mental impairment that substantially limits one or more major life activities". The following racial and ethnic groups, including African Americans, Hispanic Americans, Native Americans/Alaska Natives who maintain tribal affiliation or community attachment, Hawaiian Natives, and natives of the U.S. Pacific Islands, have been recognized to be under-represented in biomedical research. However, overseas immigrants in the nation are currently not included in the list. Due to globalization of the world and a higher public awareness of communication disorders, it is expected that clinicians in the U.S. will encounter more scenarios where they have to manage a clientele containing a wider spectrum of individuals with different cultural and linguistic backgrounds. More evidence on discourse assessment and management is needed to support clinicians' daily practice.

For example, Ulatowska et al. (2000) examined the features of repetition in narratives of African Americans as a tool to emphasize thematic contents of oral discourse or as cohesive ties within and among superstructural elements of the discourse. How the use of repeated (or duplicated) oral content could be altered and constrained by aphasia was also discussed. It was found that presence of aphasia did not limit the thematic functions served by repetitions among African Americans, but their ability to flexibly vary the semantic content and syntactic structure of the repetitions was affected. According to the authors, this study was culturally specific and clinically relevant to African Americans because this ethnic group makes extensive use of repetitions in their spoken language. One can easily realize that comparable research investigations addressing specific language characteristics of other under-represented ethnic groups are currently limited.

In addition, as illustrated in Chapter 8, clinical professionals working with the English-speaking clinical population are privileged to have a wide variety of clinical resources and evidence to manage discourse deficits. Such a rich amount of conducted research, relevant knowledge and evidence, as well as clinically useful materials are, in contrast, not available to clinicians with a multilingual clientele. To meet the growing needs of speech-and-language pathologists, bilingual therapists, and related practitioners in the U.S. and worldwide, more theoretical and clinical research about narrative-level performance in the multilingual population is needed. More channels are also needed to disseminate findings and resources from these studies to clinicians as well as to share related professional information with the general public.

Application of Existing Linguistic Models and/or Frameworks to Disordered Discourse

A linguistic model largely refers to the pattern(s) of using structural linguistics to describe the various aspects of a language, such as the phonology, semantics, morphology, syntax, and to accurately define linguistic concepts and their relationships. Many linguistic models or frameworks have been proposed by linguists for measuring and describing various aspects of the organizations of natural oral or written text. Most of them were developed based on typical speakers of a language who have no impairment in language skills. Reports of applying these linguistic models to the clinical populations are sparse.

For example, because previous investigations of discourse coherence in aphasia have mainly been conducted using a approach of qualitative assessment, the existing body of work on this subject has provided mixed results, leaving the question of whether coherence in brain-damaged speakers is impaired or intact unanswered. Kong et al. (2014) have reported the use of the Rhetorical Structure Theory (RST; Mann & Thompson, 1988; Taboada & Mann 2006) to differentiate the coherence in discourse, elicited by tasks of story-telling and sequential description, between healthy speakers and those with anomic aphasia. Given that coherent discourse contains a hierarchical, rather than linear, internal structure (Fox, 1987; Grosz & Sidner, 1986; Hobbs, 1985), the RST offers a linguistically useful method to characterize the structure of a text based on the relations that hold between parts of the oral output. According to Mann and Thompson (1988), discourse consists of elementary discourse units (EDUs) that can be defined as minimal building blocks of a discourse structure (which roughly correspond to clauses). These basic segments are connected to each other with semantic, or rhetorical, relations (such as "Consequence," "Cause," "Evaluation," or "Elaboration") forming a complete tree-like structure. The coherence of discourse is then established through the construction of discourse structures. Kong et al. found that speakers with anomic aphasia demonstrated significantly lower production fluency, fewer EDUs, smaller relation sets, and more errors (semantic, phonemic paraphasia, morphological errors, and neologisms) than their non-brain-damaged counterparts. Analysis of semantic relations employed suggested that controls used a richer set of relations, particularly those for describing settings, expressing causality, and providing elaborations. The aphasic discourse also tended to contain more reformulations, corrections, false starts, and retracing as well as a higher degree of omitting essential informational content. In addition, the aphasic output was rated by naïve listeners with a significantly lower degree of coherence and clarity than controls. It was further concluded that the use of RST to quantify discourse coherence allowed a more objective measurement on the macro-linguistic characteristics in aphasia. Specifically, as a result of the higher degree of simplified or structural disruptions but reduced proportion of information content and elaboration, speakers with anomic aphasia are poorer in their coherence in oral discourse.

The application of RST in disordered language was novel and offered an alternative approach to measuring oral discourse. It is reasonable to say that no one linguistic model or framework can fully explain how we use language. Consideration of one or more models of discourse production in relation to discourse deficits can provide us with different perspectives to examine how impaired narrative skills vary as a function of factors such as behavioral, cognitive, and social problems. More applicational investigations are, therefore, warranted in the future.

Application of Technology in Treating Discourse Production

The advancement of technology justifies the need to highlight not only the growing interest to investigate technology-based (e.g., Milman et al., 2020; Uslu et al., 2020) or simulated (Pilnick et al., 2018) discourse intervention among researchers, but also its clinical implementation among practitioners. Additional investigations to inform how technology can supplement traditional behavioral trainings and potentially improve clients' and caregivers' engagement in the rehabilitation process (inside as well as outside therapy rooms) will be of great importance.

The severe acute respiratory syndrome coronavirus 2 (SARS-CoV-2), or COVID-19, pandemic has caused unprecedented challenges to people with disabilities and there are still significant knowledge gaps regarding various short- and long-term clinical impacts (Kong, 2021a, 2021b). Amid this global pandemic, eHealth has become the most practical tool for healthcare service delivery. One obvious change was the transition from in-person to remote assessment and intervention. While further development and refinement of this existing mobile/online management is needed, Kong (2021c) has also summarized and proposed some potential opportunities to reap the eHealth benefits (such as timely remote interactions) and directions that warrant examinations to improve care of aphasia and discourse-related problems.

Concluding Remarks

The preceding overview in this chapter aims to provide a brief snapshot of some representative research on neglected topics of disordered discourse that has been reported so far. Clearly, inconsistencies and limited evidence that is conclusive are two critical drawbacks and concerns. What remains to be done is to expand the scope of relevant research to advance our understanding of problematic discourse production caused by acquired communication disorders. Until now, the majority of research on neurogenic disordered discourse production has been focused on monolingual English speakers with stroke-induced aphasia. There is room for a great deal of work to be done on discourse deficits associated with other etiologies or with other languages. The increased emphasis on discourse analyses in research concerning evaluation and remediation of narrative-level impairments in relation to linguistic and cognitive deficits is encouraging. Emergence of future studies would probably facilitate researchers and clinicians to think in new ways about manifestation of discourse symptoms as well as their management options. More importantly, results of these research investigations will have a significant impact on clinical practice in the foreseeable future.

Acknowledgement

Part of the research results presented in this chapter was supported by a grant from the National Institute of Health (NIH) "Toward a multi-modal and multi-level analysis of Chinese aphasic discourse" (R01DC010398) to the author.

References

Alyahya, R., Halai, A. D., Conroy, P., & Lambon Ralph, M. A. (2020). A unified model of post-stroke language deficits including discourse production and their neural correlates. *Brain, 143*(5), 1541–1554.

Bates, E., D'Amico, S., Jacobsen, T., Székely, A., Andonova, E., Devescovi, A., Herron, D., Lu. C. C., Pechmann, T., Pléh, C., Wicha, N., Ferdermeier, K., Gerdjikova, I., Gutierrez, G., Hung, D., Hse, J., Iyer, G., Kohnert, K., Mehotcheva, T., … Tzeng, O. (2003). Timed picture naming in seven languages. *Psychonomic Bulletin & Review*, 10(2), 344–380.

Bloom, R. L., Obler, L. K., de Santi S., & Ehrlich J. S. (1994). *Discourse analysis and applications: Studies in adult clinical populations*. Hillsdale, NJ: Lawrence Erlbaum Associates, Inc.

Borovsky, A., Saygin, A. P., Bates, E., & Dronkers, N. (2007). Lesion correlates of conversational speech production deficits. *Neuropsychologia, 45*, 2525–2533.

Braun, A. R., Guillemin, A., Hosey, L. & Varga, M. (2001). The neural organization of discourse: An H₂ ¹⁵O-PET study of narrative production in English and American Sign Language. *Brain, 124*, 2028–2044.

Caplan, D. (2009). *The neural basis of syntactic processing*. In M. S. Gazzaniga (Ed.), *The cognitive neurosciences* (4th ed.) (pp. 805–817). Cambridge, MA: MIT Press.

Cato, M. A., Moore, A. B., Crosson, B. (2001). Elucidation of semantic organization in the brain using functional neuoimaging: A review. *Topics in Language Disorders, 21*, 60–74.

Crosson, B., Rodriguez, A. D., Copland, D., Fridriksson, J., Krishnamurthy, L. C., Meinzer, M., Raymer, A. M., Krishnamurthy, V., & Leff, A. P. (2019). Neuroplasticity and aphasia treatments: new approaches for an old problem. *Journal of Neurology, Neurosurgery, and Psychiatry, 90*(10), 1147–1155.

Damasio, H., Tranel, D., Grabowski, T., Adolphs, R., & Damasio, A. (2004). Neural systems behind word and concept retrieval. *Cognition, 92*, 179–229.

Den Ouden, D. B., Malyutina, S., Basilakos, A., Bonilha, L., Gleichgerrcht, E., Yourganov, G., Hillis, A. E., Hickok, G., Rorden, C., & Fridriksson, J. (2019). Cortical and structural-connectivity damage correlated with impaired syntactic processing in aphasia. *Human Brain Mapping, 40*(7), 2153–2173.

Ding, J., Martin, R. C., Hamilton, A. C., & Schnur, T. T. (2020). Dissociation between frontal and temporal-parietal contributions to connected speech in acute stroke. *Brain, 143*(3), 862–876.

Dogil, G., Ackermann, H., Grodd, W., Haider, H., Kamp, H., Mayer, J., Riecker, A., & Wildgruber, D. (2002). The speaking brain: A tutorial introduction to fMRI experiments in the production of speech, prosody and syntax. *Journal of Neurolinguistics, 15*, 59–90.

Fox, B. (1987) *Discourse structure and anaphora.* Cambridge: Cambridge University Press.

Friederici, A. D. (2006). The neural basis of language development and its impairment. *Neuron, 52*(6), 941–952.

Gorno-Tempini, M. L. & Price, C. J. (2001). Identification of famous faces and buildings: A functional neuroimaging study of semantically unique items. *Brain, 124,* 2087–2209.

Grabowski, T. J., Damasio, H., & Tranel, D. (2000). Retrieving names of unique entities engages the left temporal pole. *Neuroimage, 11,* S262.

Grosz, B. J., & Sidner, C. L. (1986) Attention, intentions, and the structure of discourse. *Computational Linguistics, 12*(3), 175–204.

Hickok, G. (2009). The cortical organization of phonological processing. In M. S. Gazzaniga (Ed.), *The cognitive neurosciences* (pp. 767–776). Cambridge, MA: MIT Press.

Hobbs, J. (1985). *On the coherence and structure of discourse.* Retrieved from www.isi.edu/~hobbs/ocsd.pdf

Inubushi, T. & Sakai, K. L. (2013). Functional and anatomical correlates of word-, sentence-, and discourse-level integration in sign language. *Frontiers in Human Neuroscience, 7,* 681.

Keller, T. A., Carpenter, P. A., & Just, M. A. (2001). The neural bases of sentence comprehension: A fMRI examination of syntactic and lexical processing. *Cerebral Cortex, 11*(3), 223–237.

Kong, A. P. H. (2021a). The impact of COVID-19 on speakers with aphasia: What is currently known and missing? *Journal of Speech, Language, and Hearing Research, 64,* 176–180.

Kong, A. P. H. (2021b). COVID-19 and aphasia. *Current Neurology and Neuroscience Reports, 21*(11), article 61.

Kong, A. P. H. (2021c). Mental health of persons with aphasia during the COVID-19 pandemic: Challenges and opportunities for addressing emotional distress. *Open Journal of Social Sciences, 9*(5), 562–569.

Kong, A. P. H., Linnik, A., Law, S., & Shum, W. (2014, October 5–7). Measuring the coherence of healthy and aphasic discourse production in Chinese using Rhetorical Structure Theory (RST). [Poster presentation]. Fifty-second annual meeting of Academy of Aphasia, Miami, FL, USA. doi: 10.3389/conf.fpsyg.2014.64.00028

Mann, W. C., & Thompson, S. A. (1988). Rhetorical structure theory: Toward a functional theory of text organization. *Text, 8*(3), 243–281.

Milman, L., Anderson, E., Thatcher, K., Amundson, D., Johnson, C., Jones, M., Valles, L., & Willis, D. (2020). Integrated discourse therapy after glioblastoma: A case report of face-to-face and tele-neurorehabilitation Treatment Delivery. *Frontiers in Neurology, 11,* 583452.

National Institutes of Health. (2011). *Diversity definitions.* Available from www.ninds.nih.gov/diversity_programs/definitions.htm

Peelle, J. E., Troiani, V., Wingfield, A., & Grossman, M. (2010). Neural processing during older adults' comprehension of spoken sentences: Age differences in resource allocation and connectivity. *Cerebral Cortex, 20*(4), 773–782.

Pilnick, A., Trusson, D., Beeke, S., O'Brien, R., Goldberg, S., & Harwood, R. H. (2018). Using conversation analysis to inform role play and simulated interaction in communications skills training for healthcare professionals: Identifying avenues for further development through a scoping review. *BMC Medical Education*, *18*(1), 267.

Saffran, E. M., Berndt, R. S., & Schwartz, M. F. (1989). The quantitative analysis of agrammatic production: Procedure and data. *Brain and Language*, *37*, 440–479.

Schiffrin, D., Tannen, D., & Hamilton, H. E. (2001). *The handbook of discourse analysis*. Malden, MA: Blackwell Publishers Inc.

Schumacher, R., Bruehl, S., Halai, A. D., & Lambon Ralph, M. A. (2020). The verbal, non-verbal and structural bases of functional communication abilities in aphasia. *Brain Communications*, *2*(2), fcaa118.

Schumacher, R., Halai, A. D., & Lambon Ralph, M. A. (2019). Assessing and mapping language, attention and executive multidimensional deficits in stroke aphasia. *Brain*, *142*(10), 3202–3216.

Taboada, M., & Mann, W. C. (2006). Rhetorical Structure Theory: Looking back and moving ahead. *Discourse Studies*, *8*, 423–459.

Troiani, V., Fernández-Seara, M. A., Wang, Z., Detre, J. A., Ash, S., & Grossman, M. (2008). Narrative speech production: An fMRI study using continuous arterial spin labeling. *NeuroImage*, *40*, 932–939.

Ulatowska, H. K., Olness, G. S., Hill, C. L., Roberts, J. A., & Keebler, M. W. (2000) Repetition in narratives of African Americans: The effects of aphasia. *Discourse Processes*, *30*(3), 265–283.

Uslu, A., Gerber, S., Schmidt, N., Röthlisberger, C., Wyss, P., Vanbellingen, T., Schaller, S., Wyss, C., Koenig-Bruhin, M., Berger, T., Nyffeler, T., Müri, R., Nef, T., & Urwyler, P. (2020). Investigating a new tablet-based telerehabilitation app in patients with aphasia: a randomised, controlled, evaluator-blinded, multicentre trial protocol. *BMJ Open*, *10*(11), e037702.

Vigliocco, G., Vinson, D. P., Druks, J., Barber, H., & Cappa, S. F. (2011). Nouns and verbs in the brain: A review of behavioural, electrophysiological, neuropsychological and imaging studies. *Neuroscience and Biobehavioural Reviews*, *35*(3), 407–426.

Wilmskoetter, J., Fridriksson, J., Gleichgerrcht, E., Stark, B., Delgaizo, J., Hickok, G., Vaden, K., Hillis, A., Rorden, C., & Bonilha, L. (2019). Neuroanatomical structures supporting lexical diversity, sophistication, and phonological word features during discourse. *NeuroImage: Clinical*, *24*, 101961.

Wilson, S. M., Henry, M. L., Besbris, M., Ogar, J. M., Dronkers, N. F., Jarrold, W., Miller, B. L., & Gorno-Tempini, M. L., (2010). Connected speech production in three variants of primary progressive aphasia. *Brain*, *133*, 2069–2088.

Wilson, S. M., & Hula, W. D. (2019). Multivariate approaches to understanding aphasia and its neural substrates. *Current Neurology and Neuroscience Reports*, *19*(8), 53.

Glossary

Acculturation The process in which a member of a cultural group adopts the beliefs and behaviors of another cultural group. Over time with prolonged contact with another cultural group, a person demonstrates culture modification by adapting to or borrowing traits from another culture.

Adaptor A kind of gesture that is not used intentionally during communication. It is often used unconsciously, especially when a person is tense or anxious, and may occur in instances of speech failure.

Agnosia The loss of ability to recognize and identify objects, persons, sounds, shapes, or smells while the specific sense is not defective.

Agrammatism A form of expressive disorder that occurs in non-fluent aphasia and is characterized by the failure to speak in a grammatically correct fashion, usually due to misuse or omission of grammatical words or functors.

Alternating attention The ability to switch focus between two or more stimuli during a task.

Anomia An impairment in finding a target word for expression.

Anosognosia The problematic awareness or denial of the existence of an impairment or a deficit.

Aphasia An acquired deficit in understanding and using language (in verbal and/or written modalities) as a result of a brain injury.

Apraxia A problem in assembling the appropriate sequence of movements for speech production or in executing the appropriate serial ordering of sounds for speech. Its primary deficit is an inability to program articulatory movements. Significant slowness, weakness, restricted range of movement or incoordination of the articulators is often absent.

Arousal The level of wakefulness and the ability to respond to a stimulus.

Artificial Intelligence (AI) The simulation of human intelligence in machines that are programmed to think like humans and mimic human actions.

Automatic speech Verbalization of words or phrases that occurs without the conscious effort of an individual.

Automatic Speech Recognition (ASR)   A computer-driven and independent transcription of spoken language into readable text in real time. It is also known as (computer) speech recognition or speech to text.

Auxiliary verb   A verb that usually precedes a main verb and adds functional or grammatical meaning to the clause in which it appears to determine the mood, tense, or aspect of the main verb. Examples include "have", "do", or "will". (see modal auxiliary)

Avocational   An activity that one engages in as a hobby outside his or her main occupation.

Better Conversations with Aphasia (BCA)   An intensive and tailored eight-week program of conversation therapy.

Cerebrovascular accident   The medical term for stroke.

Circumlocution   A common symptom present in individuals with aphasia. In the incidence of word-finding difficulties, one may describe many features of an object, event, or action without saying the actual target word.

City Gesture Checklist (CGC)   A "quick and dirty" method to assess gesture use through different coding categories, inform therapy targets, and measure outcomes. It allows users to record observations of different types of co-gestures employed, identify factors that affect gesture use, and determine the effectiveness of using the observed gestures.

Closed-class word   A class of words made up of a finite set of items which are rarely expanded, i.e., words in a closed class, such as prepositions, determiners, or conjunctions. (see function word)

Code switching   Changing of languages over phrases or sentences by individuals who speak two or more languages (bilingual or multilingual speakers).

Code mixing   Switching of languages at the intra-phrasal level by individuals who speak two or more languages (bilingual or multilingual speakers).

Cognate   Cognate words have a common etymological origin. Congates in two languages usually share a similar meaning, spelling, and pronunciation.

Cognition   The ability to acquire and process knowledge about the world, usually involving the activities of thinking, understanding, learning, and remembering.

Cognitive-communication skills   A set of skills of understanding and using both spoken and written language, appreciating and employing both verbal and non-verbal aspects of communication, and using cognitive skills sub-serving language.

Coherence   The semantic connectedness of a text at the propositional level.

Cohesion   The semantic relations among contiguous utterances, established through the use of lexical and grammatical devices such as conjunction, reference, and ellipsis.

Content unit Defined by Yorkston and Beukelman (1980) as formation expressed to describe a key element of a picture stimulus. It may include nouns and action words.

Content validity Refers to the degree of faithfulness with which a sample or measure represents some attributes or behaviors. It estimates how much a measure represents every single element of a construct.

Conversational dyad Conversation involving two persons who interact face to face as senders and receivers.

Copula A word used to link the subject of a sentence with a predicate.

Core lexicon A lexical item that plays a critical and significant role in constructing a semantically coherent narrative.

Correct information unit (CIU) Defined by Nicholas and Brookshire (1993) as a unit of words that are intelligible in context, accurate in relation to a picture stimulus or a topic, and relevant to the information about the content of the stimulus or topic.

Delirium A disturbance in a person's mental abilities that results in a decreased awareness of one's environment and confused thinking.

Dementia A decline in mental ability in the rate beyond normal ageing that is severe enough to interfere with daily functioning.

Dementia of Alzheimer's type (DAT) The most common form of dementia that accounts for up to 80% of dementia cases.

Diadochokinetic rate (DDK) An assessment that measures how quickly an individual can accurately produce a series of rapid and alternating speech sounds.

Discourse A unit of language that is larger than a sentence.

Divided attention The ability to simultaneously and concurrently focus on two or more stimuli.

Dysarthria A group of motor speech disorders resulting from disturbances in muscular control, including weakness, slowness, or incoordination of the speech mechanism due to damage to the central or peripheral nervous system or both. The disorder encompasses co-existing neurogenic disorders of several or all the basic processes of speech production, including respiration, phonation, resonance, articulation, and prosody.

Emblems A type of referent-related or content-carrying gesture that contains a specific meaning common to a given language community.

Etiology The underlying cause of a deficit or a symptom.

Executive function A set of mental processes that permits one to plan, carry out, and monitor a sequence of actions that is intended for accomplishing a goal.

Focused attention The ability to respond or to focus on a specific stimulus.

Function word The in-between or "smaller" words used to frame the major content words in a sentence. Examples are conjunctions, pronouns, or articles. (see closed-class word)

Hemianopia   A sensory impairment that makes one unable to see something.

Hemorrhagic stroke   A stroke due to a rupture of weakened blood vessels in the brain. Its common causes include aneurysms and hypertension.

Huntington's disease   An inherited disease that causes the progressive breakdown or degeneration of nerve cells in the brain.

Illocutionary act   A complete speech act made in a typical utterance that consists of the delivery of proposition(s) of the utterance.

Illustrator   A type of functional gesture that reinforces or supplements what is being said and is used mostly in face-to-face interactions. It is often tied to the content and/or the flow of speech.

Indirect intervention   An intervention approach commonly used in dementia that utilizes strategies to modify the physical and/or linguistic environment around those with dementia.

Informative word   Defined by Kong and Law (2004) as a key lexical item of a picture stimulus. It is counted only when used accurately in a descriptive narrative.

Interlocutor   A person who takes part in a dialogue or conversation.

Ischemic stroke   A stroke due to an obstruction within a blood vessel supplying blood to the brain. It accounts for the majority (about 80%) of all stroke cases.

Jargon   A lengthy and fluently articulated utterance that makes little or no sense to a listener. It may consist of verbal and neologistic paraphasias.

Lexical diversity   The range of vocabulary deployed in a text by a speaker that reflects the capacity to access and retrieve target words from a relatively intact knowledge base (i.e., lexicon) for the construction of higher linguistic units (Fergadiotis & Wright, 2011).

Life Participation Approach to Aphasia (LPAA)   A consumer-driven service-delivery approach that supports individuals with aphasia.

Logorrhea   A language symptom found in speakers with TBI. It is characterized by the excessive production of incoherent and repetitive language that appears to be incessant and never-ending.

Macrostructure   The overall or global meanings of a discourse.

Main concept   Defined by Nicholas and Brookshire (1995) as a statement that provides an outline of the gist or essential information portrayed in a stimulus picture or an outline of the essential steps in a procedure. It should contain only one main verb.

Main event   Defined by Capilouto, Wright, and Wagovich (2006) as the mentioning of an event that is of sufficient importance to a story as a whole and independent from the other events in the story. It may contain more than one main verb.

Maintenance   The maintained or preserved treatment effect after the end of intervention.

Matrix verb The verb of a matrix clause, which is a clause that contains a subordinate clause.

Maze Hesitation phenomena, false starts, revisions, filled pauses, or sound, syllable, or word repetitions commonly found in discourse produced by speakers with traumatic brain injury.

Measure of Textual Lexical Diversity (MTLD) A measure to estimate the lexical richness of a text developed by McCarthy (2005). It employs a sequential analysis and calculates the recurrent Type-Token Ratio (TTR) of increasingly longer segments of a transcript.

Mild cognitive impairment (MCI) A transitional stage between the expected cognitive decline of getting older and the more serious cognitive decline of dementia.

Modal auxiliary A verb that usually precedes a main verb and expresses necessity, uncertainty, ability, or permission of the verb phrase. Examples include "can", "could", "may", "might", "must", "ought", "shall", or "should". (see auxiliary verb)

Monologue An extended speech that involves the speaking of only one person.

Moving Average Type Token Ratio (MATTR) First reported by Covington (2007), it is a measure used to estimate lexical diversity that is based on computing the TTR of successive non-overlapping segments of the text.

Narrative A sequence of written or spoken words to represent a series of connected events.

Neologism An error made up of an idiosyncratic new word or a new phrase. It is often used in place of a target word or phrase.

Norm-referenced assessment The process of evaluating a person's performance by judging and ranking him or her against the performance of their unimpaired peers.

Number of Different Words (NDW) The sum of all unique lexical items appearing in a transcript.

Open-class word A class of words in which new words can be added to the class as the need arises. They may include nouns or verbs in which the total inventory is potentially infinite and continually expanding.

Pantomime A type of referent-related or content-carrying gesture that describes objects and actions in a complex and sequential manner.

Paragrammatic A form of grammatical disorder that occurs in fluent aphasia and is characterized by grammatical errors such as incorrect tense markers or misuse of pronouns in the context of a wide range of syntactic organizations.

Paraphasia The production of unintended syllables, words, or phrases during the effort to speak. It can be semantically or phonologically related to the target.

Parkinson's disease   A progressive disorder of the nervous system that affects one's movement.

Perseveration   The pathological and persistent repetition of syllables, words, or phrases associated with brain damage.

Phonomotor Treatment (PMT)   An intensive treatment program that focuses on phonological processing and has been found effective to improve lexical retrieval as well as discourse production in people with aphasia.

Politeness marker   Word or words that enhance cooperativity in a dialogue and are essential to professional or work communication. Individuals with moderate or severe TBI typically underuse these markers.

Primary progressive aphasia (PPA)   A language disorder that involves progressive decline in the ability to use language. It is often associated with a disease process that causes atrophy in the frontal and temporal areas of the brain, and is distinct from aphasia resulting from a stroke.

Proposition   The key or major content of a clause or sentence.

Prosody   A complex phenomenon that pertains to the pitch, loudness, tempo, stress, intonation, and rhythm of speech.

Regulator   A type of functional gesture that supports the interaction and communication between a sender and a recipient.

Reinforcement   A method of selecting and strengthening behaviors by arranging immediate (positive) consequences under specific stimulus conditions.

Reliability   The degree of consistency about the measurement of an assessment tool.

Right hemisphere damage (RHD)   Damage to the right side of the brain that may lead to a group of deficits or changes in cognitive-communication skills.

Selective attention   The ability to selectively attend to a target stimulus and to ignore peripheral non-target stimuli.

Speech act   An utterance that has a performative function in language and communication.

Stereotypic utterance   A non-propositional utterance in the form of a syllable, word, or phrase that is repeated or overused by a subgroup of speakers with aphasia.

Sustained attention   The ability to maintain focus on a stimulus during continuous or repetitive activities.

Terminable unit (T-unit)   Defined by Hunt (1964, 1965) as a main independent clause plus all subordinate clauses and non-clausal structures (i.e., dependent modifiers of the main clause) that are attached to or embedded in it.

Topic shading   A language symptom found in speakers with TBI. It is characterized by verbal output that tends to contain frequent inappropriate shifting of conversational topic(s) that relate in some manner to previous ones.

Transcript   The end product of transcribing or translating speech, spoken language, and non-verbal aspects of human interaction from audio or video recordings to a written (or graphic) medium.

Traumatic brain injury (TBI)   A form of acquired brain injury that occurs when a sudden trauma causes damage to the brain.

Type-Token Ratio (TTR)   The ratio of the Number of Different Words (NDW) to the total number of words in a transcript.

Validity   The degree to which an assessment tool measures what it claims to measure.

voc-D   A measure to estimate lexical diversity developed by Malvern and Richards (1997) using a curve-drawing approach.

Index

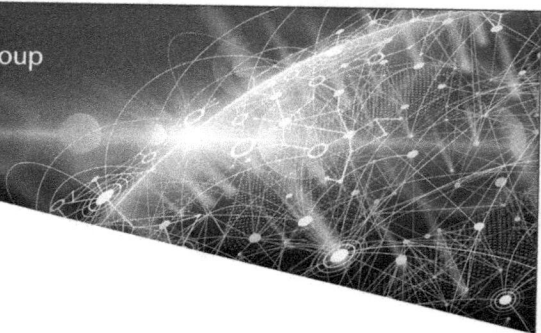

For Product Safety Concerns and Information please contact our EU
representative GPSR@taylorandfrancis.com
Taylor & Francis Verlag GmbH, Kaufingerstraße 24, 80331 München, Germany